Understanding
Fascia, Tensegrity, and
Myofascial Trigger Points

Understanding Fascia, Tensegrity, and Myofascial Trigger Points

A Roadmap for Fascia-Focused Therapists

JOHN SHARKEY

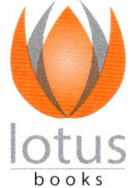

lotus
books

First published in 2026 by
Lotus Books
1607 N. Market Street, Champaign, Illinois 61820
Phone: 1-800-747-4457

Anatomy Illustrations Amanda Williams
Line Drawings Lee Lawrence
Photographs Supplied by the author, unless otherwise indicated
Text Design Medlar Publishing Solutions Pvt Ltd., India
Cover Design Chris Fulcher
Printed and Bound Versa Press, United States of America

Medical Disclaimer

This publication is written and published to provide accurate and authoritative information relevant to the subject matter presented. It is published and sold with the understanding that the author and publishers are not engaged in rendering legal, medical, or other professional services by reason of their authorship or publication of this work. If medical or other expert assistance is required, the services of a competent professional person should be sought.

Acknowledgements

I must mention, and give special thanks to, the wonderful National Training Centre (NTC) tutors. Thank you to all my students and graduates over the past forty or so years; it has been such a privilege to teach and learn from you. I also wish to thank and acknowledge the texts, and their authors, listed in the resources section, which were invaluable as reference material for the writing of this book.

A special thank you to my colleague Tom Myers, a licensed massage therapist in the USA practicing structural integration, who deserves much credit for the concept of "Anatomy Trains," a game invented to help students gain an appreciation of fascial continuity. Tom and I shared many a conversation regarding these continuities over many years, and I am delighted to see how he has managed to play an influential role in creating a global interest in fascia.

I wish to express my deepest respect and heartfelt gratitude to all body donors, along with their families and friends. Donating one's body is an unparalleled act of selflessness, a profound gift to the advancement of medical knowledge, particularly in the field of anatomy. As a clinical anatomist, I am dedicated to ensuring that every image I utilize holds significant educational value, honoring the invaluable contribution made by donors. Their generosity leaves an indelible mark, shaping the future of medical understanding.

British Library Cataloging-in-Publication Data
A CIP record for this book is available from the British Library

ISBN: 978-1-7182-3750-6 (print)
10 9 8 7 6 5 4 3 2 1

E9900

Contents

Dedication

To my beloved wife, Fidelma, whose unwavering love, friendship, and support have been the cornerstone of my life journey. Your strength and kindness inspire me every day.

To our two extraordinary daughters, Xsara and Katie, your vibrant spirits illuminate my world. Watching you both grow into remarkable young women fills my heart with immense pride and joy. May these pages serve as a small tribute to the love and inspiration you have bestowed upon me. This book is dedicated to our shared journey, a roadmap for understanding and healing, guided by the profound connections that bind us as a family.

Finally, I dedicate this book to Doctor Tom Findley, whose spirit of love and sharing endures.

We are formed in tubes, pockets, pouches, and helices that never fail to be part of the multidimensional wholeness from which we form, in and around.

—J. Sharkey, 2024

Foreword

This roadmap caters to the curiosity and learning journey of anyone eager to delve into the profound understanding of the complex processes and interconnected workings of the human body.

The book you are holding in your hands delivers exactly what it promises and more. If you are a manual or movement practitioner—it is *treasure*.

I don't write that lightly, or because it's kind to write nice things in a foreword. It is to describe the depth and breadth of usable wisdom within these pages that *any* practitioner—especially one who cares about their clients and the significance of the fascial matrix in the story of their wellbeing—must have in their collection.

This is not a book to gather dust on a shelf, either, after you've read it once. It's much more likely that you will be deeply grateful (as I am) to have it by your side every day—whatever the modality you work in, as a movement, manual, or medical practitioner. It will continue to provide you with references, resources, and rich templates that make sense to you and your client in practice.

The pages explain the what, the why, and the where of the underlying logic and practical applications of working with fascia, through the lens of any discipline, to take into practice. This book provides the most essential and authoritative bridge across the Great Divide from twentieth- to twenty-first-century anatomy, bravely built by a rare and valuable combination of experience, education, and practiced—as well as practical—wisdom.

The authority comes from a clinical anatomist, an exercise physiologist, and a manual therapist who is a teacher, author, and educator who deeply appreciates what it is to have learning difficulties. Each of these fields is enough as a career path for any one human being to put into practice and teach. John Sharkey is that rare combination of all three: a pioneer, consummately capable of weaving all these subjects together—so that you and

I don't have to. It is frankly a privilege to read this work and be among the first in the world to enjoy having it on my desk and behind my repertoire. (You'll see why shortly.) John takes us by the hand and leads us through all the questions and wondering about how we can best put our own practices into practice, with the advantage of his wisdom beside us.

Through his decades of experience in the anatomy laboratory, teaching medical students the classical medical syllabus and specialist surgeons the more contemporary interventions that honor the fascia, John has served us all. That dedicated service to educate specialists and practitioners around the world called him to write a book that identifies and applies all that we need to know about making sense of fascia-focused work and evolving with it. More than that, John somehow compels us all to collaborate in its evolution. His words welcome us in to learn with him, however we best do that.

Whether it is in the movement classroom, at the manual therapy table, or for medical assessment—this book simplifies and makes accessible how twenty-first-century anatomy can transcend and include all that precedes it, as the science evolves. The book consciously and conscientiously provides us with the means to evolve with it ourselves, whatever practice we are dedicated to. Indeed, in my humble opinion, no one should be in practice without this wisdom to hand.

Why?

Because you will have at your fingertips the full underlying logic of why we need to cross

this Rubicon (from classical to contemporary anatomy), and you will have the means to enhance your method, whatever it is, in practice. John doesn't dumb it down, yet he organizes the language and the logic we all struggle with, to provide deep insight and guidance. As the understanding of fascia expands exponentially and explodes the reasoning behind our inherited understanding of the human body (reduced to the functioning of a biological movement machine), he demonstrates why that doesn't serve us—and why understanding fascia does. John does not simply ditch the old and demand the new, to make his personal case. Rather, there is huge respect for our scientific history and growth and a calling for common sense to gain traction as the research into fascia grows and sheds new light in the hallowed halls of learning. That new light illuminates how we work.

In this book, John provides a vehicle for each one of us to cross the bridge from twentieth- to twenty-first-century anatomy as we shift paradigms from one era to the next and navigate the journey for ourselves, with reliable research and key information. That vehicle invites each one of us to adapt the knowledge to our own modality. Adapt we must—from the outdated notion that the human body is made up of parts, based in the theory of mechanical logic and hard-matter physics.

John does the impossible. He takes us into the science, uses the classical tenets to build the vehicle, then drives us elegantly across the chasm from old, hard-matter physics to new, soft-matter physics as the foundation of wholeness in the living human body. You soon realize you are riding inside a new model of continuity, connection, and collaboration—with the old wisdom firmly and reassuringly distinguished, so you get the keys to drive the vehicle yourself. I'll let you discover how that happens by reading it. I will add one caveat.

It is not just for you.

Your clients will love you for having this book on your desk, because it gives them such a powerful resource to describe the aches and pains that they can't account for when they see the beautifully illustrated pain referral patterns that can guide you both. Everyone wins with this particular manual. It is based on (but not limited to) a bodywork therapy that works—over and over again—for people, whatever their age and stage of health and healing.

John offers some essential and super-valuable assets to every reader, before this thoughtfully written material even begins:

• The knowledge of anatomy that a clinical anatomist must have and impart to the undergraduate medical student to be able to bestow the title of doctor
• The level of knowledge of exercise physiology required to translate that anatomy into application for anyone teaching movement
• The essential knowledge of therapeutic fascia-focused application in real life for all types of manual practitioners
• The educational experience to coach others in those applications, so that they gain those abilities, both for themselves and, ultimately, for their clients/patients

• The grace to explain in language everyone can understand and tell their own story—whatever their own learning ability

John is a storyteller and a compassionate man who loves to help others succeed, whatever their modality or vocation. He constantly challenges his own profound knowledge and experience by working in private practice, by teaching practitioners of all stripes, by presenting around the world to all different modalities, and by researching and writing scientific discussion papers to support the work and stimulate further research.

From his extensive studies, John has had to make sense between the academic pursuit of anatomy and physiology and the practical demands of educating therapists in applied practice. A careful distinction had to be made between the therapies and the techniques. The therapy has to have an ethos, an education modality, and a profound reach—it includes a great deal more than the techniques. The techniques have to have tried and tested applications and the means to learn them, so they show up as a benefit to the client receiving the treatment. Bringing these aspects together has been a life-long practice—the essence of which is condensed into these pages.

Indeed, in this book, John has gone one huge step further—he takes the specific focus of fascia (and all it implies) and APPLIES it into generalized practice, making it relevant whichever therapy you have chosen to undertake. You do not have to be a doctor to understand it. Yet every doctor I have met loves the clarity and support this work offers in understanding pain referral patterns and the value of referring a patient to a suitable practitioner, given the information found here. It is an asset.

John has devoted his life's work to researching, learning, and then teaching what he has discovered. Integrating neuromuscular techniques (NMTq) from his mentors, such as Doctor David Simons, and colleagues, including Leon Chaitow, John has created a fascia-focused therapy with a wide application in all manual therapy. However, it also includes a unique integration using medical exercise, which can anchor the results in the clients' ability to live them in their everyday lives. There are no genuine practitioners who will not benefit from the way this book provides the explanation and deeper logic to support optimum movement and pain management through any kind of therapeutic or practical intervention.

John has been a leading protagonist in the world of fascia science over the last forty years, forming a kind of connective tissue of fundamental logic and guidance that any practitioner can use. As a movement and manual therapist, I treasure such a book in my practice room, and reach for it often, for reasons that you too will enjoy:

- It is an excellent reference book for many practical questions about anatomy and pain—why pain can be referred and where to look.
- It is an instant resource that provides the logic behind neural patterns.
- The illustrations of pain referral patterns provide an instant guide for clients to point at and help explain what they might find difficult to describe.

- The client has an immediate sense of being heard, listened to, and understood!
- There is no need to feel alone in a world of practitioners who might not share your fascination with the wholeness of the fascial matrix and the new science of body architecture.
- It consciously holds the practitioner's hand as an authoritative guide.

To briefly summarize:

The introduction expounds on the history of and recent discoveries about fascia. The term *fasciategrity* is explained, to describe the way in which fascia acts in the human body architecture, from embryo to elder. That principle sits quietly and potently behind the logic of all the therapeutic methods described in the book. Backed by research and the variety of beautiful images that John can include from the anatomy laboratory, the introduction builds the means to bridge the Rubicon from classical anatomy to contemporary "anatomy for the twenty-first century," so every practitioner can benefit.

In part I we have the theory, to learn the logic we need to navigate whatever therapeutic journey we are on as practitioners. The language becomes our friend in understanding anatomy and how to navigate everything that follows.

Part II is practical and provides some profound and valuable keys to understanding why fascia impacts how we practice; specifically, through myofascial trigger points and site-specific fascia tuning pegs. These become keys in assessment and treatment. There are also a variety of applied techniques and treatment protocols.

In part III we find the clearly illustrated resource of pain referral patterns that is so valuable in practice. It ties the whole book together and makes sense of how to apply the wisdom and logic with our clients.

Most practitioners love being practical (rather than reading about practices), because that is where they can make a difference to their clients. For all the anatomy atlases and tomes of techniques I have on my shelves, this book is the one I use every single day in practice.

It really is a treasure trove and feels like a practical best buddy to have sitting beside me!

May it bless you with curiosity, insight, and confidence to make an even bigger difference to those you serve.

In gratitude and grace,

Joanne Avison
Brighton, England, 2024

Introduction

Why This Book Is Important for Fascia-Focused Therapists

The content within these pages elucidates the fundamental principles and concepts underpinning fascia-focused therapies. This book serves as a valuable resource for instructors and a supportive study companion for students engaged in the realm of fascia-focused therapies, irrespective of their therapeutic backgrounds.

The information contained here transcends the confines of a traditional manual on fascia science. Instead, what unfolds is a comprehensive guide for practitioners of diverse therapeutic backgrounds, inviting therapists of every stripe to explore and grasp the nuanced intricacies of the human body through the fascia lens. Throughout these pages, readers will uncover insights into the elaborate tensegrity-based architecture, revealing a harmonious interplay of unified systems and tubes within tubes. This roadmap caters to the curiosity and learning journey of anyone eager to delve into a profound understanding of the complex

processes and interconnected workings of the human body.

Human dissection studies highlight the repetitious constructive nature of form reflected by the "tubes within tubes" analogy. Blood vessels, nerves, lymphatics, muscle fibers, bones, hair, ducts, digestive tract, interstitium, bronchioles, and ureters are all examples of cylindrical, tubular structures of varying shapes. This tubular helical architecture reflects the first principles of tensegrity constructs. I wish to draw the reader into a world of exploration and discovery to set the foundations for a better understanding of what it is to be a self-constructed, unified, living tensegrity.

Fascia-focused integrated therapeutic approaches encompass a diverse range of hands-on manual techniques employed to address soft-tissue pain and injury comprehensively, with a primary emphasis on chronic pain and alterations in sensation. These methods include fascia therapy, centering on specific fascial considerations. The inclusion of medical exercise, which employs graded physical activities and motor learning sequences to restore functionality, mitigates the risk of injury. What sets these approaches apart is their innovative, fascia-focused nature, bringing together a rich tapestry of hands-on techniques. The amalgamation of soft-tissue approaches can easily be integrated into a wide range of manual and movement therapies. This collaborative effort results in a holistic and adaptable framework that caters to the diverse needs of individuals seeking therapeutic intervention.

Centered on what can be termed "anatomy for the twenty-first century," this book delves into the crucial aspects of neurophysiology necessary for a comprehensive understanding of the science and hypotheses associated with the myriad techniques and physical activities integrated into fascia-focused therapies. While acknowledging that the explanations rooted in classical anatomy have persisted for centuries, the approach here is one of balanced evolution. Rather than dismissing established concepts outright, the book encourages an appreciation of historical origins and insertions, while fostering an awareness that these are linguistic conveniences, not reflective of a unified body and rooted in hard-matter physics.

By embracing this perspective, readers are guided to navigate beyond traditional anatomical constructs, recognizing the intricacies of the human body as a dynamic, interconnected whole based on soft-matter physics.

A liver cannot survive outside a body, and without the liver the body would no longer be whole and, likewise, would not survive.

Like a liver sustaining the body's vitality within, therapists play a crucial role in the interconnected web of manual therapy methods. Just as a liver is indispensable to the body's wholeness and survival, therapists, regardless of their chosen manual therapy approach, contribute to the well-being of the human form. As you delve into these pages, consider the continuity of human anatomy, opening your mind to the notion that addressing indurated, spastic, or adhered tissue in one area can reverberate throughout the body.

This book delineates recommended applications of diverse techniques, offering a spectrum of approaches. It outlines a rationale for the sequential integration of manual therapy and medical exercise interventions. This descriptive hierarchy provides a framework for making informed choices, guiding patients back to pain-free movement. In the hands of a skilled therapist, whether practicing neuromuscular techniques (NMTq) or other fascia-informed methods, the alleviation of acute or chronic myofascial or osseofascial pain is possible. Through NMTq, a restoration of homeostasis occurs across unified fascial systems, encompassing the nervous, skeletal, and other soft-tissue elements. The fascia-focused therapist seeks to optimize joint function, myofascial health, and overall arthrokinematics, while fostering healing by reinstating core myofascial function throughout the soma.

The focus extends to treating fascial adaptations, myofascial trigger points (MTrPs), local ischemia, neural interferences, postural and biomotional dysfunctions, nutritional factors, and emotional well-being.

Acknowledging the evolving understanding of MTrPs, I emphasize that they can emerge anywhere within a muscle or muscle fiber. The outdated practice of marking their location with an "X" has been dispelled, reflecting a more accurate understanding.

For instance, the third edition of the widely recognized "bible" on MTrPs, *Myofascial Pain and Dysfunction: The Trigger Point Manual* (2018), no longer employs an "X" to signify MTrP locations. It is imperative for therapists to hone sensorial palpation skills, adapting to this updated knowledge in the pursuit of effective and compassionate care.

What This Book Is Not About

This book does not aim to exhaustively cover every modality variation within the realm of manual therapy. It refrains from offering intricate instructions on therapist positioning or hand placements tailored to specific anatomical locations, myofascial structures, or groups of fascial tissues.

Rather than suggesting that sole reliance on this text can furnish readers with complete sensorial skills and knowledge for the precise application of fascia-focused techniques, I encourage a broader perspective. Sensorial palpatory proficiency and comprehensive understanding necessitate active engagement in a recognized course of studies, guided by qualified tutors.

This book serves as a valuable complement to formal education. It offers insights and perspectives that can enhance the practitioner's overall comprehension and

approach, irrespective of their chosen manual therapy method. It acknowledges the diversity of therapeutic practices and encourages readers to integrate the knowledge gained within the broader context of their ongoing professional development.

The History and Genesis of Fascia-Focused Therapies

While European anatomists adopted the term "fascia" as early as the fifteenth century, fascia—as understood in the context of medieval medicine (eighth to tenth century)—was an integral component of a traditional healing system that encompassed various aspects of the body's structure and function. This system of medicine—often referred to as the "Canon of Medicine" by its most famous Persian practitioner, Avicenna (Ibn Sina)—had a holistic approach to understanding the human body.

Medieval Persian physicians may have been the first to recognize fascia as a connective tissue that was an essential component of the so-called musculoskeletal system, providing support and integrity to the body's overall structure. Their description of fascia included bones, cartilage, blood vessels, dura mater, lymphatic vessels, nerves, ligaments, and tendons made up of thin, rigid, and woven fibers. Fascia could be thin and fragile, such as that surrounding the abdominopelvic organs, or it could be tough and impenetrable, offering protection from harmful pathogens. Fascia was reported to contain channels and pathways, which were believed to be essential for the flow of various fluids supporting overall health and well-being, all of which is confirmed by current research.

In modern European anatomy (circa eighteenth century), anatomists and physicians—including Giovanni Alfonso Borelli and Antonio Maria Valsalva—described fascia primarily as a membranous structure that provided support and protection to various organs and tissues. During the nineteenth century, modern anatomy began to take shape, with the work of anatomists such as Andreas Vesalius and, later, Henry Gray, whose *Gray's Anatomy* became a seminal reference. However, *Gray's Anatomy* paid little attention to the topic of fascia.

In the early nineteenth century, efforts by anatomist John D. Godman to shine new light on the importance of fascia were largely ignored. In the 1960s, therapist John Barnes emerged, among others, as a trailblazer in the realm of fascia-focused methodologies, coining the term "myofascial release." Barnes's approach zeroes in on liberating fascial restrictions through a methodical application of gentle, sustained pressure. Recent studies have shed light on the efficacy of stimulating C-tactile afferent fibers, achieved through delicate tactile interaction. This requires the sensory touch provided by the therapist and necessitates conscious awareness from the patient, guided by the therapist's intention. This intricate interplay activates specific brain regions, yielding noteworthy therapeutic outcomes.

The Fascia Research Congress, first held in 2007 in Boston, USA, played a significant role in the popularity of fascia-focused research and therapies. The congress served as a critical platform for scientists, healthcare professionals, and practitioners of various sorts to share and disseminate knowledge about fascia and its importance in the human body. The fact that the Fascia Research Congress has become a recurring event underscores the legitimacy and importance of fascia research. This validation has encouraged more researchers to investigate fascia, leading to a deeper understanding of its functions and potential clinical applications.

The information and research shared at the congress and through the *Journal of Bodywork and Movement Therapies* have contributed to the growth and genesis of fascia-focused therapies and techniques. Such approaches include myofascial release, neuromuscular therapy, fascia therapy, fascial stretch therapy, osteopathy, structural integration, fascia integrated technique, fasciategrity in motion, Fascial Manipulation®, and Myofascial Induction®. These fascia-focused approaches have gained greater recognition and popularity among healthcare professionals, medical specialists, and the public.

Surprisingly, the most recent edition of *Gray's Anatomy* offers an extensive and thorough exploration of fascia. The past sixteen years have witnessed a surge in cadaveric studies focusing on fascia, led by Carla Stecco, Gil Hedley, myself, Thomas Myers, and Andrej Pilat. This research has imparted a novel perspective on the human body's interconnectedness and the integration of fascia.

A noteworthy moment in medical anatomy occurred in London in 2019, when a team of clinical anatomists (figures 0.1 and 0.2) presented the inaugural fascia forum during the Fifth Congress of the International Federation of Associations of Anatomists (IFAA).

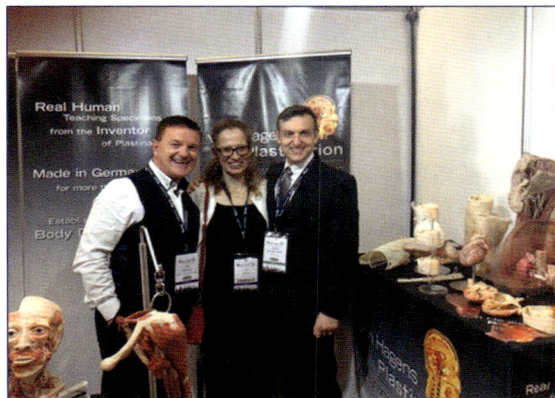

Figure 0.1. Members of the team delivering the first fascia forum at the Fifth International Congress of the IFAA, London, 2019. (L to R) John Sharkey, Carla Stecco, and Vladimir Chereminskiy.

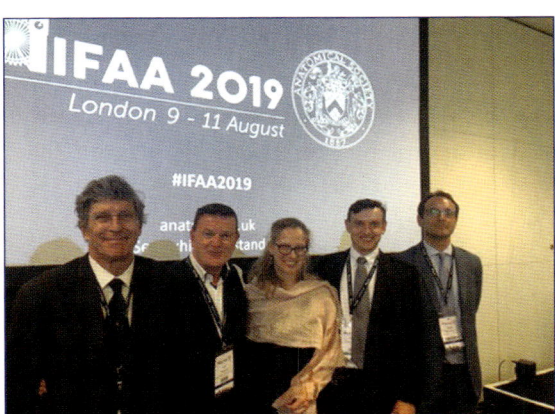

Figure 0.2. The team of clinical anatomists presenting at the first fascia forum as part of the Fifth International Congress of the IFAA. (L to R) Raffaele de Caro, John Sharkey, Carla Stecco, Vladimir Chereminskiy, Andrea Pozianato. Present but missing from the photo was Doctor Veronica Macchi.

A pivotal figure driving the surge of interest in fascia science is Professor Robert Schleip, whose groundbreaking research delves into fascia's contractile and physiological aspects. Schleip's research contributes to our comprehension of fascia's crucial role in movement, pain modulation, and overall well-being.

Professor Carla Stecco, an esteemed anatomist, and her team at the University of Padua in northern Italy are a central force propelling the burgeoning fascination in fascia science. Their dedicated efforts in the field of anatomy deserve special mention and commendation, adding anatomical investigative insights to the intricate study of fascia. More recently, a superb textbook, in two volumes, by Doctor Andrej Pilat, is essential reading for all fascia-focused therapists. Pilat's book was described by Professor Andry Vleeming as a convenient "go-to resource." But more than that, these volumes by Pilat add, in a significant way, to the growing body of research and practical applications of fascia-focused interventions. Fascia therapy, as a distinct therapeutic approach, has emerged because of the evolving understanding of fascial dynamics. The therapeutic application of fascia-focused interventions seeks to address imbalances, restrictions, and dysfunctions within the fascial system, acknowledging its crucial role in maintaining overall physiological integrity.

Consciousness

Consciousness, from both the patient's and the therapist's perspective, assumes a significant role in the practice of fascia therapy. The patient's awareness and perception of their own body, sensations, and movements are pivotal elements in the therapeutic process. Mindfulness, a heightened state of awareness, encourages patients to actively engage with their bodily experiences, facilitating a deeper connection with the fascial system.

Consciousness is integral to the therapeutic interaction. A heightened awareness of your own motion and emotion, touch, and responsiveness to the patient's feedback allows you as therapist to navigate the intricacies of the fascial network with precision and sensitivity. The therapist's attunement to the patient's verbal and nonverbal cues creates a dynamic interplay that enhances the therapeutic effectiveness of fascia-focused interventions. Furthermore, the therapeutic encounter becomes a shared journey of exploration, where both patient and therapist collaborate in unraveling the depths of fascial tension, addressing somatic imbalances and promoting overall well-being. The integration of consciousness into fascia therapy aligns with a holistic approach to healthcare, acknowledging the inseparable connection between mind and body.

In conclusion, the genesis of fascia therapy stems from an enhanced understanding of the dynamic role played by the fascial system in the human body. The integration of consciousness into the therapeutic process, from both the patient's and therapist's perspective, underscores the significance of a holistic approach to fascia-focused interventions. As the field continues to evolve, further research and exploration of the intricate interplay between consciousness and fascial dynamics will undoubtedly contribute to the refinement and advancement of fascia

therapy as a therapeutic modality. Innovative ideas and perspectives in the realm of fascia-focused therapies are essential for advancing our understanding of the role of fascia in human anatomy, and I hope the book you are holding in your hands will also prove to have added in a small way to the history and genesis of fascia-focused therapies.

Note: While our comprehension of fascia remains a dynamic and evolving field, within the pages of this book I designate bone as a distinctive facet of fascia. I recommend therapists to employ low intensity techniques precisely designed at addressing osseofascial elements. This targeted approach proves invaluable in addressing persistent chronic pain issues, often stemming from trauma within the more robust fascial structures commonly recognized as bone.

MTrPs—Welcome Home

As a practicing therapist, I ardently embraced exploring the intricate realm of fascia, referred to as "the orphan tissue," and the phenomena known widely as myofascial trigger points (MTrPs). Janet Travell, David Simons, and Lois Simons, among others, have contributed to our understanding and treatment of MTrPs. Simons (Lewit and Simons 1984) described the evolution of MTrPs in the following way:

> *In the core of the trigger lies a muscle spindle that is in trouble for some reason. Visualize a spindle like a strand of yarn in a knitted sweater. … [A] metabolic crisis takes place, which increases the temperature locally in the trigger point, shortens a minute part of*

the muscle (sarcomere)—like a snag in a sweater—and reduces the supply of oxygen and nutrients into the trigger point. During this disturbed episode, an influx of calcium occurs, and the muscle spindle does not have enough energy to pump the calcium outside the cell where it belongs. Thus, a vicious cycle is maintained, and the muscle spindle can't seem to loosen up, and the affected muscle can't relax (figure 0.3).

Having tested his concept, Simons found an oxygen deficit at the core of an MTrP relative to the muscle tissue surrounding it. Travell and Simons (1983) confirmed that the following factors all help to maintain and enhance

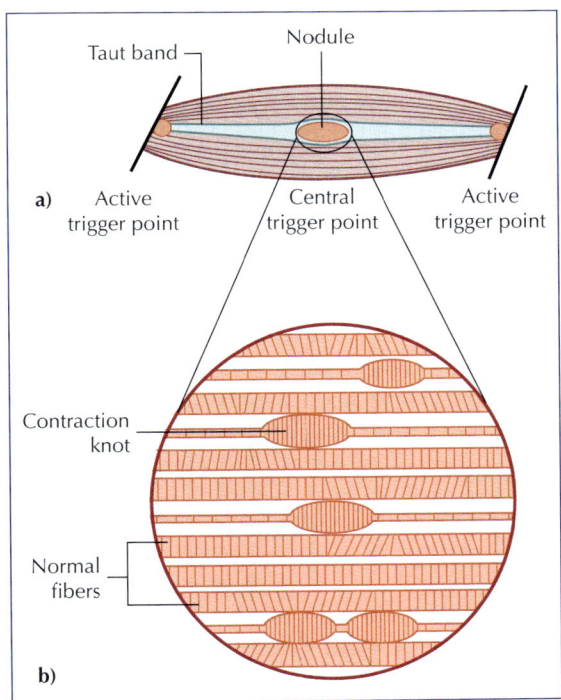

Figure 0.3. Travell and Simons (1983) described a trigger point as *"a highly irritable localized spot of exquisite tenderness in a nodule in a palpable taut band of (skeletal) muscle."*

MTrP activity: nutritional deficiency (esp. vitamin C, B-complex, and iron), hormonal imbalances (e.g., low thyroid, menopausal, or premenstrual situations), infections (bacteria, viruses, or yeast), allergies (esp. wheat and dairy), and inadequate oxygenation of tissues (aggravated by tension, stress, inactivity, and poor respiration).

A primary focus of any fascia-focused therapist is to understand the pathophysiology, formation, etiology, and treatment of MTrPs. A special effort is made to locate the source of referred pain and any perpetuating influences (overuse, misuse, and disuse) and eliminate them, while paying attention to correct negative postural patterns. To facilitate that focus, chapter 5 provides the classical anatomical descriptions of the so-called *origin*, *insertion*, and *primary movements* of muscles, together with the referral pattern of MTrPs associated with each muscle (i.e., myofascial structure) and a unique comment on the kinetic system involvement. Inappropriate movement and the functional adaptations that emerge as a result are offered as significant contributing elements in the genesis of the MTrP.

From the viewpoint of clinical anatomy, I vividly characterize the MTrP as a state of rigor contraction comparable to the profound muscular stiffness observed in the finality of death. This analogy delves into the intricate physiology of an MTrP, offering a poignant perspective.

In the realm of MTrPs, my depiction parallels the postmortem rigidity witnessed by anatomists. Much as the finality of death initiates an irreversible contractile state in muscles, an MTrP manifests a sustained and unyielding contraction within a specific muscle region during its active state. The physiology unfolds with a cascade of events reminiscent of the inevitability of rigor mortis.

Within the core of the MTrP, a muscle spindle—the sensory organ responsible for muscle length and tension regulation—is ensnared in a metabolic crisis. This disturbance triggers a local rise in temperature within the MTrP, initiating a process that echoes the metabolic chaos in death's aftermath. A minute part of the muscle—the sarcomere—experiences shortening, resembling the tightening of a thread within a fabric. Simultaneously, the supply of vital oxygenated blood and nutrients to the trigger point is curtailed, akin to the cessation of life-sustaining processes postmortem. In this disturbed episode, calcium influx surges within the affected area. The muscle spindle—normally entrusted with regulating calcium levels—falters in expelling this surplus calcium, perpetuating a vicious cycle. The muscle spindle remains trapped in a persistent state of tension, impeding its ability to inhibit contraction. This unrelenting contraction extends to the broader muscle, creating a palpable and enduring felt nodule, a myofascial trigger point.

It is crucial to grasp the distinctive nature of this characterization, underscoring that an MTrP operates independently of neural input or an external energy supply. The intricacy lies in the understanding that the conventional pathways of neural signaling or the reliance on a continuous energy source does not govern the contraction at the heart of an MTrP. Instead, it emerges as a manifestation of electromagnetic phenomena.

This distinctive feature challenges conventional processes in muscle physiology, emphasizing that the perpetuation of an MTrP is not contingent upon the typical neural commands regulating muscle activity. Unlike the traditional muscle contractions, which hinge on neural impulses, the MTrP engages in an electromagnetic dance, wherein the forces at play transcend the conventional bounds of neuromuscular communication. In essence, the MTrP operates in a realm of its own, tapping into electromagnetism's subtle yet potent forces.

This departure from the norm underscores the complexity of this phenomenon, prompting a reevaluation of the traditional models, which predominantly rely on neural and energy-driven mechanisms. By recognizing the electromagnetic underpinnings of MTrPs, we open a gateway to a deeper comprehension of the intricate forces governing myofascial physiology. This unique perspective prompts further exploration into the interplay between electromagnetism and the myofascial system, ushering in a paradigm shift that enriches our understanding of the nuanced mechanisms at play within the realm of myofascial trigger points.

A Chicken or Egg Dilemma

It is worth noting that some or all of the pain and changes in sensation attributed to MTrPs may be a result of secondary hyperalgesia of peripheral neural origin. The difficulty here is that MTrPs mimic everything from neural pain to headaches. MTrPs could be located in or around an adjacent hyperalgesic nerve trunk, or be the cause of it. For example:

- The discrete upper-limb pain syndromes attributed to MTrPs in the middle finger extensor, the extensor carpi radialis, or the supinator muscles could be due to nerve-generated pain in the radial or posterior interosseous nerve trunks, or a secondary effect as a direct result of compression due to the MTrP.
- MTrPs situated in the pronator teres muscle coincide with the median nerve. The median nerve refers pain into the thenar muscles, which follow the course of the median nerve in the forearm. MTrPs in the flexor digitorum referring pain into the hand could represent a compressed median nerve in the proximal forearm.
- Myofascial pain in the shoulder girdle could represent entrapment of the suprascapular nerve, the long thoracic nerve, the axillary nerve, or the dorsal scapular nerve. This is a worthwhile consideration as the pain-reference zone of these MTrPs follows the course of these nerves.
- In the lower limb, myofascial pain has been attributed to MTrPs close to the sciatic, tibial, superficial, and deep fibular nerves.

The earliest therapeutic sessions should typically be spent learning from the patient, watching (visual input) the patient's breathing pattern and facial expressions, and listening (with your ears, hands, fingers, elbows, etc.) to their unique and individual story. Taking the time to listen to each personal story to assess the fascia while considering possible changes and migrations, the type of pain, and referral pattern directs the fascia-focused therapist to locate and treat the true source of insult. The modern NMTq employed can immediately affect pain, sensation, and quality/range of motion. Such results are often the foundation for further treatment to ensure a lasting return to homeostasis. Focus on correct breathing supports the body's physiological and psychological well-being, contributing to pain relief and cognitive health while promoting a state of relaxation and balance. Simple nose breathing exercises that are easy for patients to integrate into their daily routine should be encouraged (see p. 25).

Limiting the amount of therapeutic intervention provided in any session (especially in the early stages of treatment) is recommended, to allow an appropriate period of time to witness changes and facilitations. Changes require energy, and the central nervous system must have the capacity to facilitate such energy-demanding changes, so you are encouraged to work slowly and take time (the patient requires the energy to accept and integrate such changes).

If a patient lacks the energetic capacity, too many changes could set them back and compound their problems. Conversely, inadequate intervention could aggravate the patient's symptoms when MTrPs are involved.

Therapists must ensure due diligence and professional practice. It is paramount that the patient is fully informed of any therapeutic interventions and what they involve, and that permission is sought and gained from the patient. Although it is rare, NMTq can result in tissue soreness immediately after a treatment session or in the hours following treatment, and the patient must be made aware of this possibility both verbally and in writing, and you must have their signed consent stating that this possibility has been clearly explained to them and that they understand the likelihood, although small, of such a possibility.

Medical Exercise

Medical exercise has a focus on health-related functional fitness, appropriate breath control, and neuromuscular efficiency, with a view to reducing the risk of injury, and includes post-rehabilitation exercise, including:

- Assessment (functional capacity, including respiratory efficiency)
- Spinal stabilization (core efficiency/ kinetic)
- Corrective exercise (may include water-based training)
- Range of motion training (flexibility training)
- Cardiorespiratory training (heart/lung function)
- Functional conditioning (neuromuscular efficiency, work, sport, life specific)
- Strength training (this is included later in the program)
- Specialist (hypertension, diabetes, arthritis, chronic fatigue syndrome, etc.)

Medical exercise is best provided two to three times a week under strict supervision.

Of course, physical activity should be for life, and patients should be encouraged to remain active after the rehabilitation period. At all times, exercise should be supervised by a qualified professional medical exercise specialist. Medical exercise involves developing and implementing physical activity programs for patients within special populations or with post-rehabilitation needs. It does not include the specialist providing any form of medical diagnosis or medical treatment.

Combining fascia-focused techniques with medical exercise, emphasizing neuromuscular reeducation and efficiency, and neuromuscular reactive training, and using tasks based on functional movement encourages body-wide muscular contractions in their appropriate neurological, synergistic sequence.

The groundbreaking efforts of pioneers such as Bernarr Macfadden, Joseph Pilates, Moshe Feldenkrais, Ida Rolf, and others were centered around achieving optimal postural alignment through purposeful movement. This approach is effective, assuming no existing myofascial imbalances are caused by spasms or MTrPs. Initial intervention is necessary to restore the neural activity and chemical equilibrium of muscles operating at the sarcomere level. Once this therapeutic milestone is reached, the focus can shift toward progressively challenging movements, emphasizing neuromuscular efficiency and reeducation. It is imperative to underscore the significance of performing most functional activities standing. Given that life predominantly unfolds in an upright posture, transitioning from lying to sitting to standing is a fundamental functional requirement. Integrating this transition into a range of physical activities tailored to an individual's life and specific needs is paramount for comprehensive well-being.

A crucial component, often overlooked, is integrating breath work with targeted fascia interventions and medical exercise. This synergy could serve as the missing link, enhancing the overall effectiveness of therapeutic strategies.

Recommended Breath Exercises Suitable for All Patients (and Therapists)

Nose-breathing exercises can be effective in reducing anxiety, myofascial stiffness, and pain by promoting normal pH of myofascial tissues as a result of enhanced oxygen intake and cellular uptake.

Here are a few simple exercises to share with patients, family, and friends:

Deep Belly Breathing (Diaphragmatic Breathing)

1. Sit or lie down in a comfortable position.
2. Place one hand on your chest and the other on your abdomen.
3. Inhale slowly through your nose for a count of 4, expanding your abdomen as you breathe in.
4. Exhale through your nose for a count of 4, allowing your abdomen to contract.
5. Repeat this process for several minutes, focusing on the rise and fall of your abdomen with each breath.

4-7-8 Breathing

1. Sit in a comfortable position with your back straight.
2. Close your mouth and inhale quietly through your nose for a count of 4.
3. Hold your breath for a count of 7.
4. Exhale slowly and completely through your nose for a count of 8.
5. Repeat this cycle for a few minutes. It can help reduce anxiety and induce relaxation.

Alternate Nostril Breathing

1. Sit comfortably with your back straight.
2. Use your right thumb to close off your right nostril and inhale through your left nostril for a count of 4.
3. Close your left nostril with your right ring finger and release your right nostril. Exhale through your right nostril for a count of 4.
4. Inhale through your right nostril for a count of 4, then close it off and release your left nostril. Exhale through your left nostril for a count of 4.
5. Repeat this pattern for several cycles, focusing on your breath and calming your mind.

Box Breathing

1. Sit or lie down comfortably.
2. Inhale through your nose for a count of 4.
3. Hold your breath for a count of 4.
4. Exhale through your nose for a count of 4.
5. Pause and hold your breath again for a count of 4.
6. Repeat this sequence for a few minutes, adjusting the count as needed.

PART I

THEORY

Fascia and Tensegrity—A Fasciategrity Perspective

T his chapter sets the stage by providing a concise overview of fascia and tensegrity.

The "speaks for itself" term *fasciategrity* is a portmanteau of *fascia* and *tensegrity* coined by Avison and myself and used for the first time at the 2018 British Fascia Symposium. Combining fascia research and tensegrity science into a single term provides a rich syntax for describing human form and function.

> *An astoundingly wide variety of natural systems, including carbon atoms, water molecules, proteins, viruses, cells, tissues and even humans and other living creatures, are constructed using a common form of architecture known as tensegrity. The term refers to a system that stabilizes itself mechanically because of the way in which tensional and compressive forces are distributed and balanced within the structure.*
> (Ingber 1998, 48–49)

Fasciategrity speaks about the distribution of tensional and compressional force

relationships of balance and integrity within a unified fascial system or body-wide fascial net. From the intricate architecture of beehives to the majestic Giant's Causeway, from the resilience of trees to the detailed design of invertebrates and vertebrates, from the microscopic realm of plankton to the unseen world of viruses, and, of course, within the complex structures of the human body, all embody the principles of tensegrity constructs.

Embryologically, we emerged from the fundamental embryonic soup within the oocyte and morphed into one multifunctional original fabric called *fascia*. The temporal dance of genetic and epigenetic self-assembly navigates through a labyrinth of developmental transformations invaginating, twisting, permeating, folding, and spiraling, culminating in a diverse array of tissues ranging from more stiffened bone to the supple leptomeninges, representing a spectrum from hardness to softness. Soft, hard, stiff, fluidic, turgid, puffy, and everything in between.

This journey through softness, hardness, stiffness, fluidity, turgidity, and all the nuances in between unfolds against the backdrop of time, where self-organization follows a hierarchical, time-dependent sequence. Tendons, aponeuroses, epineuria, muscle fibers, retinacula, ligaments, cartilage, and bodily fluids occupy the intermediate realms of this spectrum, manifesting in the delicate balance between harder and softer elements of soft matter.

Bodily fluids—including lymph, blood, mucus, cerebrospinal fluid, and synovial fluid—are all liquid crystal matrices, with viscosities along a spectrum that could be compared to thick paint (e.g., emulsions or colloids). Notably, the ground substance of these liquid crystalline matrices is bound water. A crucial point to consider is that connective tissue naturally expresses nonlinear behavior. In other words, forces are shared in an omnidirectional manner.

In the face of compelling evidence to the contrary, characterizing human beings and all living entities as mere mechanical constructs is not only unsatisfactory but also fundamentally untrue, discordant, and disharmonious. Despite the seeming elegance of mechanistic theories, a closer examination reveals that they fail to resolve inherent issues.

The mechanistic perspectives of historical figures such as Vesalius, Descartes, Newton, and Borelli—particularly in the realm of anatomy—have significantly contributed to the pervasive tendency to view all living forms through a mechanical lens. Over the centuries, we have lauded biomechanical insights derived from concepts like pin joints, lever systems, bone-to-bone origin-insertions, and the reduction of the living

body to distinct "parts," all intricately explained and compounded by the principles of hard-matter physics. As our understanding of the "body as a machine" has evolved from the Renaissance period to the present day, modern technology has advanced, enabling medical specialists to substitute body parts using an array of materials, including acrylic resin, silicone, aluminum, titanium, copper, magnesium, iron, stainless steel, superglue, screws, metal plates, and notably, cement.

Yet it seems paradoxical that these materials, derived from external, nonbiological sources, are deemed the most appropriate replacements for components of a self-constructed life form. The journey from the Renaissance to the contemporary era has indeed ushered in technological marvels, but viewing the intricate, dynamic, living organism merely in terms of its mechanical parts and materials remains a reductionist perspective that fails to capture the true essence and complexity of life (figure 1.1).

As the world's population ages, demand for knee and hip replacements continues to rise. Replacement joints have traditionally

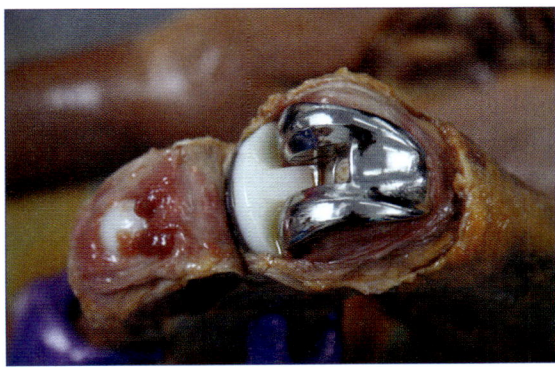

Figure 1.1. Modern technology helps create a knee replacement.

been made from hard-matter materials such as metal or ceramic, which have a high risk of wear and tear over time, leading to further complications and repeated surgeries.

I advocate for using tensegrity principles to guide the design of soft-matter materials for hip and knee replacements. By designing replacements that adhere to tensegrity principles, the body's natural and appropriate tensional-compressional forces can be more closely maintained, reducing the risk of complications while improving therapeutic outcomes. Such materials include hydrogels, which are highly absorbent and can retain water, making them ideal for mimicking the natural lubrication found in joints. Additionally, hydrogels have a similar stiffness to cartilage and can provide a more natural feel than traditional joint replacements. Other soft-matter materials such as elastomers, polymers, and fibrous composites have also shown promising results in preclinical studies, offering improved kinematic properties and providing a more nature-inspired solution to chronically painful joints.

What Is Tensegrity? A Fuller Explanation

What is tensegrity and why is knowledge of tensegrity so important to the fascia-focused movement and manual therapist? For nonliving constructs tensegrity reflects an architectural approach that uses tension and compression to create stable structures, where components are held together in equilibrium through the balance of these forces, resulting in elegant and efficient designs that are both lightweight and resilient.

Put simply, living tensegrity is the harmonious interplay of tension and compression within a continuous self-constructed structure, facilitating stability, fluidity, and motion without reliance on levers, pin joints, screws, or mechanical interventions (figure 1.2).

Living tensegrities represent intricate frameworks that weave together their tiniest tensegrity structured building blocks—such as DNA, proteins, carbohydrates, and lipids—across various organizational tiers, spanning from organelles to cells, tissues, organs, and the entire organism. This prompts the question, in light of the diverse molecules involved, of how they engage, come together, and autonomously structure themselves to form a cohesive entity with emergent properties beyond the summation of individual component traits. Tensegrity is a model that provides the answers. *Tensegrity* is a word constructed by architect Buckminster Fuller by compressing together the words *tension* and *integrity*.

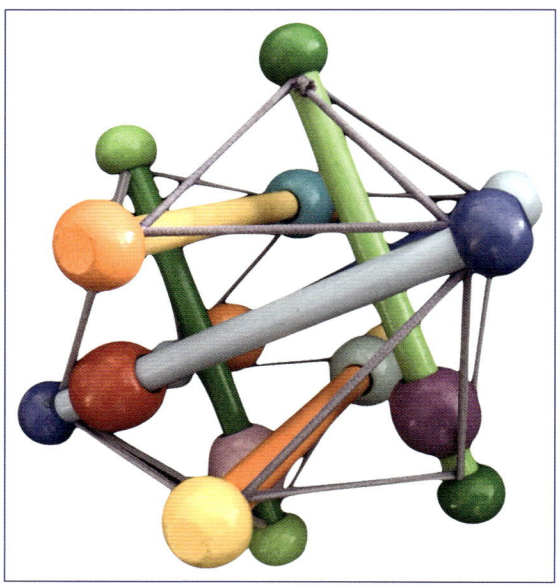

Figure 1.2. The icosahedron.

Fuller wanted to provide a word that encompassed the basic first principles of a geometric construct known as the *icosahedron*. Fuller was correctly convinced that if properly understood, the tensegrity icosahedron would provide an explanation for how atoms, molecules, humans, animals, insects, viruses, bacteria—in fact, the entire cosmos—is architecturally constructed. Similar to the simplicity of Albert Einstein's most famous equation $E = mc^2$, Fuller reduced the complexities of life and form to tension and compression. A tensegrity icosahedron model should be viewed as a simplistic mathematical attempt at explaining the complexity of living constructs (figure 1.3).

A simple mathematical model cannot reflect the complex behaviors of living tensegrities. Such simplistic models are void of life forces, breath, fluidic dynamics, thoughts, emotions, and consciousness.

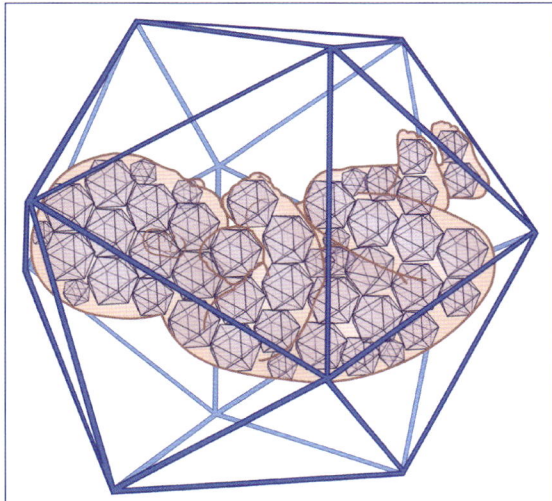

Figure 1.3. The icosahedron baby reflects the premise that we are scale-free icosahedra from micro to macro.

There is no better model than the human body to represent and explain living tensegrity.

A tensegrity icosahedron is typically made up of two types of component: *isolated compression* members and *infinite tensional* members. As everything is connected to everything in human tensegrity, there is, and can only be, one member providing both tension and compression as required in any given moment. To build a biological organism on the principles of tensegrity, the tensegrity truss must reflect continuity within a hierarchical construction, starting at the infinitely small subcellular component. Importantly, it must have the potential to build itself and provide self-stability.

The structure would be one integrated tensegrity that includes an integrated series of *trusses* (a truss is a structure composed of interconnected triangles) that evolved from infinitely smaller trusses that could be both structurally independent and interdependent at the same time. The triangulated arrangement of a truss offers stability without movement, and for movement to be facilitated, we need one or more additional three-bar trusses, essentially constrained by the lengths of the links and the angles between them. Therefore, living tensegrities consist of multiple-bar, closed kinematic systems of trusses. Donald Ingber aptly described this intricate truss system as the icosahedron.

Employing "anatomy for the twenty-first century" as a lens to understand self-constructed living forms introduces a novel paradigm and vision. This perspective significantly influences therapeutic interventions and guides the selection of appropriate movement modalities, aiming to facilitate greater ease of movement and alleviate or eliminate pain among individuals in our communities.

In navigating the intricate landscape of human biology, scientific understanding, grounded in the principle of uncertainty, has advanced to a level of maturity and sophistication. This progress empowers us to explore and gain confidence in various domains, encompassing evolution, embryology, ontology, phylogeny, biomechanics, and our subjective experience of reality. The journey of exploration is far from concluded. The scientific process remains dynamic and ever evolving. Our comprehension of the intricacies of human form and function is continually expanding, emphasizing the perpetual nature of scientific inquiry.

Tensegrity science coupled with fascia research is providing satisfactory explanations for the transient dynamics of human movement and stability. The take-away message for therapists is that tension and compression coexist as a necessary dual personality of the living tensegrity. This nonmechanical symbiosis of tension and compression permeates living tensegrities, manifesting in intricate fibrous fascial networks juxtaposed with compartmentalizing fascial specialities (e.g., cranial, diaphragmatic, muscular, abdominal, neural, interstitial) responding to tension and compression dancing in tandem. Delving deeper, one encounters the cellular realm, where cell dynamics must contend with and respond to the intracellular milieu, including inhomogeneous, anisotropic molecular microtubules and microfilaments within the cytoskeleton shaping and informing the internal protein architecture through their binding geometry. In my 2021 paper in the *International Journal of Anatomy and Research*, I referred to this as a *unified systems conception*. In this nature-inspired tensegrity-based model, fascia is a process providing the unitality of continuity and acts as a universal singularity permeating the whole soma. Thus, the living tensegrity or fasciategrity model is a model of wholeness, and the tensegrity icosahedron serves as the fundamental structure, behaving akin to a liquid crystal, thanks to the geometric limitations imposed by the close arrangement within living three-dimensional shapes.

The intricate framework of cellular tensegrity, woven from biopolymers, integrates dynamic elements such as contractile cytoskeletal microfilaments and osmotic components. Together, these elements orchestrate the conversion of mechanical forces within the extracellular matrix and cytoskeletal networks into the intricate dance of biochemical processes, physiological responses, and fluid motion. This cohesive web, which I call *fasciategrity* (combining the words *fascia* and *tensegrity*), forms the foundation of a coherent continuum stretching from the microscopic realm of cells to the unified entity of the organism.

Within this framework, myofascial force transmission plays a pivotal role, with structures like septa, tendons, and ligaments serving as key nodes in a body-wide network of mechanosensitive signaling. These tensegrity-based structures act as finely tuned regulators, ensuring the optimal tension required for the integrity of the fascial system.

This book does not require the reader to be the intellectual equivalent of Einstein to comprehend or appreciate the new anatomical narrative of human form and function. In its most unabridged form, this book wishes to make it abundantly clear that humans are not machines. Brains, muscles, nerves, lymphatics, and blood vessels are not mechanical nor mechanistic. The paradigm in medicine and anatomy of defining and describing humans, and all life on earth, as mechanical constructs has, in my opinion, through misguided belief and injudicious personal opinion, been smuggled past the customs officers guarding the medical and anatomical borders and led us down the wrong epistemological path. This has resulted, at best, in inaccurate descriptions and models of human form and function, and at worst set us back years in our search for the truth. Based on a seventeenth-century view, we currently embrace a body consisting of disconnected parts, pin joints, levers, hard-matter physics, and, most worryingly, linear explanations for a complex, nonlinear, unified system. Put simply, there are no straight lines in the human body, and everything is in continuity.

Tensegrity is therefore important to the fascia-focused therapist for several reasons.

The tensegrity-informed model confirms that wriggling your big toe is a full-body, complex engagement and coordination of the entire fascial system. Instead of focusing solely on localized symptoms or areas of pain, therapists can consider how tension and compression patterns throughout the body contribute to a patient's condition. This allows for more effective and targeted interventions that address underlying issues rather than simply treating surface-level symptoms. When the body maintains proper tension and compression relationships, it can move with greater ease and stability while minimizing strain and energy expenditure. Fascia-focused therapists can leverage this understanding to help clients improve their movement mechanics, enhance performance, and reduce the risk of injury. Tensegrity underscores the body's dynamic adaptability and capacity for self-regulation, including the physical and nonphysical attributes of human form and function. By acknowledging the body's inherent ability to respond and adapt to internal and external stimuli, fascia-focused therapists can support processes of healing and rehabilitation. This involves incorporating movement-based therapies, manual fascia-focused techniques, and interventions that encourage the body to restore balance and function.

What Is Fascia?

Fascia is a connective tissue that plays a crucial role in providing structural support and integrity throughout the human body. Comprising a complex network of collagen fibers, elastin, and ground substance, fascia forms a continuous web that surrounds and penetrates muscles, organs, nerves, and blood vessels (figure 1.4). This three-dimensional matrix not only encases individual muscle fibers but also forms them into functional units.

Fascia serves as a dynamic system, allowing for movement and flexibility while maintaining stability. Fascial continuity means it is everywhere, wrapping

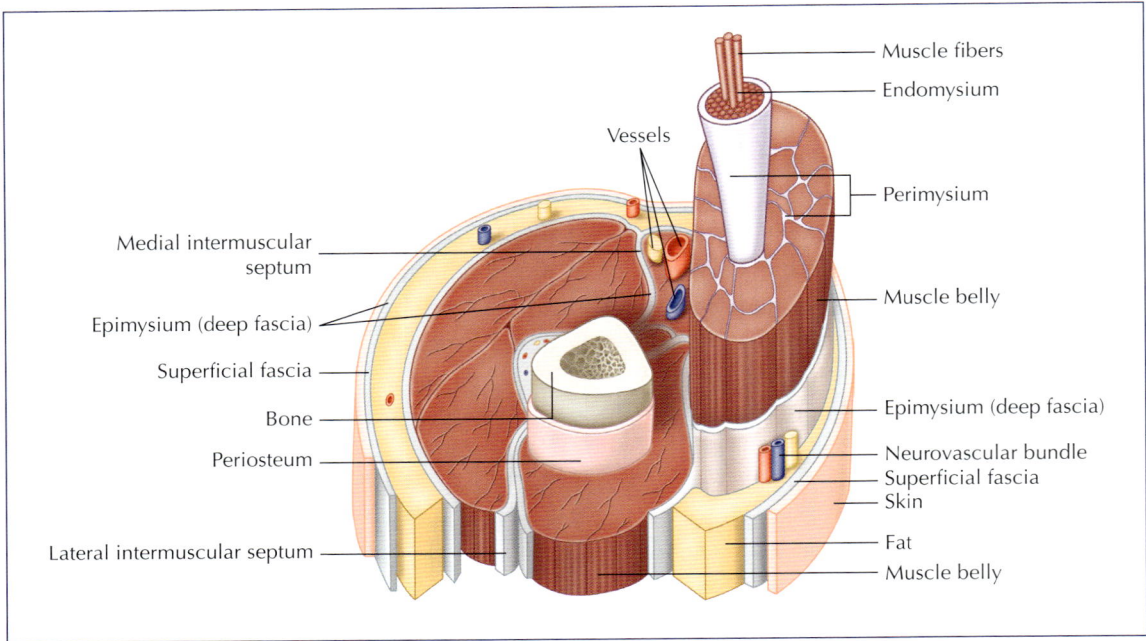

Figure 1.4. The many layers of fascia, which allow for movement and flexibility while maintaining stability.

internal fat, organs, nerves, blood vessels, viscera, muscle fibers, muscle bellies, and osseous (i.e., bone) tissues. It facilitates communication between local and more distant body parts, influencing coordination, interoception, and proprioception. Beyond its mechanical functions, fascia is involved in various physiological processes, such as nutrient exchange and waste removal. Its responsiveness to stress and strain highlights its importance for understanding and addressing issues related to posture, movement, and overall well-being. In essence, fascia is an intricate and interconnected system that contributes significantly to the body's form, function, and overall holistic health.

Medical professionals, including surgeons and neural block specialists, should have a thorough understanding of fascia at multiple levels, including its macroscopic and microscopic anatomy. With an embryological understanding of the process of fascia migration, the clinical anatomist can provide surgeons with the shortest, bloodless path via specific embryological fascial plains. This ensures surgical approaches can be minimally invasive, reducing tissue disruption, the need for cauterization, and reducing bleeding, while improving healing, therefore restoring function more rapidly. However, as there are no spaces in the human body, it is creating the space during surgery to allow cameras and surgical tools to carry out a procedure that causes the most significant structural damage to the fascial tissues. The functional and morphological variations of this one unifying connective tissue in the body are site-specific—reflecting its particular local function and based on environmental influences. Fascia has specialized cells that produce a lubricant (hyaluronan), which if not produced in exactly the right amount can result in an increased stiffening and aggregation of the tissue, loss of gliding between the planes, resulting in afferent receptors within the fascia plane becoming irritated, leading to peripheral sensitization. So, tela subcutanea and deep fascia share the name *fascia*, but they have very different functions.

While a strict definition of fascia has been established, although not universally agreed upon, what is not included in the medical curriculum is a focus on the ubiquitous nature and continuity of this omnidirectional tissue.

When Is a Connective Tissue Not Fascia?

The Federative International Programme for Anatomical Terminology (FIPAT) serves as the governing body for anatomical terminology within the International Federation of Associations of Anatomists (IFAA), the preeminent global entity in the field of anatomy. Given the diverse array of perspectives and vested opinions, achieving consensus on precise, delimited definitions is fraught with discord and controversy. The challenge of defining "fascia" is particularly pronounced, and compounded by the complexities introduced by translating terms into myriad languages.

The linguistic richness of Europe further exemplifies the intricacies inherent in anatomical terminology. *Ethnologue*, which publishes statistics and other information on world languages, catalogs over two hundred languages in Europe alone. The interpretation of anatomical terms can vary among languages, precluding a direct one-to-one correspondence for anatomical words. While certain languages may share etymological roots and possess overlapping vocabularies, each language invariably incorporates distinctive nuances, idioms, and cultural contexts that contribute to the nuanced meanings of anatomical terms.

From the French standpoint, the widely utilized term *fascia superficialis* omits reference to the panniculus adiposus and the textus connectivus laxus situated beneath the stratum membranosum. Consequently, these tissues do not fall under the classification of fascia according to that perspective. Anatomists recognize the necessity of precise dissection to separate the skin from the tela subcutanea, underscoring the continuous nature of the skin and the underlying fascia. However, it is imperative to note that the skin itself does not qualify as fascia.

Practitioners who adhere to a fascia-centric therapeutic approach emphasize the preliminary engagement of the skin to exert therapeutic influence on deeper tissues. This perspective highlights the therapeutic significance of the skin as a gateway to access and affect underlying fascial structures.

It is fitting that the FIPAT have constructed a definition of fascia specifically for the world of medical anatomy and professionals involved in medical studies. However, such a definition may not meet the needs of manual and movement therapists, who require a more holistic appreciation of the human form. What about skin, blood, and bones; how do they fit into the nature of wholeness? Investiagting the embryological development and origin of fascia supports a less reductionist view. In the realm of embryonic ontogenesis, a captivating narrative unfolds, elucidating the genesis of fascia amid the intricate differentiation processes of mesodermal and ectodermal cellular populations. Within this developmental tableau, fascia emerges as a pivotal connective tissue, gradually imbuing the evolving embryonic form with structural integrity and dynamic interconnectivity. As the embryonic journey progresses, the fascial network intricately intertwines with diverse anatomical substrates, encompassing muscle fibers, osseofascial elements (bones), nerves, blood vessels, and visceral organs. All tubes within tubes within tubes. This developmental orchestration culminates in the establishment of a vast cellular landscape, comprising an estimated thirty trillion cells, serving as the scaffolding upon which subsequent physiological processes unfold.

Embryologically, the inception of fascia is heralded on the twenty-first day of embryonic development, marking a seminal milestone in the continuum of cellular differentiation. Subsequent to its establishment, fascial maturation unfolds through a meticulously orchestrated series of temporal events, the precise coordination of which remains a subject of inquiry. The elucidation of the mechanisms governing these dynamic interactions finds resonance in the realm of epigenetics, with particular attention directed toward the conceptual framework of tensegrity architecture.

Doctor Donald Ingber, a prominent figure in this domain, has proffered a paradigmatic perspective, positing the responsiveness of the genetic code to extrinsic stimuli and the architectural constraints of cellular tensegrity. Through his seminal investigations, Ingber has unveiled a vista wherein the genetic landscape of cells manifests plasticity, engendering adaptive responses to environmental cues and cellular milieux. This theoretical framework provides a cogent lens through which to comprehend the intricate dance of cellular dynamics underlying fascial development and adaptation.

Recent strides in scientific inquiry have illuminated the nexus between fascia and the cognitive-emotive domain, unveiling a realm wherein the omnipresent connective tissue serves as a conduit for bidirectional neurological communication. Specialized sensory cells ensconced within the hypothalamus and anterior brainstem emerge as pivotal mediators in this dialogue, orchestrating the transmission of neural signals imbued with affective and cognitive valence. This intricate interplay engenders a nuanced interoceptive landscape, wherein physiological sensations interface with affective experience, creating a tapestry of emotions and consciousness.

The confluence of these interdisciplinary insights underscores the burgeoning potential for fascia-focused therapeutic modalities in the amelioration of chronic pain syndromes and mental health disorders. As researchers endeavour to unravel the enigmatic interplay between fascia and mind, the prospect of harnessing fascia-based interventions to modulate affective states and mitigate pathological conditions comes ever closer, heralding a new frontier in the realm of integrative medicine and holistic healthcare paradigms.

Fascia—It Is What You Think

While fascia has traditionally been considered in the context of physical mechanics and structural support, emerging research suggests that it also plays a significant role in our mental and emotional experiences, as well as our interoceptive and emotional processes.

Interoception is the awareness of the internal state of your body, which includes sensations such as heart rate, breathing, and feelings to and from the gut. The interoceptive nervous system, a component of the autonomic nervous system, is responsible for monitoring and regulating our internal physiological states. Fascia, with its pervasive presence throughout the body, is now understood to be involved in transmitting and modulating these internal signals, influencing our perception of emotions and feelings. Fascia acts as an information highway for interoceptive signals, with its sensory receptors conveying information about tissue tension, pain, and pressure. This connection between fascia and interoception underscores the idea that fascia *is what you think*—our thoughts and emotions are intimately connected to the sensations and information relayed by fascia (figure 1.5).

So the way we think and feel is not solely a function of our brain but involves a complex interplay between our mental and emotional states and the information transmitted through our body's fascial network. Fascia doesn't only support our physical structure, it influences our emotional experiences, and the two are inseparably linked. Our thoughts and emotions are not confined to our brains but are intertwined with the sensations and

signals carried by fascia, ultimately shaping our subjective experiences and feelings.

There is nothing simple about attempting to define fascia: it is one thing for those who see the body as a whole and another for those who deal in parts. Fascia is one thing and many. It can be described as a unified system,

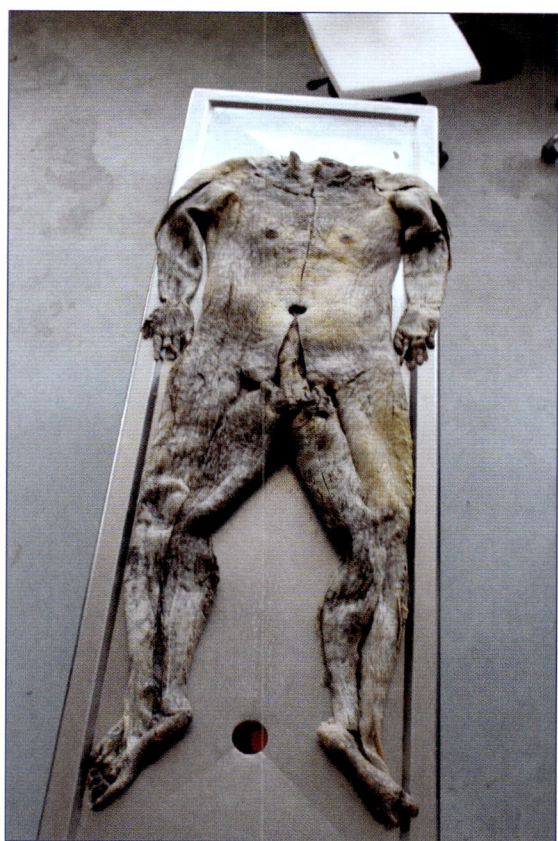

Figure 1.5. Research suggests that fascia plays a role in our mental and emotional experiences. As the superficial fascia (tela subcutanea), shown here as one continuous structure, is now recognized as the most sensory tissue in the human body it prompts a re-evaluation of how our bodies process and transmit sensory information, potentially revolutionizing our comprehension of mind-body interactions.

a net, a connective tissue, a sensory organ, a dissectible sheet (or sheath), a tendon, a ligament, interstitium; some have even been bold enough to include bone in the spectrum of specialized fascia. We could, in the spirit of Buckminster Fuller, come up with a definition suited specifically for fascia-focused movement and manual therapists. In fact, as mentioned previously, we have already done so—*fasciategrity*.

As this three-dimensional connective tissue was seen to wrap around or tie together structures at varying depths, one can appreciate why the name *fascia* was chosen by anatomists four hundred years ago: *fascia* is Latin for *bandage* (figure 1.6). However, this one, unifying connective tissue in the body has functionally and morphologically different variations, which are site-specific—reflecting a particular function and based on environmental influences. A widely accepted definition of fascia is a collagen-rich pliable sheet or sheath or any aggregation of connective tissue that one can dissect (this should also include osseofascial tissues such as cartilage). The inclusion of the word *dissect*, unfortunately, rules out blood and other bodily fluids as being included within a fascial system. Fascia-focused therapists should appreciate that blood and lymph are associated with every cell in the body and should be considered a special subclassification of fascia. Fascia continuity means it is everywhere—wrapping the internal fat, organs, nerves and blood vessels, viscera, muscle fibers, muscle bellies, and osseous tissues.

Fascia is typically divided into plains of varying thickness and classified by number

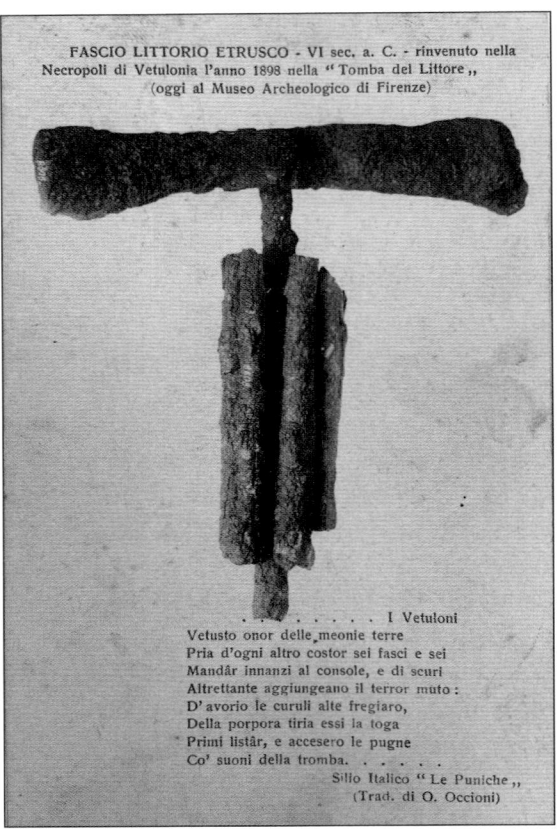

Figure 1.6. Postcard from 1937 showing a fasces-like decorative element, a bundle of rods 60 cm in length with a two-headed axe, all in iron—an ancient Roman symbol of auathority and power—found in 1898 in the Tomb of the Lictor at the Etruscan site of Vetulonia. (Image: T. C. Brennan).

of plains, fat content, protein variation, nerve accommodation, and innervation. The fascia located immediately beneath the skin is the most superficial *tela subcutanea* (also called *fascia superficialis* or *panniculus adiposus*), which is a predominantly fatty fascia (figure 1.7). The fat associated with this fascia needs to be understood in relation to posture, nerve compression, and overall morphology. The deep fascia (*fascia profunda*) wraps around

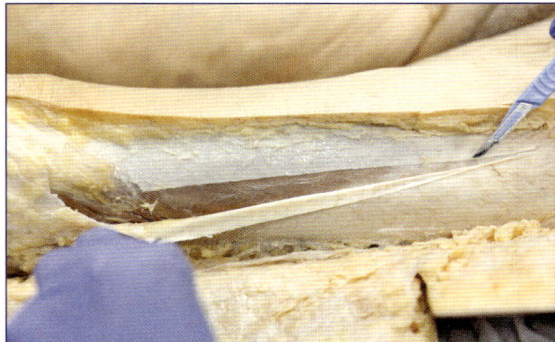

Figure 1.7. Fascia continuity in a sagittal section showing skin; the fatty superficial fascia, tela subcutanea, with differing levels of fat deposition depending on location; and the very dense, deep fascia profunda, with a rich network of blood vessels visible.

and permeates our muscles, providing us with a protective, force-transferring facility. The skeletal fascia is the *periosteum*. The visceral fascia (*subserous fascia*) wraps around all our organs and plays a significant role in thermal regulation, energy dynamics, perception, emotional response, and metabolism.

Muscle-associated fascia manifests distinct morphological variations throughout the body. In the limbs, both upper and lower, tendons for the most part exhibit a cord-like structure, while muscles in the torso, such as the rectus abdominis, feature flat tendons known as *aponeuroses*. The fascia aponeurosis enables the omnidirectional transmission of forces—allowing, for instance, the transfer of muscle-generated force from the lower limbs to the upper limb through the thoracolumbar aponeurosis. This intricate transmission is finely tuned by associated fascia tuning pegs, including deep pelvic myofascial units (figure 1.8).

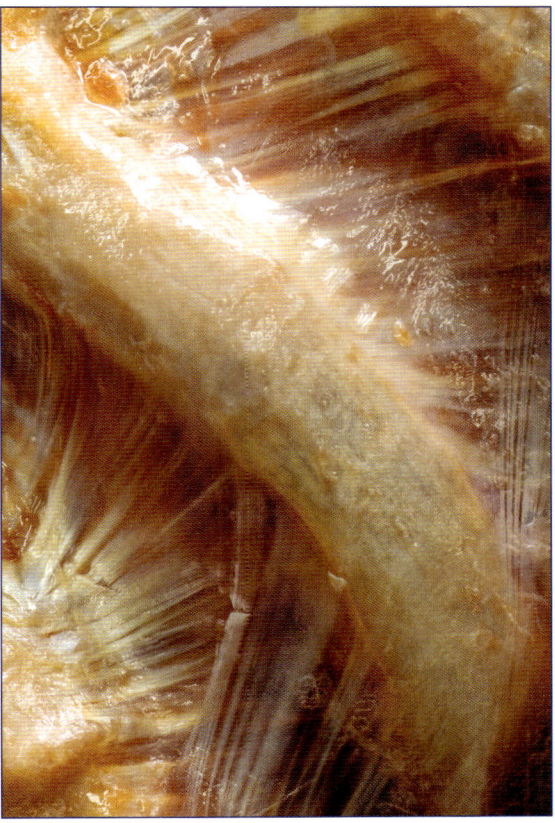

Figure 1.8. In this non-embalmed specimen, note the lattice-based decussation of the collagenous fibers crossing at angles over the red protein we call muscle and continuing to criss-cross providing a structural embrace called decussation.
This beautiful image is a two-dimensional representation of what is a three-dimensional process, omnipresent in the entire soma.
Decussation seems to be a fundamental building principle in nature.

It is crucial to acknowledge that muscle forces are inherently nonlinear, and resist the simplistic, even comforting, notion of linearity. The forces shared are not equally distributed in every direction owing to factors such as normal dampening, fascia condensation, pathological adhesions, or tears, as well as the arrangement and number of specialized ligaments tasked with coordinating forces for translation into appropriate metabolism, physiology, motion, and emotion.

Beneath the superficial fascia, fascia tuning pegs encompass structures such as the quadratus femoris, piriformis, obturator internus, obturator externus, superior gemelli, and inferior gemelli, as well as paraspinal myofascial units such as spinalis, longissimus, iliocostalis, multifidus, and serratus posterior inferior. In the realm of neuromuscular-associated fascia, the muscle epimysium, perimysium, and endomysium work synergistically to translate forces seamlessly, minimizing friction, unless pathology leads to friction, excess heat, inflammation, nerve insult, and pain.

The force exchange, or *mechanotransduction*, facilitated by the superficial fascia through the associated retinacula cutis and the fascia profunda is poorly understood. Extramuscular force pathways include the neurovascular tracts, lymphatics, and the interstitium. These provide an expansive or reductive hydraulic effect on fascia locally or at a distance, as demonstrated in fascia-focused dissections carried out at the University of Dundee by this author (Sharkey 2020 (Tensegrity informed observations)).

The morphology and histology of fascia vary by location, reflecting the local operating forces and epigenetic influences informing its formation. Fascia-focused Thiel soft-fixed dissections have provided unique insights into fascial anatomy, which could provide a new functional classification based on hierarchical functional categories, including:

- Gliding
- Restraining
- Containing
- Force-transductive
- Communicating
- Septal
- Invaginating
- Osseous

Integrated "Anatomy for the Twenty-First Century"—Building Blocks

The historical exploration of anatomy shaped a reductionist perspective on what is essentially a "global" or "holistic" organism. Traditionally, anatomical studies were specialized, homing in on particular processes or applications. Anatomists saw their role as delving into the body's structure, studying the configuration of elements, microscopic organization, and the developmental processes therein. The intricate interplay between structure and function wasn't always fully comprehended. This book aims to guide readers in grasping fundamental concepts of human anatomy (including embryology), physiology, exercise science (via medical exercise), and applications focused on fascia, all from an integrated standpoint.

Embryology—Being Human

Embryology is the study of the development of an organism from the fertilized egg to its fully formed state. According to professor of anatomy Jaap van der Wal, the embryological origins of fascia can be traced back to the mesenchyme, or mesodermal germ layer,

during early embryonic development. Mesoderm is one of the three primary germ layers (along with ectoderm and endoderm) that forms during gastrulation, a crucial stage in embryogenesis (figure 2.1).

During gastrulation, the embryonic disc undergoes a process where cells migrate and differentiate to form the three germ layers. Within the mesoderm, a population of cells differentiates into mesenchyme, which is a loosely organized, undifferentiated embryonic connective tissue. Mesenchymal cells are multipotent, meaning they have the capacity to differentiate into various cell types, including fibroblasts, the cells responsible for producing the extracellular matrix (ECM) that forms the structural basis of fascia.

As embryonic development progresses, these fibroblasts within the mesenchyme further differentiate and organize themselves to form the more specialized connective tissues, including the numerous variations of fascia found throughout the body. The ECM they produce is rich in proteins such as collagen and elastin, and glycosaminoglycans,

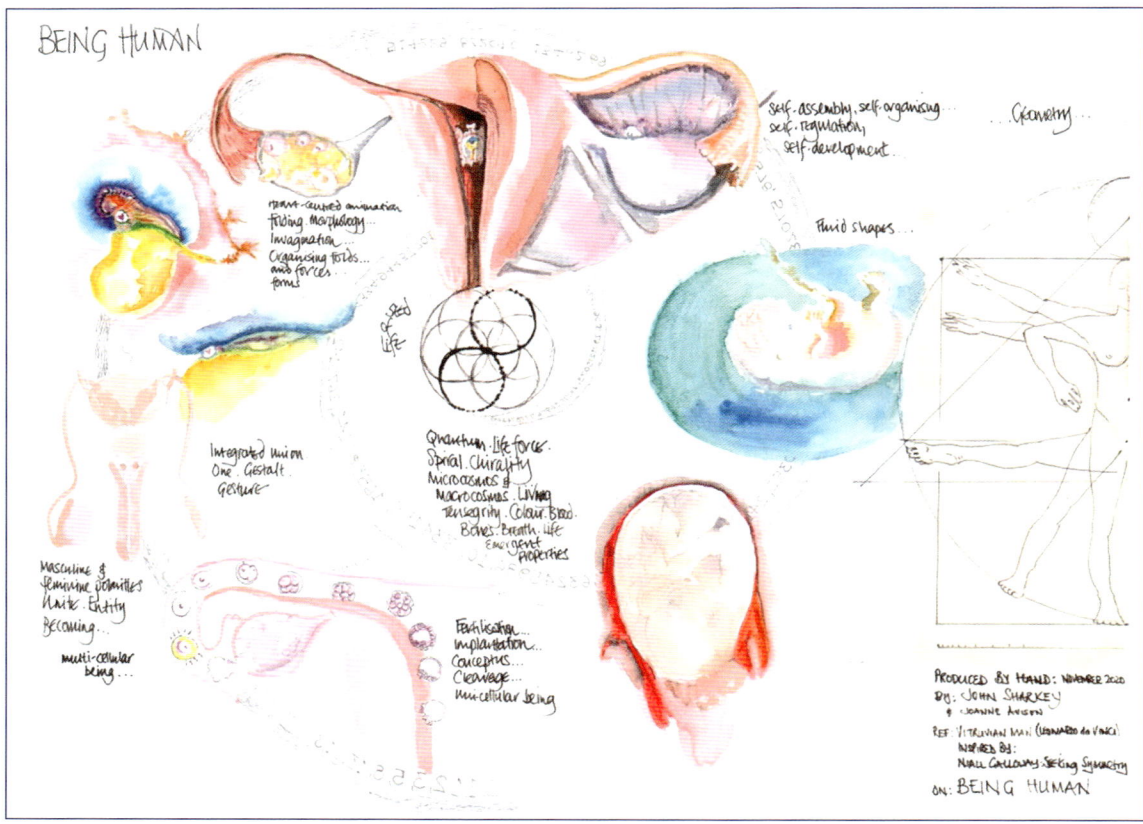

Figure 2.1. A beautiful watercolor depicting the various stages of the self-developing embryo from fertilization through implantation, conceptus (zygote plus its associated membranes), and cleavage, to the multicellular conscious human being. (Produced by hand, November 2020, by the author and Joanne Avison).

which give fascia its characteristic strength, flexibility, and resilience. The differentiation and organization of mesenchymal cells into fascia are tightly regulated by genetic signals and molecular cues, ensuring the proper development of fascial structures in the correct locations within the body.

Genetics plays a crucial role in embryonic development. Epigenetics, the regulation of gene expression without changes to the underlying DNA sequence, also plays a significant role. Epigenetic processes, such as DNA methylation and histone modification, regulate when and where genes are turned on or off during embryonic development. Epigenetic forces contribute to cell differentiation and the formation of specialized tissues. These mechanisms influence the fate of mesenchymal cells, determining whether they differentiate into fibroblasts and subsequently form ligaments or tendons. This, in effect, explains why you have an iliotibial tract on the lateral aspect of your lower limb and why your spine is contained within a tube we call the posterior and anterior longitudinal ligaments.

Tensegrity influences and guides embryonic development and structural stability through a balance of tension and compression. Tensegrity provides the framework to understand how emerging forces influence embryonic development, leading to chirality in tissues and the formation of a tubular network, or tubes within tubes (see figures 1.8 and 2.2). *Chirality* refers to the property of asymmetry or handedness in a molecule or structure, where there are two distinct forms that are mirror images of each other, much like the left and right hands. In biology, chirality is often observed in the spatial arrangement of molecules or the asymmetry of structures during development, and influences various physiological processes. Chirality is a fundamental characteristic of fascia and fascial structures (see figures 1.8 and 2.3). Cells and tissues experience tensional and compressional forces as they undergo morphogenesis and organogenesis. Tensegrity can influence chirality in fascia by exerting mechanical forces that impact cell orientation, migration, and tissue organization—for example, such forces contribute to the establishment of the left-right asymmetry of the heart and gut.

The development of blood vessels is influenced by tensional forces within the developing vessel, along with compressive forces from surrounding tissues and the pulsatile nature of blood flow. This environment influences cellular behaviors, affecting cell shape, alignment, and organization. Alignment is critical as if fascia or any fascial structure, such as a blood vessel, had only one fiber orientation it would have little or no structural integrity.

Eric Blechschmidt, a German embryologist, contributed significantly to our understanding of embryonic development. While he did

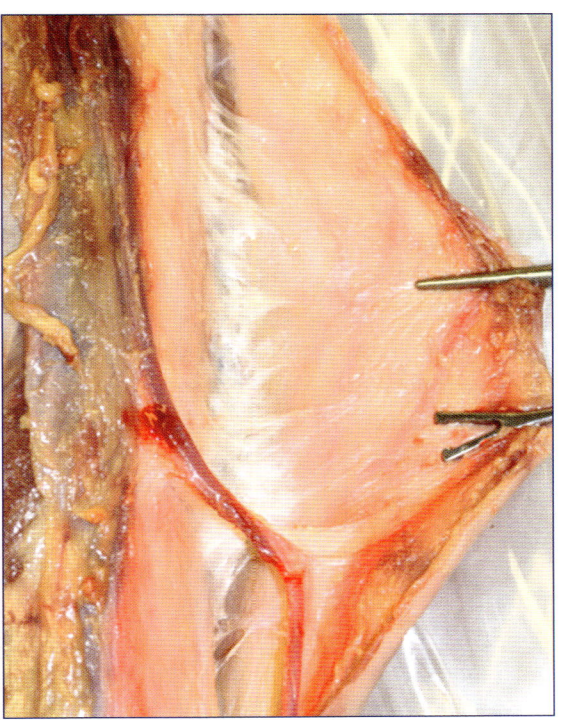

Figure 2.2. Living tensegrities are tubes within tubes within tubes. Bones are tubes, arteries and veins are tubes, nerves are tubes, muscle fibers are tubes, and fascia comprises a microtubular network, primarily responsible for the transportation of electromagnetic particles, ions and fluids.

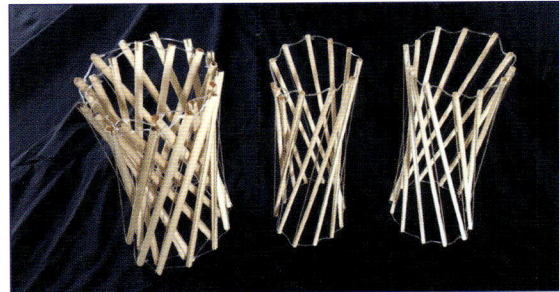

Figure 2.3. Right: A chiral structure with both right- and left-handed arrangements. Left: The fusion of right and left chiral configurations of collagen fibers, contributing to the integrity and stability of the tube. As a result of this chirality, any stress applied to micro- or macro-tubules would manifest as a spiral force rather than a longitudinal one.

not specifically focus on chirality in the same way it is discussed in molecular and structural biology, he did observe and describe asymmetry and handedness in developing embryos, and his work laid a foundation for appreciating the complexity and interconnectedness of embryonic development. Taking a phenomenological approach to embryology, Blechschmidt sought to understand the unfolding of life by closely observing and documenting the intricate processes involved. His emphasis on the dynamic and holistic nature of embryonic development deviated from the reductionist approaches prevalent in some areas of biology. Instead of isolating individual components, Blechschmidt acknowledged the interconnectedness of many factors, including movement, nutrient exchange, and regional interactions within the developing embryo. His observations extended beyond the anatomical structures to include the temporal dimension of development. By studying the sequential stages of embryogenesis, he provided a comprehensive framework for understanding how asymmetry and differentiation manifest over time.

With his phenomenological approach, Blechschmidt aimed to capture the essence of the developmental experience, considering not only the physical changes but also the qualitative aspects of embryonic life. This perspective allowed him to explore the unfolding narrative of embryonic development, highlighting the importance of the embryo's interaction with its environment. His holistic approach continues to influence the study of embryology, reminding researchers to consider the multidimensional aspects that contribute to the formation of a new life.

The Language of Anatomy

Exploring the realms of anatomy and physiology presents an exhilarating challenge. Even as a perpetual student in this lifelong journey of learning, my initial foray into the study of anatomy left me with awe and a touch of trepidation. The prospect of delving into the intricacies of how the human body functions was daunting, compounded by the necessity to embrace a new language, the language of anatomy. Yet, it was within this very linguistic realm that I discovered my greatest ally. Delving into the etymology and significance of each unfamiliar word or term, deconstructing them into their elemental components, dissolved the intimidation factor and granted me a profound understanding.

The term *anatomy* itself signifies dissection— the meticulous exploration of an organism's regions, deemed to be its "parts." Rooted in Latin *anatomia*, and stemming from the Greek *anatomē*, where *ana* means "up," and *temenos* means "to cut," *anatomy* encapsulates a centuries-old tradition of studying the body through dissection, as vividly depicted in Rembrandt's iconic (but anatomically inaccurate) *Anatomy Lesson of Dr. Nicolaes Tulp* (figure 2.4).

Unraveling the linguistic tapestry further, the term *muscle* finds its origin in the Latin *musculus*, the diminutive of *mus*, meaning "mouse." This imaginative association arises from the movement of muscles beneath

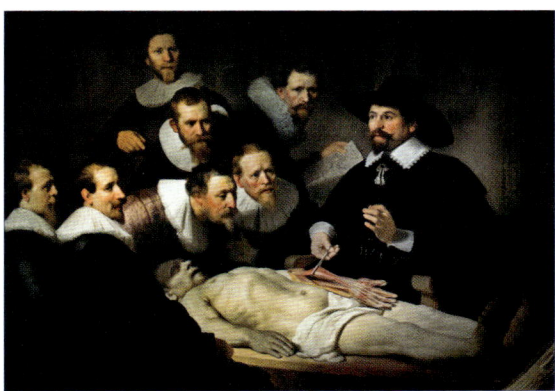

Figure 2.4. **The Anatomy Lesson of Dr. Nicolaes Tulp**, *by Rembrandt (1632). Courtesy of Shutterstock.*

the skin, resembling the subtle motion of a mouse beneath a sheet. This linguistic journey not only unveils the historical methods of anatomical exploration but also enriches our comprehension of the intricacies that govern the human form.

The language of anatomy has a wonderful history. Early anatomists, including the father of medicine, Hippocrates (460–377 BC, figure 2.5), and Aristotle (384–322 BC), used Latin and Greek terms to describe body parts, prominent structures, muscles, and so on. It should be noted that the word *part* is a language of convenience, as a "part" could never survive without the whole (i.e., there are no parts until the anatomist cuts them apart). Hippocrates was a great surgeon, while Aristotle made accurate observations of animal embryos.

Greek and Latin terms are not the only ones used in anatomy. At around the same time, the medical school in Alexandria, Egypt, was providing public dissections of human bodies to reveal their internal structures.

And even then, many centuries had passed since the birth of the anatomical sciences in Egypt, around 3000 BC; the earliest surviving papyruses recording the practice of anatomy are from a few hundred years later, notably the *Ebers Papyrus*, which dates to around 1550 BC (Persaud 1984, figure 2.6).

In the sixteenth century, Andreas Vesalius played a pivotal role in the revival of anatomy with his seminal work, *On the Fabric of the Human Body in Seven Books*. During the Renaissance, Vesalius and other anatomists introduced a standardized nomenclature, although muscles were initially designated by numbers as a method of study, rather than individual names. The practice of numbering

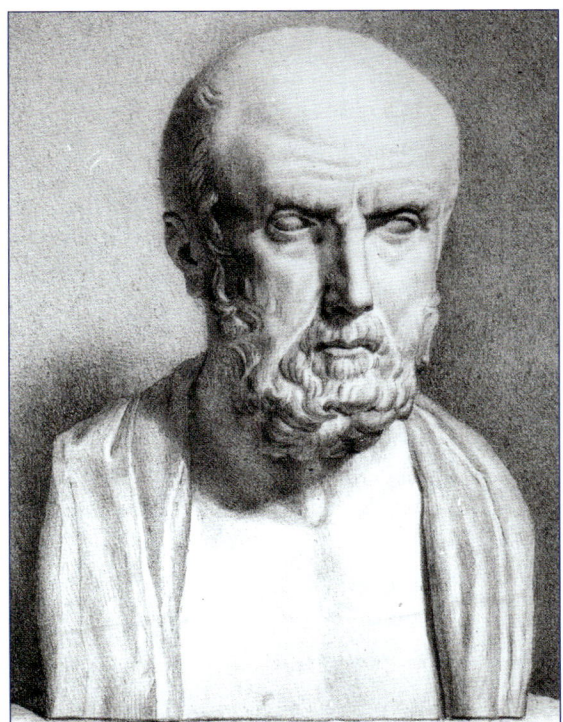

Figure 2.5. Hippocrates, the father of medicine. Image © Archives Charmet/Bridgeman Images.

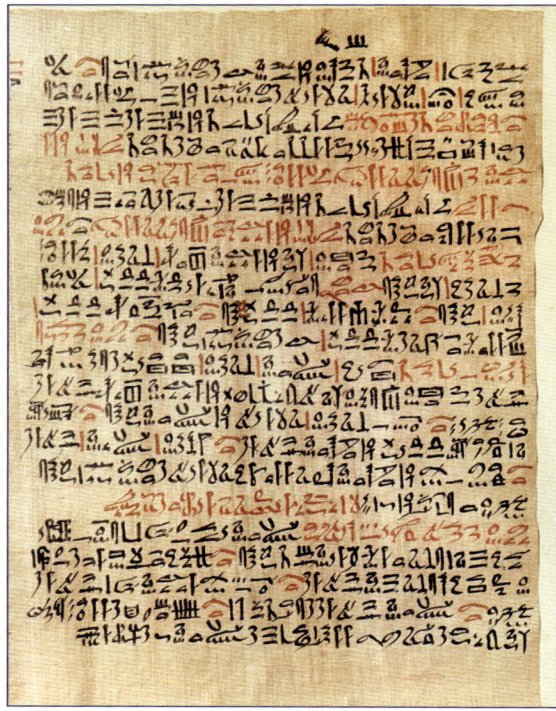

Figure 2.6. The Ebers Papyrus. Image © Archives Charmet/Bridgeman Images.

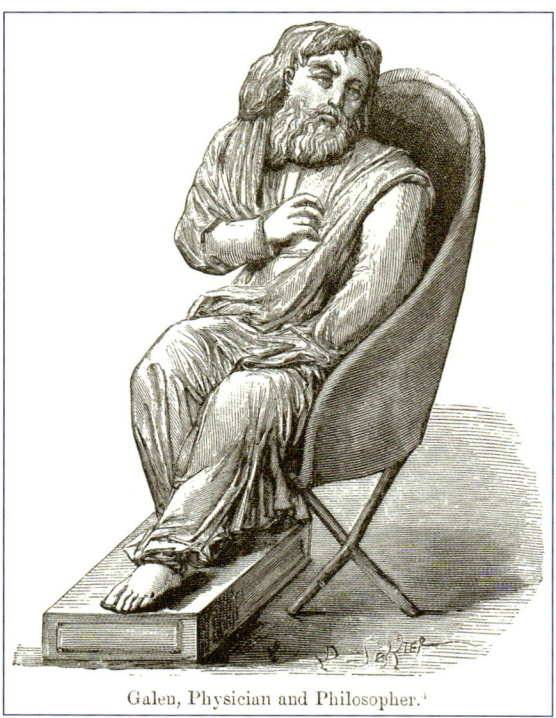

Galen, Physician and Philosopher.

Figure 2.7. Galen introduced the method of numbering muscles. Image © Archives Charmet/ Bridgeman Images.

muscles can be traced back to the eminent physician and anatomist Galen (130–200 AD, figure 2.7), and this method persisted until the late seventeenth and early eighteenth centuries. Significant changes occurred during this later period, when specific myological terminology began to replace the numerical system. Notably, British anatomist William Cowper and Scottish anatomist James Douglas played pivotal roles in the naming of muscles, contributing to the evolution of anatomical language and understanding.

Anatomy was progressed during the Middle Ages by the work of medical students and teachers at universities and medical colleges throughout Europe, particularly in Salerno, Padua, and Bologna in Italy, and at this

time the ingenious work of Leonardo da Vinci was born. Also around this time the study of anatomy in Persia was unfolding as a rich and distinct intellectual tradition, contributing valuable insights alongside the parallel advancements in Europe and the USA. Persian anatomists emphasized the importance of direct observation and dissection, aligning with the principles of empirical inquiry.

While the European and American anatomical traditions were evolving concurrently, they often drew inspiration from Greco-Roman sources and later embraced the Renaissance spirit of inquiry. Notably, the European and American approaches tended to involve an even greater emphasis on human cadaver dissection, building on the legacy of figures like Vesalius.

The study of anatomy in countries such as India, Pakistan, Australia, and elsewhere developed within their own cultural and educational contexts. In India, a rich historical tradition of Ayurveda and traditional medicine incorporated anatomical knowledge, with ancient texts describing bodily structures and functions. Modern anatomical education in India evolved with the establishment of medical colleges during the British colonial era, blending traditional knowledge with Western anatomical approaches. In Pakistan, a similar fusion of traditional and Western anatomical teachings occurred, reflecting the country's diverse medical education landscape.

Anatomical knowledge among indigenous peoples in the central and southern Pacific before the arrival of Westerners, particularly in Australia, was rich and diverse, although specific details are challenging to ascertain due to limited written records from that time period. Indigenous cultures in these regions had developed intricate understandings of human anatomy over generations through observations, practical experiences, and cultural traditions. This knowledge was often passed down orally from generation to generation and was deeply intertwined with spiritual beliefs, traditional healing practices, and cultural ceremonies.

In Australia, Aboriginal peoples had a sophisticated understanding of human anatomy, which was essential for activities such as hunting, gathering, tool-making, home building, and healing. They possessed detailed knowledge of the structure and function of various organs, bones, muscles, and bodily systems, which they used for medicinal purposes and surgical procedures. Aboriginal healers, known as *ngangkari*, or "clever people," employed this knowledge to treat illnesses, injuries, and ailments within their communities. Similarly, in other parts of the central and southern Pacific, such as Polynesia, Micronesia, and Melanesia, indigenous peoples had their own unique systems of anatomical knowledge. Traditional healers and practitioners in these regions employed a variety of methods, including massage, herbal medicine, and ritualistic practices, to address health issues and maintain well-being.

While much of this traditional anatomical knowledge was not recorded in written form before the arrival of Europeans, archaeological evidence, oral histories, and anthropological studies provide insights into the depth and breadth of indigenous anatomical understanding in the central and southern Pacific. These cultures' holistic perspectives on the human body often encompassed not only physical aspects but also spiritual, emotional, and social dimensions, reflecting the interconnectedness of individuals with their environment and community.

In Oceania generally and Australia specifically, the study of anatomy went on to follow the Western biomedical model, with a focus on human cadaver dissection and alignment with global medical standards. The diverse population and commitment to international collaboration in this region have contributed to a multifaceted approach in anatomical research and education. In other regions of the world, the study of anatomy has seen unique trajectories. Different countries have adopted a mix of traditional practices and contemporary anatomical methods, influenced by cultural, historical, and educational factors.

The global exchange of anatomical knowledge continues to foster a comprehensive understanding of the human body, enriching the collective endeavor to advance the medical sciences worldwide. Despite variations in methodology, the collective pursuit of anatomical understanding across the world has ultimately enriched the global discourse on the intricacies of the human body. The history of anatomy is ancient and fascinating. If we were to provide names for our muscles today, we could say *the muscle with two tendons on the upper part of the upper limb*. Of course, history has provided us with the term *biceps brachii*, which even sounds poetic. In anatomy, words are often modified by adding a prefix or suffix. For example, the suffix *-itis* means inflammation. Tendonitis is therefore the swelling or inflammation of a tendon, although it is more correctly spelled *tendinitis* (note the change of letter from *o* to *i*).

By breaking down the words, we can work out the meaning of anatomical terms, or at least have fun trying.

Prefixes, Suffixes, and Combining Forms

A good example of a word root, used as a base, is *brachii*, which means "of the arm." Technically the arm is only from the elbow to the shoulder, and below the elbow is the forearm. By adding a prefix at the beginning of a base or a suffix to the end of a base, you will change its meaning (table 2.1).

One can also add a vowel to combine one root to another or to join it with a suffix, known as a *combining form*. To assist you to that end, here is a table listing common prefixes, suffixes, and combining forms with English translation. This will help to remove the threat of learning anatomy. This list is by no means exhaustive but offers some useful examples.

Table 2.1. Common Prefixes, Suffixes, and Combining Forms.

Prefix/Suffix/Combing Form	Translation	Example
a-	without or lacking	avascular
ab-	away from	abduct
ad-	to, toward	adduct
aden-, adeno-	gland	adenoid
adip-, adipos-	fat	adipose tissue
aer-, aeros-	air	aerobic metabolism
af-, ad-	add, move toward	afferent, adduct
-al-	pertaining to	brachial

Table 2.1. Common Prefixes, Suffixes, and Combining Forms. (Continued)

Prefix/Suffix/Combing Form	Translation	Example
alb-	white	albino
-algia	pain	neuralgia
andro-	male	androgen
angio-	vessel	angiogram
ante-	in front or before	anterior
anti-	against or opposed	antibody
arter-	artery	arterial
arthro-	joint	arthrokinetics
-asis	state	homeostasis
aur-, auri-	ear	auricle
auto-	self	automatic
bi-	two/double	biceps
bio-	life	biology
blast-	precursor	blastocyst
brachi-	arm	brachialis
bronch-	windpipe/airway	bronchial
bucc-	cheek	buccal
calc-	pertaining to the heel	calcaneus
capit-	head	capitate
carcin-	cancer	carcinoma
cardi-, cardio-	heart	cardiac
carpal-	wrist	carpal tunnel
cata-	down	catabolism
caud-	tail	caudal
cerebr-	brain	cerebrospinal
chondr-	cartilage	chondrosis
-cide	destroy, kill	bactericide

(Continued)

Table 2.1. Common Prefixes, Suffixes, and Combining Forms. (Continued)

Prefix/Suffix/Combing Form	Translation	Example
-clast	broken, break, destroy	osteoclast
con-	together	connective tissue
contra-	against, opposite	contralateral
corn-	hard	cornea
corp-	body	corpse
cost-	rib	costal
cranio-	skull	craniology
-crine	to separate	endocrine
cyst-	sac	cystoblast
-cyte	cell	erythrocyte
cyto-	cell	cytoplasm
de-	away from, down	detract, depress
dendr-	tree	dendrite
-derma-	skin	dermabrasion
di-	twice, two	disaccharide
dia-	through, between, apart, across	diameter
digit-	finger, toe	digital
dis-	apart, away from, reversal or separation	discharge
-duct	draw	abduct
dys-	painful, difficult, bad	dysmenorrhea
e-	without, away from	emit
ec-	out from	eccentric
ecto-	outside (or outer side)	ectoderm
-ectomy	to remove (cut out)	vasectomy
-edema	swelling	lymphedema
-emia	presence of substance in blood	lipidemia

Table 2.1. Common Prefixes, Suffixes, and Combining Forms. (Continued)

Prefix/Suffix/Combing Form	Translation	Example
en-	in, into	endemic
endo-	within, inside	endomysium
epi-	on, over, above	epidermis
erythro-	red	erythrocyte
ex-	out, away from	exhale
exo-	outside	exoskeleton
extra-	outside, beyond, in addition	extracellular
-ferent	carry	efferent
fila-	thread	filament
-form	having shape or form	fusiform (expressing resemblance)
gastro-, gaster-, gastr-	stomach, belly	gastrointestinal
-genesis	origin, production, formation	pathogenesis
glu-	sugar, sweet	glucose
glyco-	sugar	glycogen
-gram	a drawing, record of	myogram
-graph	to write, record	electrocardiograph
hem-	blood	hematology
hemi-	half	hemisphere
histo-	tissue	histology
homeo-	same	homeostasis
hydro-	water, hydrogen	hydromassage
hyo-	u-shaped	hyoid
hyper-	above, more	hyperactive
hypo-	under, less	hypoactive
-ia	pathological condition	pneumonia
-iatr	cure, treat, medical treatment	pediatrics

(Continued)

Table 2.1. Common Prefixes, Suffixes, and Combining Forms. (Continued)

Prefix/Suffix/Combing Form	Translation	Example
infra-	beneath	infraorbital
inter-	between	intervertebral
intra-	within	intracapsular
ipsi-	itself, same	ipsilateral
-ism	condition, process	dimorphism
iso-	equal, alike, uniform	isometric
-itis	inflammation	gastritis
kino-, kine-	move, movement	kinesiology
-lemma	husk, sheath around structure	sarcolemma
leuko-, leuco-	white	leukocyte
liga-	to bind	ligament
lipo-	fat	liposuction
macro-	large	macrophage
mal-	abnormal, bad	malalignment
-malac-, -malaco-	soft	osteomalacia
mega-	big, great	megacolon
melano-	black	melanocyte
meso-	middle	mesoderm
meta-	next, change, after	metastasis
micro-	small	microscope
mito-	thread-like, filament	mitochondria
mono-	one or single	monosaccharide
morph-	form	morphology
multi-	much, many	multicellular
myelo-	marrow, spinal cord	myeloid
myo-	muscle	myocardium
nas-	nose	nasolacrimal duct

Table 2.1. Common Prefixes, Suffixes, and Combining Forms. (Continued)

Prefix/Suffix/Combing Form	Translation	Example
neo-	new	neonatal
neuro-	nerve, nervous system	neuromuscular
-oid	form, resemblance	epidermoid
-ology	science, branch of knowledge	physiology
-oma	tumor, swelling	carcinoma
onco-	mass, tumor	oncology
orb-	circle	orbicularis oris
-ory	referring to	olfactory
-ose	full of	adipose
-osis	state, condition, abnormal condition	neurosis, osteoporosis
osteo-	bone	osteoblast
-ous	expressing material	serous
para-	near to, beside	paraplegia
patho-	disease	pathology
per-	through	permeate
peri-	around	periosteum
phag-, phago-	to eat	phagocyte
-phobia	fear	hydrophobia
pneumo-	air, lungs, gas	pneumonia
pod-, podo-	foot	podiatry
poly-	many, much	polymer
post-	after, behind	postpartum
pre-	before, in front of	prenatal
pseudo-	false	pseudocyst
pterygo-	wing	pterygoid
pulmo-	lung	pulmonary

(Continued)

Table 2.1. Common Prefixes, Suffixes, and Combining Forms. (Continued)

Prefix/Suffix/Combing Form	Translation	Example
quadr-	four, one quarter	quadriceps
re-	back, again, contrary	reabsorption
retro-	backward, located behind	retroperitoneal
-rrhagia	burst forth, pour	menorrhagia
-rrhea	flow, discharge	amenorrhea
sarco-	flesh	sarcomere
-sclero-	hard	arteriosclerosis
-sect	to cut	dissect
semi-	half	semitendinosus
som-, somat-	body	somatic
spino-	spine	spinous process
-stalsis	contractile	peristalsis
-stasis	stop, stand still	hemostasis
steno-	a narrowing, contracted	stenosis
sub-	below	subcutaneous
super-	above, beyond	superficial
supra-	above, upon	supraglenoid
sym-, syn-	together	symphysis pubis, synthesis
therm-, thermo-	heat	thermoregulation
-thorax	chest	pneumothorax
-tomy	to cut	anatomy
trans-	through, across, beyond	transection
tri-	three	triceps
uni-	one	unicellular
vas-	vessel	vascular
vene-	vein	venesection
viscer-	internal organ	viscera

Terms Used in Anatomy

Anatomical Localization

Understanding anatomical localization terms is easier if you consider an organism with a straight central nervous system (CNS), such as a lizard. In this context, *rostral*, *caudal*, *ventral*, and *dorsal* correspond to movements respectively toward the nose or face (rostrum), the tail, the belly, and the back. However, in humans and other primates, the CNS axis bends, altering these orientations. For the brain, *caudal* now refers to the back of the head, *ventral* to the body, and *dorsal* to the top of the head.

Anatomical study often involves examining the intricate three-dimensional organization of the CNS through slices, or planes, employing the "stereotactic approach" (*stereo*, "solid object," and *tactic*, *tactus*, "touch"). Common slice orientations include axial (horizontal), coronal (vertical, revealing both ears), and parasagittal (vertical, showing from the nose to the back of the head). A sagittal slice bisects the head into equal left and right sides, while a parasagittal slice is one parallel to the sagittal plane. This nuanced understanding enhances the comprehension of anatomical relationships in three-dimensional space.

Glossary of Commonly Used Directional Terms

All references to human movement are considered to begin from the internationally accepted reference point known as the *anatomical position*. The anatomical position is one of a person standing erect with the face forward, the arms hanging by the side, the fingers extended, the palms of the hands facing forward, and the feet flat on the ground and slightly turned out.

In the anatomical position, joints are said to be in the *neutral position*.

Abduction	Movement away from the midline (or to return from adduction)
Adduction	Movement toward the midline (or to return from abduction)
Anterior	Toward the front of the body (as opposed to posterior)
Caudal, caudad	Toward the tail, inferior
Cephalad	Toward the head, superior
Contralateral	On the opposite side
Deep	Away from the surface (as opposed to superficial)
Distal	Away from the point of origin of a structure (as opposed to proximal)
Dorsal	Relating to the back or posterior portion (as opposed to ventral)
Extension	Movement at a joint resulting in separation of two ventral surfaces (as opposed to flexion)
Flexion	Movement at a joint resulting in approximation of two ventral surfaces (as opposed to extension)
Inferior	Below or furthest away from the head
Ipsilateral	On the same side

Lateral   Located away from the midline (opposite to medial)

Medial   Situated close to or at the midline of the body or organ (opposite to lateral)

Posterior   Relating to the back or the dorsal aspect of the body (opposite to anterior)

Proximal   Closer to the center of the body or to the point of attachment of a limb

Rotation   Movement around a fixed axis

Superficial On or near the surface (as opposed to deep)

Superior   Above or closest to the head

Ventral   Anterior part of body (as opposed to dorsal)

Glossary of Commonly Used Anatomical and Other Terms

Acetabulum   Meaning "vinegar bowl"; on the coxal bone, the outer surface presents as a rounded cavity

Acute   Of recent onset (hours, days, or a couple of weeks); short-term

Adhesions   Fibroblast formation caused by tearing, or disruption of collagen fibers from trauma, immobilization, or as a result of surgical treatment

Afferent   Conveying a fluid or a nerve impulse toward an organ or area (as opposed to efferent)

Analogous   Similar in function or appearance but having a different origin or structure (cf. homologous)

Anomaly   Structure that is unusual or abnormal

Anterior tilt Rocks the cephalad portion of the pelvis anteriorly with an increase in lumbar lordosis

Aponeurosis Fibrous sheet of collagenous bundles serving as a connection between a muscle and its attachment

Articulation Joint or junction between two or more bones

Chronic   Long-lasting (two weeks or more)

Contract   Shrink or decrease in size, shorten

Coronal plane Vertical plane at right angles to the sagittal plane that divides the body into anterior and posterior portions

Cranial   Relating to/or toward the skull/head

Decussation Fibers crisscrossing, sometimes from one side of the body to the other

Dermatome   Area of skin supplied by a single spinal nerve

Efferent   Conveying a fluid or a nerve impulse away from a central organ (as opposed to afferent)

Evagination To protrude from; an out-pouching, forming a sac or tube

Fascia — Connective tissue lying beneath the skin enveloping muscle groups and investing various organs

Foramen — Natural opening, found primarily in bones

Fossa — Pit or depression

Friction — Back and forth movement (using digits or other) creating heat in the tissues

Frontal plane — Same as coronal plane

Ganglion — Collection of nerve cell bodies located outside the brain or spinal cord

Greater trochanter — Broad flat process at the top of the lateral femur

Horizontal plane — Transverse plane at right angles to the long axis of the body

Insertion — Site of an attachment of a muscle, tendon, or aponeurosis to bone

Intermediate — Between two structures

Joint — Meeting of two or more bones

Ligament — Band of fibrous connective tissue joining two or more bones

Lumen — Cavity or passageway within a tubular organ or vessel

Meatus — Tube-like opening within a bone

Median — Centrally located, situated in the middle of the body

Motor — Of axons, conveying impulses from the CNS to muscles or glands, producing movement or secretion (as opposed to sensory)

Palmar — Anterior surface of the hand

Palpate — To examine by pressing or touching

Patent — Open or exposed

Plantar — Sole of the foot

Plexus — Network of nerves or vessels

Postganglionic — Situated distal to a ganglion

Preganglionic — Situated anterior or proximal to a ganglion

Prevertebral — In front of the vertebral column or vertebrae

Process — Marked prominence protruding from a bone, marking site of attachment of muscles

Prone — Position of the body in which the ventral surface faces down (as opposed to supine)

Sagittal plane — Vertical plane extending in an anteroposterior direction dividing the body into right and left parts

Sensory — Of axons, conveying information from the periphery into the CNS (as opposed to motor)

Septum — Partition dividing two cavities or masses of soft tissue

Supine	Position of the body in which the ventral surface faces up (as opposed to prone)
Tendon	Fibrous band of dense regular connective tissue that attaches a muscle to a bone
Transverse plane	Same as horizontal plane
Tubercle	Small, rounded elevation on a bone
Tuberosity	Relatively large protuberance from the surface of a bone
Valgus position	Relates to the alignment of segments of the upper and lower limbs—position in which the distal bone is abducted with respect to the proximal bone
Varus position	Relates to the alignment of segments of the upper and lower limbs—position in which the distal bone is adducted with respect to the proximal bone

Regional Areas

The human body can be divided into the *axial* and *appendicular* regions (see p. 66). The axial division is made up of the head, neck, and trunk. The appendicular division comprises the limbs, which are attached to the axis of the body. An *axis* is a point around which movement takes place. Figure 2.8a and b show terms used to indicate specific body areas.

A Few Words on Decussation

The principle of decussation holds a paramount role in tensegrity-informed anatomical construction because of its inherent capacity to enhance strength and integrity in biological structures. Decussation refers to the crossing or interweaving of fibers, creating a crisscross pattern, which contributes to increased stability and resilience.

This principle is notably evident in the organization of nerves and fascia throughout the human body. Nerves often exhibit decussation, where fibers cross over from one side to the other (this is also known as a *commissure*), facilitating efficient communication between different regions of the nervous system. This arrangement not only promotes redundancy but also protects against localized damage.

Similarly, fascia, the connective tissue that surrounds muscles and organs, often displays a decussate pattern, reinforcing structural integrity and providing essential support. Through decussation, anatomical structures gain a remarkable ability to withstand forces and stresses, ensuring the overall robustness of the human body.

Cellular Level Organization of the Human Body

The basic unit of animal life is the *cell*, whose name derives from its microscopic resemblance to a small room. Some specialized cells, such as muscle and nerve cells, possess

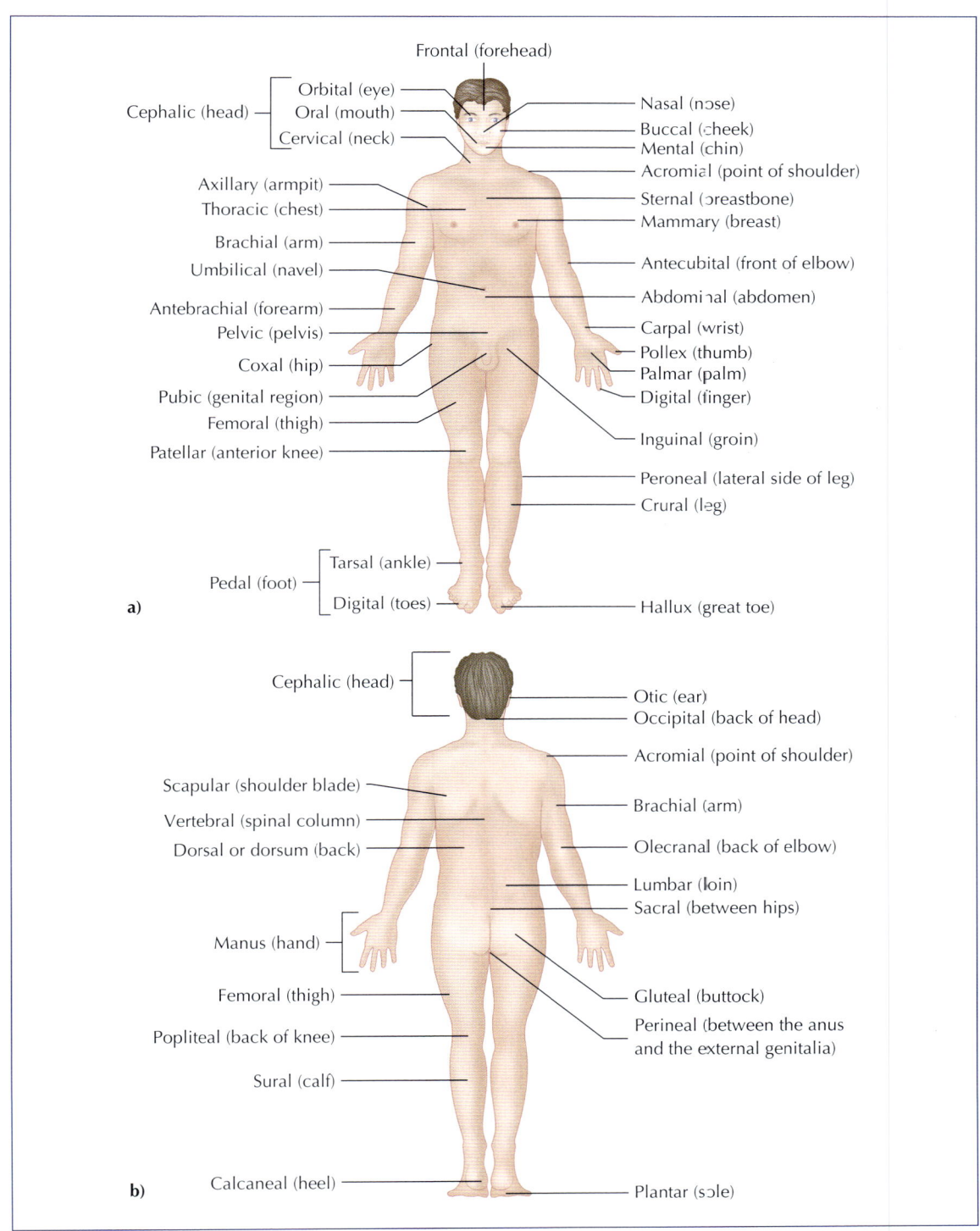

Frontal (forehead)

Orbital (eye)
Cephalic (head) — Oral (mouth)
Cervical (neck)

Nasal (nose)
Buccal (cheek)
Mental (chin)
Acromial (point of shoulder)

Axillary (armpit)
Thoracic (chest)
Brachial (arm)
Umbilical (navel)
Antebrachial (forearm)
Pelvic (pelvis)
Coxal (hip)
Pubic (genital region)
Femoral (thigh)
Patellar (anterior knee)

Sternal (breastbone)
Mammary (breast)
Antecubital (front of elbow)
Abdominal (abdomen)
Carpal (wrist)
Pollex (thumb)
Palmar (palm)
Digital (finger)
Inguinal (groin)
Peroneal (lateral side of leg)
Crural (leg)

Pedal (foot) — Tarsal (ankle)
Digital (toes)

Hallux (great toe)

a)

Cephalic (head)

Otic (ear)
Occipital (back of head)
Acromial (point of shoulder)

Scapular (shoulder blade)
Vertebral (spinal column)
Dorsal or dorsum (back)

Brachial (arm)
Olecranal (back of elbow)
Lumbar (loin)
Sacral (between hips)

Manus (hand)
Femoral (thigh)
Popliteal (back of knee)
Sural (calf)

Gluteal (buttock)
Perineal (between the anus and the external genitalia)

Calcaneal (heel)
Plantar (sole)

b)

Figure 2.8. Terms used to indicate specific body areas: (a) anterior view, (b) posterior view.

unique characteristics and are nondivisible, making them indispensable. Connective tissue cells, on the other hand, divide slowly but can undergo rapid growth when stimulated.

The human body contains more than twenty different cell types, each tailored to its specific function. While anatomy textbooks often feature a generalized cell diagram (figure 2.9), the reality is that no such universal cell exists. Although cells share a basic structure, their distinct shapes and contents align with the specific tasks they are required to perform. For instance, all cells can digest, yet stomach cells and those of the larger digestive system excel in this function.

Similarly, while all cells can facilitate nerve signals, nerve cells are particularly adept as a consequence of evolution.

In essence, each cell is like a "mini me" or "mini you." Like humans, cells have certain essential requirements, such as oxygen for respiration, a source of energy, and a way to eliminate excess heat and water. Thus, cells have a parallel need for sustenance and maintenance, mirroring vital aspects of human physiology.

All human cells are *eukaryotic*, meaning they have a *nucleus*, which is surrounded

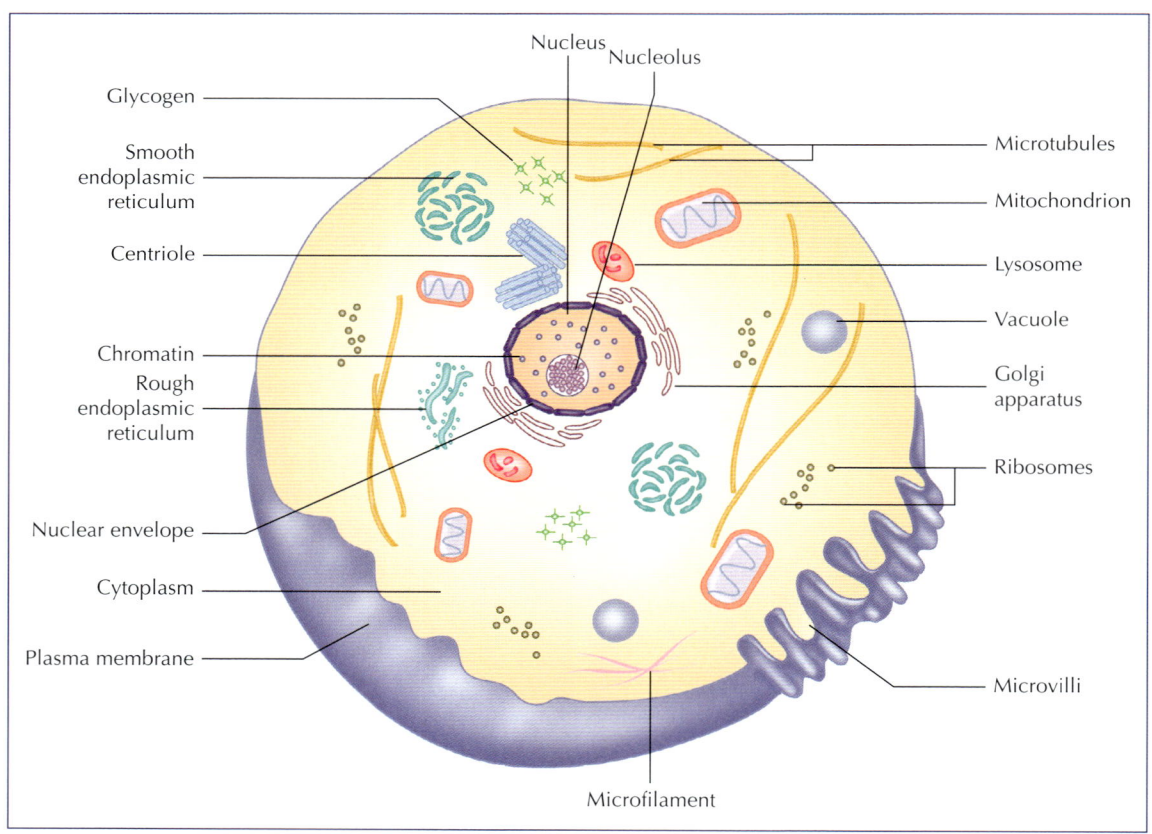

Figure 2.9. A generalized animal cell.

by a *nuclear membrane*, or *nuclear envelope*. The *plasma membrane*, or *cell membrane*, surrounds the cell and provides protection, selectively allowing nutrients to enter and waste products to leave. The plasma membrane keeps the outside out and the inside in.

Cells contain numerous units called *organelles*, each surrounded by a membrane. Organelles include the nucleus, which contains the genetic information; mitochondria, which produce energy for the cell; the endoplasmic reticulum and Golgi body, which synthesize, process, and sort selected molecules; and lysosomes, which digest waste materials.

Animal cells demonstrate several vital processes, which include:

Respiration   All cells need oxygen for combustion with food, which provides the energy to carry out cellular activities. Once energy has been produced by this combustion, carbon dioxide, heat, and water will be released.

Excretion   By-products and waste products are formed during metabolism. Excretion is the removal of these products from the cell.

Growth   Cells can increase size by producing additional cellular constituents or making the size of their organelles larger.

Movement   Animal cells can move.

Irritability   Cells can become excited in response to an external stimulus.

Reproduction   Cells can replicate themselves by dividing to produce new cells.

Cells are grouped together to form tissues. Tissues group together to form organs. Organs are grouped together to form organ systems. In anatomy we may speak about the heart, lungs, or digestive system as separate things, yet none can function without the others. There is of course an interlinking of all systems, a spillover from one to another.

Our focus will be on activities of the mitochondria because they are so important in the production of adenosine triphosphate (ATP).

Cellular Metabolism

All cells require energy to carry out their activities. Energy can be described as the ability to do work. Albert Einstein gave us the most famous equation in the world in an effort to explain what energy is, $E = mc^2$, or energy equals mass times the speed of light squared. That simple equation tells us that energy and mass are interchangeable.

When you eat something, whether it is celery, milk, chocolate, meat, or bread, the food must first be broken down into its constituent parts—fats, carbohydrates, and proteins—which can then be utilized within the body as building materials. After all, you are what you eat. The fats, carbohydrates, and proteins can also be further broken down chemically, to provide energy for cells. The main energy source used in the cell is ATP, adenosine triphosphate. It is mostly produced by the breakdown of glucose to carbon dioxide and water. Readers requiring a unique description of this process, based on Brownian motion and disorder, are encouraged to read the brilliant book by my friend and colleague Doctor Neil Theise, entitled *Notes on Complexity: A Scientific Theory of Connection, Consciousness, and Being* (New York: Spiegel and Grau, 2023).

As mentioned, cells are microscopic versions of you. They do not have teeth, so they require that food be broken down into a smaller digestible source. The process begins in the mouth, where chewing breaks food down into smaller and smaller particles and enzymes begin its chemical breakdown. Further chemical breakdown is catalyzed by enzymes in the stomach and small intestine. The products of this breakdown are absorbed in the small and large intestines. The main energy source for the body is glucose, which comes mostly from dietary carbohydrates. Cells break down glucose gradually in a series of reactions, through the processes of glycolysis, the Krebs cycle (citric acid cycle), and the system of electron transport. During these reactions small amounts of energy are used and large amounts of ATP are produced—it takes energy to make energy. There is a net gain of 30–32 molecules of ATP per molecule of glucose. Among other things, energy released from these reactions can be used for active transport (figure 2.10), synthesis, and muscle contraction. ATP is required in large amounts by cells, so they must ensure a continuous supply.

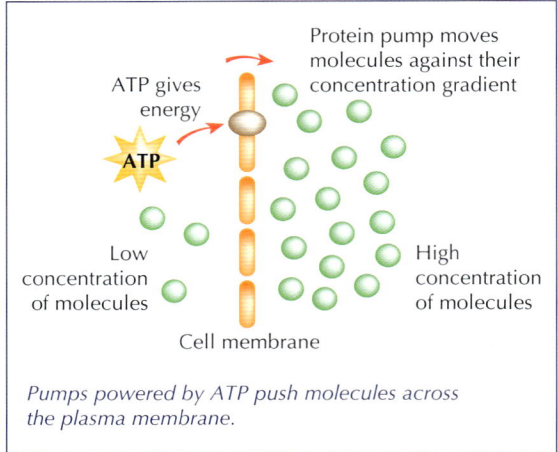

Pumps powered by ATP push molecules across the plasma membrane.

Figure 2.10. Active transport.

Let's look at how glucose is broken down to produce ATP (figure 2.11).

Glycolysis

The glucose supplied to cells from the blood is used to create energy in a process known as *glycolysis*, which takes place in the cytoplasm. It is the first step in cellular respiration. During glycolysis glucose is oxidized, with each molecule of glucose producing two molecules of pyruvate. The process consumes two molecules of ATP but produces four of them, so there is a net gain. It also produces reduced coenzymes, which contribute to ATP production.

Under aerobic conditions, the pyruvate enters the Krebs cycle and then undergoes oxidative phosphorylation, leading to the net production of thirty-two molecules of ATP. Under anaerobic conditions, pyruvate is converted to lactate, resulting in just two ATP molecules. Lactates are muscle inhibitors.

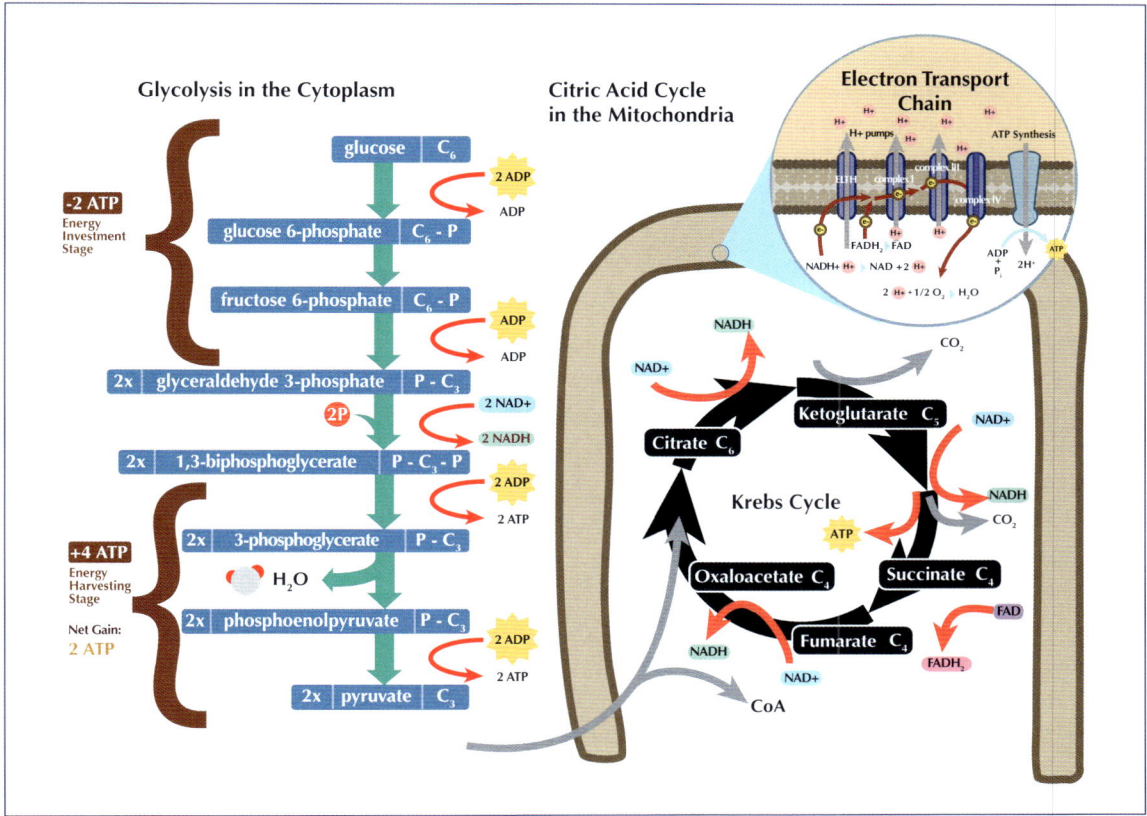

Figure 2.11. Cellular respiration. Courtesy of Shutterstock.

Of course, if we did not produce lactic acid we would not know when to slow down or stop. The production of lactic acid could well be seen as a feedback mechanism to protect us from overexertion and even heart attack.

The Krebs Cycle

The Krebs cycle, or citric acid cycle, is a circular series of reactions. Pyruvate is first converted into citric acid, and then successively into seven other molecules, which brings the cycle back to the beginning. At each step a molecule of reduced coenzyme is produced.

The Krebs cycle takes place in the matrix of mitochondria. The reduced coenzymes go on to the electron transport chain, which takes place on the inner mitochondrial membrane.

Electron Transport Chain

The electron transport chain entails a series of coupled reduction/oxidation (redox) reactions, during which electrons are transferred from one molecule to the next, creating an electrochemical gradient that is used to create a large amount of ATP, in a system called oxidative phosphorylation. The transfer of electrons produces energy that may be dissipated as heat or used to pump hydrogen ions (protons) across the mitochondrial membrane, creating a proton gradient. The proton gradient is used by the enzyme ATP synthase to convert ADP (adenosine diphosphate) and phosphate into ATP.

In this process, fuels are completely broken down with only heat, carbon dioxide, and water as the final end products of energy production. Fats, proteins, and carbohydrates can all be used as fuels to provide ATP, but only when oxygen supplies are sufficient. When oxygen supplies do not meet the current physiological needs of the cell, ATP is produced by anaerobic means. The lack of oxygen means that the Krebs cycle and the electron transport chain cannot function. In this scenario, only glycolysis occurs, producing small amounts of ATP, and only glucose is the energy source. Mitochondria are involved only when there is a sufficient supply of oxygen.

If blood glucose levels are high, excess glucose can be converted into glycogen for storage, in a process known as *glycogenesis*, which occurs in the liver and skeletal muscles. The glycogen can be converted back into glucose if needed, by the process of *glycogenolysis*. These two systems maintain blood glucose levels.

It is noteworthy that very young children have an immature and still-developing nervous system, and they lack the capability to engage in anaerobic activity with optimal efficacy. As a corollary, this means they produce less lactic acid—and they therefore lack the pivotal negative feedback mechanism designed to mitigate the risk of overexertion within the body. It is imperative to dispel the misconception that children, from a physiological perspective, are essentially diminutive adults, as such a characterization is markedly inaccurate.

Homeostasis

The maintenance of a healthy human internal environment is an intricate process involving continuous adjustments in response to external environmental changes, a phenomenon encapsulated within the framework of *allostasis*. It is important to differentiate allostasis and *homeostasis*. Allostasis is a physiological concept that refers to the active process by which the body achieves stability, or homeostasis, through adaptive changes. Unlike traditional homeostasis, which is the maintenance of a constant internal environment, allostasis is the active process of maintaining or reestablishing homeostasis by adapting to the dynamic nature of the external environment, to environmental and psychological stressors. In allostasis, the body anticipates and responds to changes by actively adjusting its physiological set points, allowing for flexibility in response to stressors, challenges, or varying demands.

This adaptive process involves the regulation of various physiological parameters, including but not limited to hormones, neural activity, and the autonomic nervous system. Allostasis is crucial for the body to effectively respond to stress, maintain internal balance, and ensure optimal functioning under different conditions. However, chronic or excessive activation of allostatic mechanisms can lead to wear and tear on the body over time, potentially contributing to various health issues. *Homeostasis*, derived from the

Greek roots *homoio* meaning "same" and *stasis* meaning "standing still," delineates the intricate mechanisms orchestrating the preservation of a consistent internal environment within specified physiological parameters. This equilibrium, however, is susceptible to disruption by various stressors, including but not limited to injury, myofascial trigger points (MTrPs), illness, exercise, emotional states, and diseases.

To ensure the preservation of homeostasis, intricate control mechanisms come into play, featuring feedback systems that incorporate proprioceptors. These sensory receptors play a pivotal role in providing the body with information about its internal state, enabling precise adjustments to maintain stability. Essential facets of homeostatic regulation include the equilibrium of fluid levels, temperature, gases, and blood sugars. The orchestration of these elements is paramount for fostering positive health and ensuring the optimal functioning of muscles, bones, fascia, and joints, thereby contributing to a state of pain-free physiological well-being. Consequently, a nuanced understanding of the interplay between external and internal factors is imperative for comprehending the complexities of human health and physiological harmony.

Overview of the Skeletal (Osseofascial) System

Functions

The osseofascial system consists of a harder fascia whose principal functions are to provide supportive lift, movement potential, fat storage, calcium homeostasis (including storage), and hematopoiesis in the bone marrow. These functions can be upset in a variety of ways, leading to various conditions encompassed by the general term *metabolic bone disease*. Bone is the hardest tissue in the human body, composed of 20 percent water, 30 percent organic matter, and 50 percent inorganic matter. Bones are extremely dense connective fascial tissue, they come in various shapes and sizes, and they provide protection to the softer tissues, including the brain and internal organs.

Osteoporosis is the most common metabolic bone disease, characterized by low bone mass and microarchitectural deterioration of bone tissue, leading to bone fragility.

Females who have a total body fat of less than 17 percent with accompanying amenorrhea should seek medical advice to ensure the best possible medical care and ensure they don't have elevated levels of serum hormone binding globulins (SHBGs). High levels of SHBGs are associated with increased risk of reduced bone health and place even young people at risk of osteoporosis.

Bone (Osseofascial Tissue)

Bone cells are contained in cavities known as *lacunae* surrounded by circular layers of bone matrix, which contains collagen and calcium salts (figure 2.12). These are needed for healthy bone.

Cartilage

Cartilage is similar to bone as it is made up of cells embedded in an extracellular matrix.

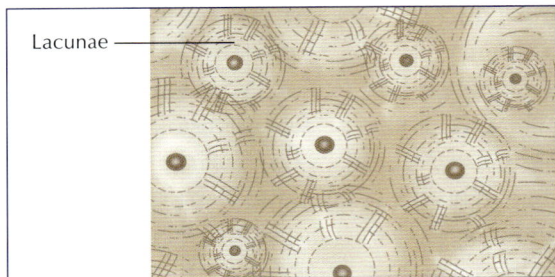

Figure 2.12. Structure of bone.

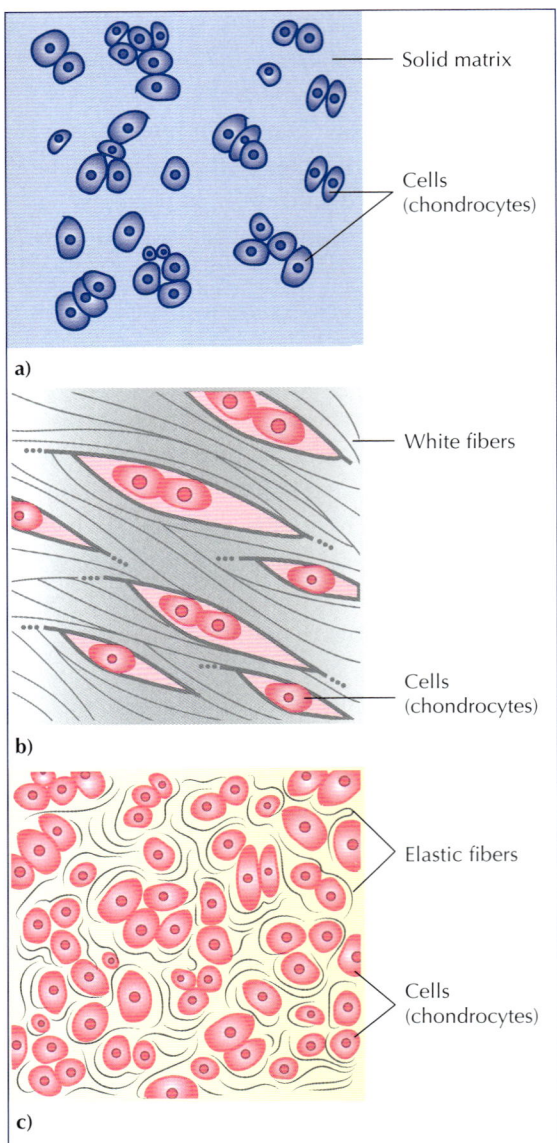

The nature of its matrix differs, though, in being thin, avascular, flexible, and resistant to compression, where that of bone is highly vascularized, hard, and inflexible. There are three main types of cartilage in the body: hyaline, fibro-, and elastic (figure 2.13).

Classification of Bones

The skeletal system is divided into the axial skeleton—the 80 bones that form the skull, ribs, sternum, and vertebrae—and the appendicular skeleton, which consists of the 126 bones of the upper and lower limbs and the shoulder and pelvic girdles (figure 2.14).

Bones come in many different shapes and sizes—for example, irregular, flat, short, sesamoid, and long (figure 2.15).

Irregular bones have complicated shapes, consisting mainly of spongy bone enclosed by thin layers of compact bone. Examples include some skull bones, the vertebrae, and the hip bones.

Flat bones are thin, flattened bones, and frequently curved; they have a layer of spongy bone sandwiched between two thin layers of

Figure 2.13. Structure of cartilage: (a) hyaline cartilage; (b) white fibrocartilage; (c) yellow elastic cartilage.

compact bone. Examples include most of the skull bones, the ribs, and the sternum.

Short bones are generally roughly cube-shaped and consist mostly of spongy (cancellous)

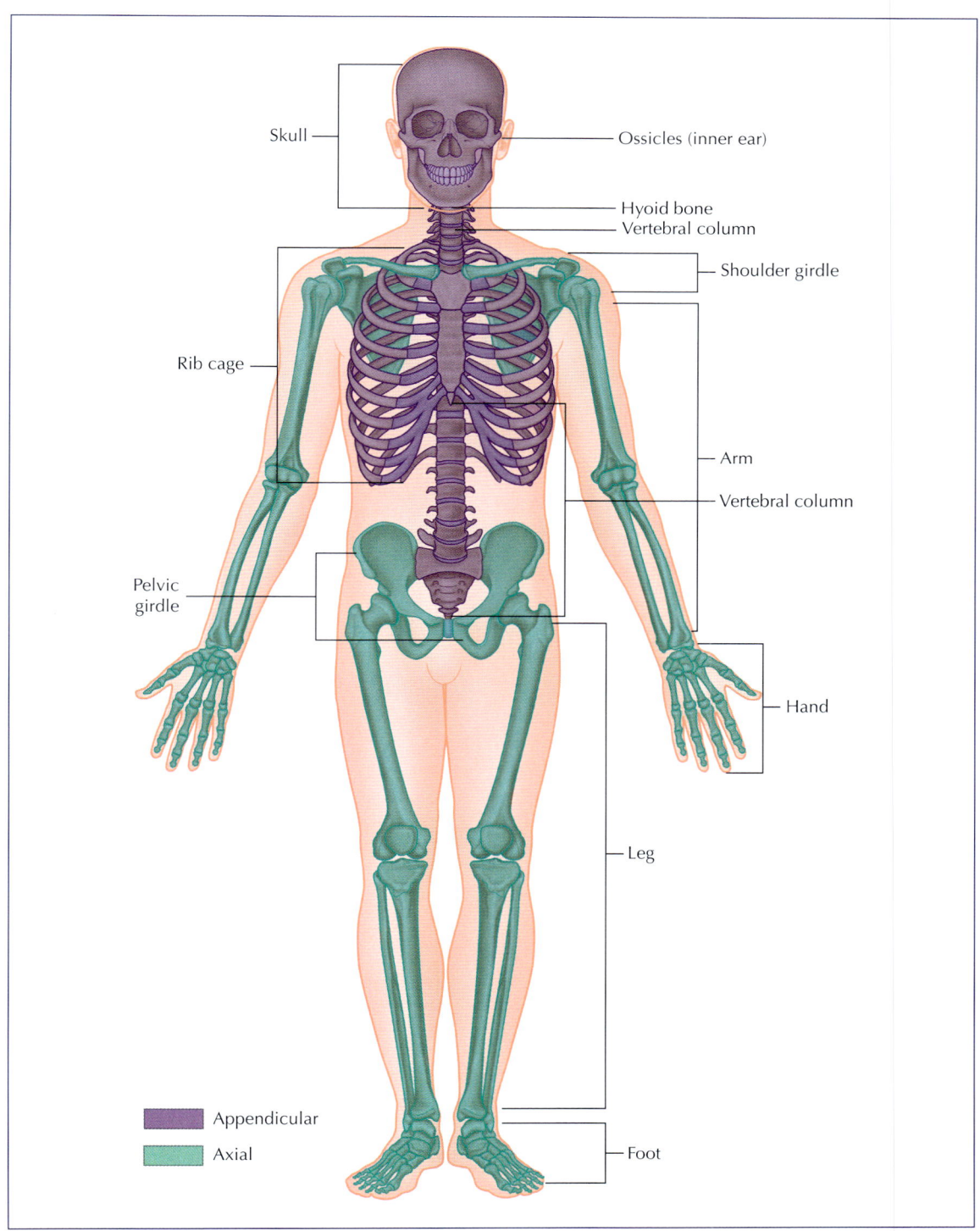

Figure 2.14. The axial and appendicular skeleton.

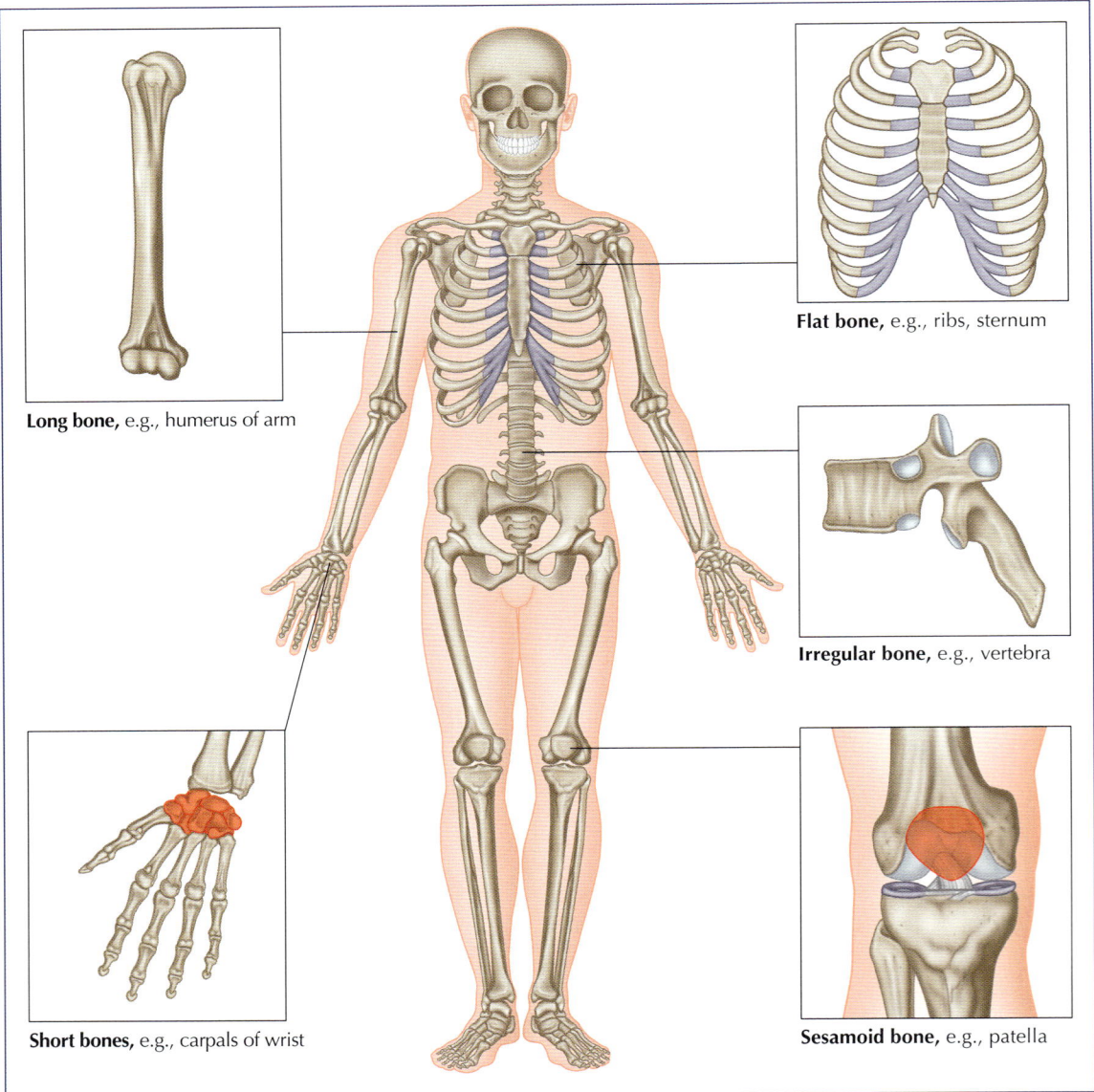

Long bone, e.g., humerus of arm

Flat bone, e.g., ribs, sternum

Irregular bone, e.g., vertebra

Short bones, e.g., carpals of wrist

Sesamoid bone, e.g., patella

Figure 2.15. Bone shapes.

bone. Examples include the carpal bones in the hand and tarsal bones in the ankle.

Sesamoid bones are a special type of short bone that is formed and embedded within a tendon. Examples are the patella (kneecap) and the pisiform bone at the medial end of the wrist crease.

I view all bones in the body as sesamoid, floating within the ubiquitous fascia.

Long bones are longer than they are wide, have a shaft in the middle and heads at both ends, and consist mostly of compact bone. Examples include the arm and thigh bones.

Classification of Joints

The categorization of articulations as *joints* is not solely contingent upon the extent of mobility inherent in each anatomical articulation but is predicated upon a nuanced consideration of the specific anatomical features characterizing the joint in question. The spectrum of joint functionality spans from immobility to limited mobility to a broad range of motion; however, that is not how joints are classified (although you would be forgiven for thinking so based on the terminology). It is imperative to acknowledge the historical derivation of the term, where the original nomenclature was *pin joint*, which has evolved over time to the more generalized term *joint*.

The concept of a pin joint presupposes the juxtaposition of two bony structures with a pin-like structure inserted to secure their alignment. It is noteworthy that this conceptualization, while linguistically encapsulated in the term *joint*, does not precisely mirror the anatomical realities of human anatomy and physiology. Inherent in the concept of a pin joint is the notion of bony overlap, which is not a characteristic feature of normal human anatomical articulations. In the physiological state, bones within the human body generally do not directly overlap with morphology suitable to accommodate a pin. Rather, they maintain a complex and dynamic relationship, either in proximity or with the presence of synovial structures facilitating articulatory movements. The occurrence of bone overlap, with the exception of the elbow joint, is typically associated with pathological conditions where the normal spatial relationships between bones are disrupted, resulting in an aberrant juxtaposition. Consequently, the conventional usage of the term *joint* should be understood within this broader context, acknowledging both its historical roots and the anatomical intricacies inherent in the diverse range of articulations observed within the human body.

Synarthrotic (nonmovable) joints may have some movement, but not enough to see with the naked eye. These joints are found mostly in the axial skeleton, where joint stability and firmness are important for the protection of the internal organs. Good examples are the joints or sutures in the cranium, sacrum, and pelvis.

Amphiarthrotic (slightly movable) joints have a layer of fibrous or cartilaginous tissue between the bones. Examples include the pubic symphysis and sternocostal joints.

Diarthrotic (freely movable or synovial) joints have an individual blood and nerve supply, a joint capsule (ligaments), and a synovial membrane with articulating cartilage or meniscus tissue (figure 2.16). Examples include ball-and-socket joints like the shoulder (glenohumeral) joint and hinge joints like the knee.

Six Types of Synovial Joints

There are six types of synovial joint: plane (or gliding), hinge (or ginglymus), condyloid (or ellipsoid), saddle, pivot, and ball-and-socket (figure 2.17).

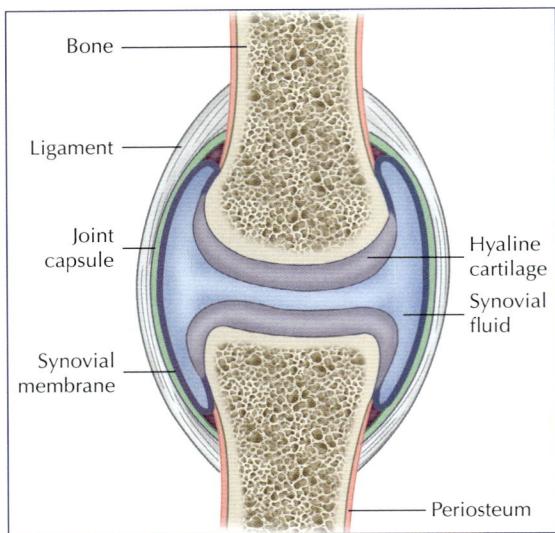

Bone

Ligament

Joint capsule

Synovial membrane

Hyaline cartilage

Synovial fluid

Periosteum

Figure 2.16. Shock absorbing and friction-reducing structures of a synovial joint.

In *plane* (or *gliding*) *joints*, movement occurs when two, generally flat or slightly curved, surfaces glide across one another. Examples: acromioclavicular joint, intercarpal joints, intertarsal joints, facet joints between the vertebrae, sacroiliac joint.

In *hinge* (or *ginglymus*) *joints*, movement occurs around only one axis—a transverse one—as in the hinge of the lid of a box. A protrusion of one bone fits into a concave or cylindrical articular surface of another, permitting flexion and extension. Examples: interphalangeal joints, elbow. The knee is a *modified hinge joint*, allowing for flexion, extension, but also rotation with a flexed knee.

In common with ball-and-socket joints, *condyloid* (or *ellipsoid*) *joints* have a spherical articular surface that fits into a matching concavity. As in the case of ball-and-socket joints, condyloid joints also permit flexion, extension, abduction, adduction, and

circumduction. Examples: radiocarpal joint, metacarpophalangeal joints of the fingers (but not the thumb).

Saddle joints are similar to condyloid joints, except that both articulating surfaces have convex and concave areas, which fit together like a saddle and a horse's back, and allow flexion, extension, adduction, abduction, circumduction, and "controlled" rotation, i.e., opposition. Example: carpometacarpal joint of the thumb.

In *pivot joints*, movement takes place around a vertical axis, like the hinge of a gate. A more or less cylindrical articular surface of bone protrudes into and rotates within a ring formed by bone or ligament. Examples: atlanto-axial joint, proximal radioulnar joint.

Ball-and-socket joints consist of a "ball" formed by the spherical or hemispherical head of one bone, which rotates within the concave "socket" of another, allowing flexion, extension, adduction, abduction, circumduction, and rotation. Thus, they are multiaxial and allow the greatest range of movement of all joints. Examples: shoulder and hip joint.

Important Bony Landmarks

As muscle is continuous with bone by means of the periosteum, the pulling forces caused by the growth of the bones and the pulling or contractile forces of the muscles and ligaments lead to bumps, lumps, and protrusions (figure 2.18). Anatomy has provided special names to describe these, and this language helps to establish the origins and insertions of the muscles and ligaments. Examples are listed below.

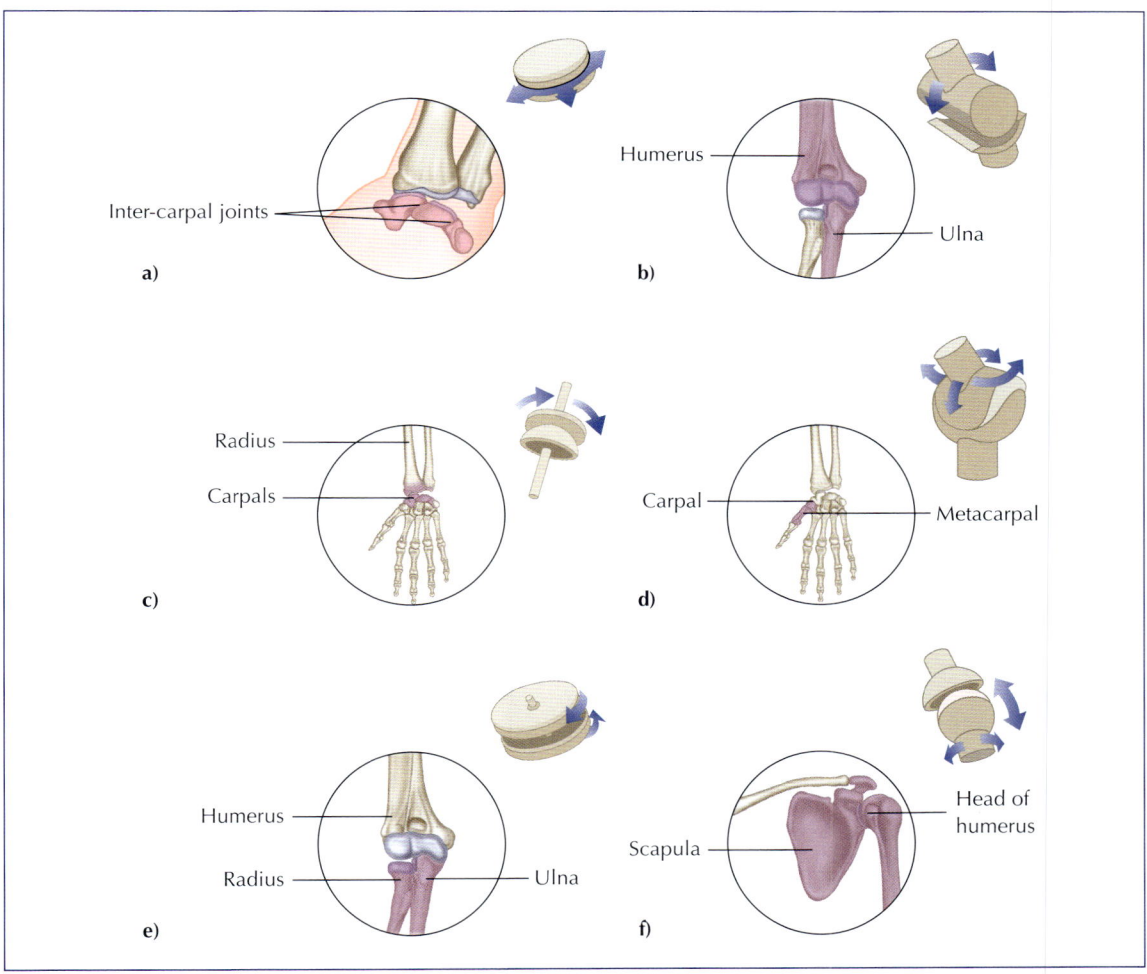

Figure 2.17. Types of synovial joint: (a) Plane or gliding (intercarpal); (b) hinge (elbow); (c) condyloid (radiocarpal); (d) saddle (carpometacarpal); (e) pivot (proximal radioulnar); (f) ball-and-socket (shoulder).

Border	Narrow ridge of bone	**Foramen**	Hole or opening in bone (or other tissues)
Condyle	Rounded projection forming a joint	**Fossa**	Shallow depression in a bone
Coracoid	Bony projection resembling a crow's beak	**Mastoid**	Breastlike or nipplelike
		Notch	Narrow gap in a bone
Crest	Border or ridge provided by a linear elevation	**Process**	Bony prominence
Epicondyle	Projection over a condyle	**Ramus**	Long, branch-like bony continuation of a bone

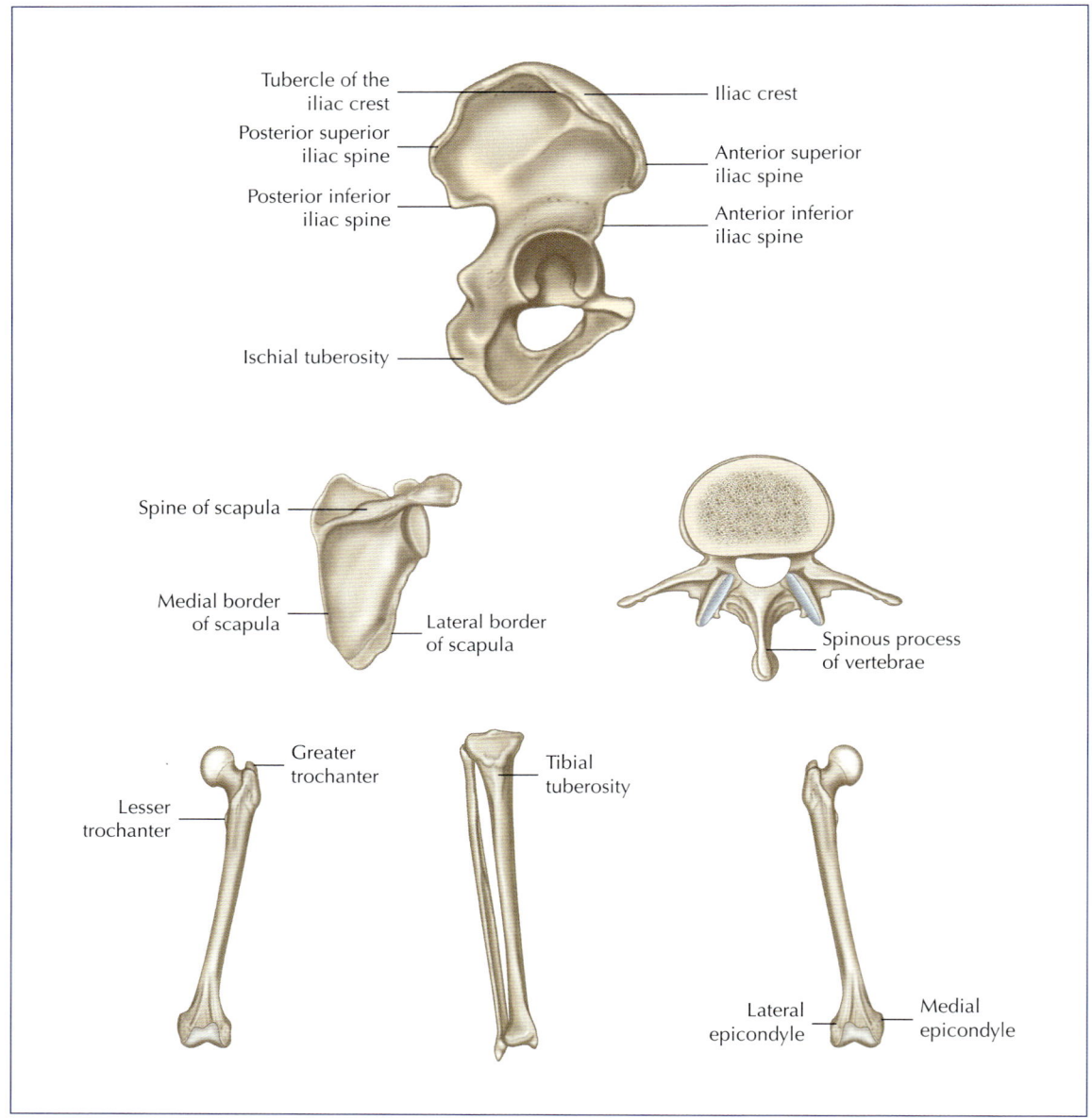

Figure 2.18. Projections on bones that are the sites of muscle and ligament attachment.

Spine	Sharp, slight projection	**Tubercle**	Rounded blunt and irregular projection
Styloid	Slender, pointed bony projection		
Trochanter	Large process on the femur	**Tuberosity**	Large rough and rounded projection

Anatomy of Bones

Although bone is the hardest fascia in the human body, it maintains a certain level of pliability, made possible by its structure and composition. Bone is generally enclosed—except in the joint regions where it transitions to articular cartilage—in an outer fibrous, dense, and vascular fascial membrane called the *periosteum*. Periosteum is composed of two laminae, an outer fibrous lamina and a deeper elastic lamina containing *osteoblasts* (bone-making cells). These cells are capable of proliferating rapidly when a fracture occurs.

In the interior of long bones is a cylindrical cavity (*medullary cavity*) filled with bone marrow and lined with a membrane composed of highly vascular tissue (*endosteum*). Between these laminae is the compact bone, or the so-called "calcium layer." The ends of long bones (*epiphyses*) are filled with red and yellow marrow.

Bones are, in general, richly supplied with blood. Blood is supplied by means of periosteal vessels. These vessels enter close to the articular surfaces and include nutrient

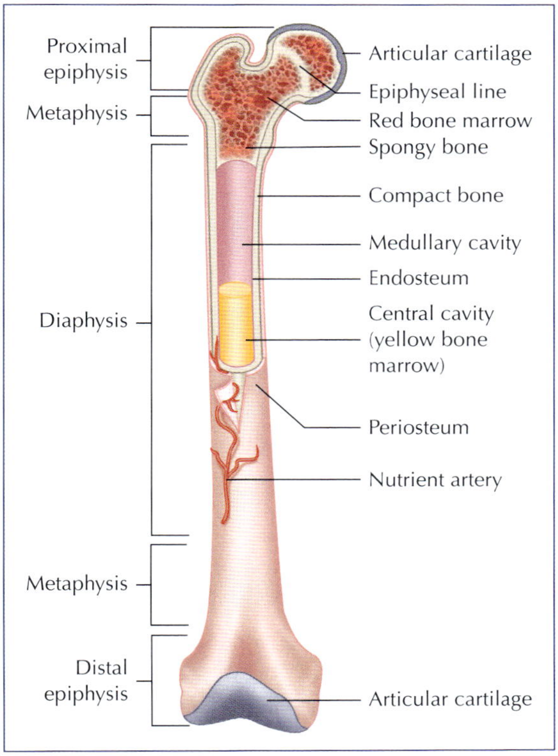

Proximal epiphysis
Metaphysis

Articular cartilage
Epiphyseal line
Red bone marrow
Spongy bone

Compact bone

Medullary cavity
Endosteum
Central cavity (yellow bone marrow)

Diaphysis

Periosteum

Nutrient artery

Metaphysis

Distal epiphysis

Articular cartilage

Figure 2.19. Components of a long bone.

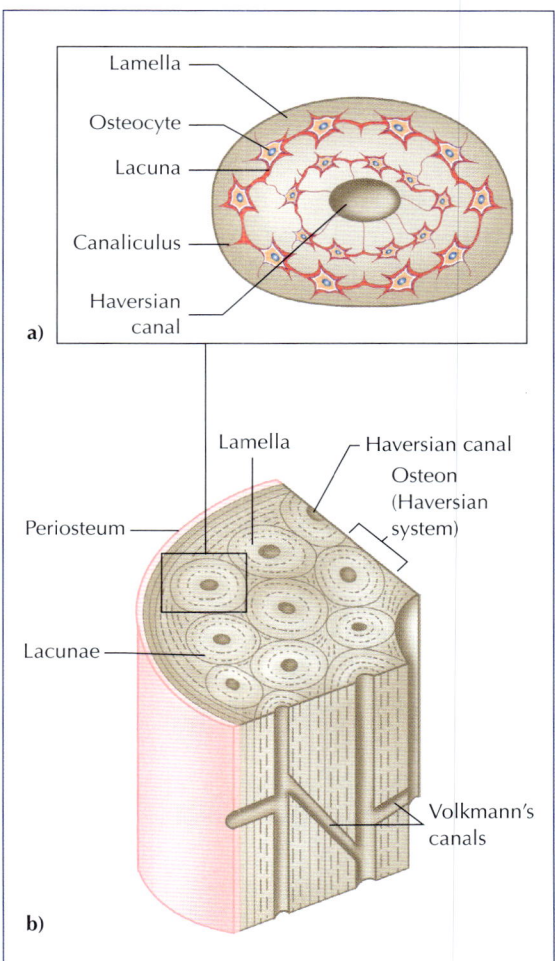

Lamella
Osteocyte
Lacuna
Canaliculus
Haversian canal

a)

Lamella
Haversian canal
Osteon (Haversian system)
Periosteum
Lacunae
Volkmann's canals

b)

Figure 2.20. Structure of compact bone.

arteries. *Perforating* or *Volkmann's canals* run at a ninety-degree angle to the long axis of the bone, connecting nerve and blood supply within the bone to the periosteum. These canals complete the system of vascular canals in osseous tissue.

Loss of the arterial supply to parts of a bone results in death of bone tissue, usually called *avascular necrosis* or *osteonecrosis*. Numerous bones in the body are prone to this complication, usually after injury, including the head of the femur, the scaphoid bone in the wrist, the navicular in the foot, and the tibial plateau. Nutrient arteries to the scaphoid bone are large and numerous at the distal end but become sparse and smaller toward the proximal end. Fractures of the scaphoid—especially of the waist or proximal pole—may result in insufficient blood being supplied, leading to necrosis and later secondary osteoarthritis.

In the foot, the navicular bone is the last tarsal bone to ossify, and its ossification center may be dependent on a single nutrient artery. Compressive forces are thought to be the cause of avascular necrosis of the ossification center. MTrPs could be another worthwhile consideration as a causative factor.

Athletes tend to have greater bone mineral density than nonathletes, although this is often site-specific. For example, tennis players have increased bone density in their dominant arm, while weightlifters have greater femoral bone density than other athletes. This illustrates the local effect of exercise on bone. Of course, you do not have to be an athlete or a weightlifter—even mild exercise offers many health benefits.

Dietary Influences on Bone Health

Although most body calcium is stored in the skeleton, there has been controversy about the influence of dietary calcium intake in the etiology and prevention of osteoporosis. Published data support a role for dietary calcium in the attainment of peak adult bone density. Poor bone health affects the muscular system and may be a source of MTrP formation. There are numerous dietary factors that play a role in skeletal homeostasis.

Sodium intake may have an important effect on bone and calcium metabolism. Sodium loading results in increased renal calcium excretion. This has led to the suggestion that lowering dietary sodium intake may reduce age-related bone loss.

Excessive protein and caffeine intake is associated with bone loss, and smoking exposure also has a negative effect on bone health. Avoidance of dairy products may lead to a low dietary intake of calcium, and an overall poor diet may have a negative effect on bone health. Low fat products are not recommended, although fish, vegetables, and appropriate hydration are important.

Professional advice should always be sought from a qualified nutritional expert.

A Little about Connective Tissue

All connective tissue consists of cells and extracellular matrix (ECM). The ECM contains insoluble protein fibrils and soluble complexes made up of carbohydrate polymers linked to protein molecules that

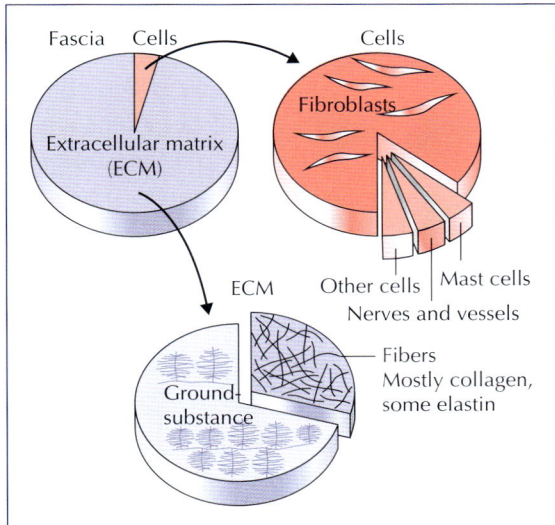

Figure 2.21. Extracellular matrix. Courtesy of fascialnet.com.

bind water (figure 2.21). From a mechanical viewpoint, the ECM allows the stresses of force and gravity to be appropriately distributed, ensuring the integrity of the shape of the different components of the body. The cells are primarily mast cells and fibroblasts—the latter secreting the ECM; it also contains macrophages and histiocytes.

The ECM of connective tissue consists of three fiber types and ground substance. The fiber types are collagen (mostly type I), elastin and reticulin, and fibronectins, and these are accompanied by the glycoprotein laminins, crucial for cell adhesion, migration, and signaling. (figure 2.22). The ground substance is gel-like and contains the insoluble protein fibrils and soluble complexes made up of carbohydrate polymers linked to protein molecules, which bind water. When the ground substance dries out (due to some stress, overuse insult, injury, etc.) the distance or space between the collagen fibers becomes reduced, allowing adherence to occur, resulting in restricted movement. The correct, healthy distance is known as the *critical fiber distance*; below that, adhesion can occur. Dehydration reduces the piezoelectric activity of cells and thereby compromises many cell processes (e.g., contraction, transmission of nerve impulses, reproduction, digestion, secretion). There are three main types of connective tissue: loose, dense regular, and dense irregular connective tissue (figure 2.22).

Loose Connective Tissue (e.g., Areolar Tissue)

Cellular Composition

Areolar tissue contains a loose arrangement of cells, including fibroblasts, macrophages, mast cells, and some white blood cells.

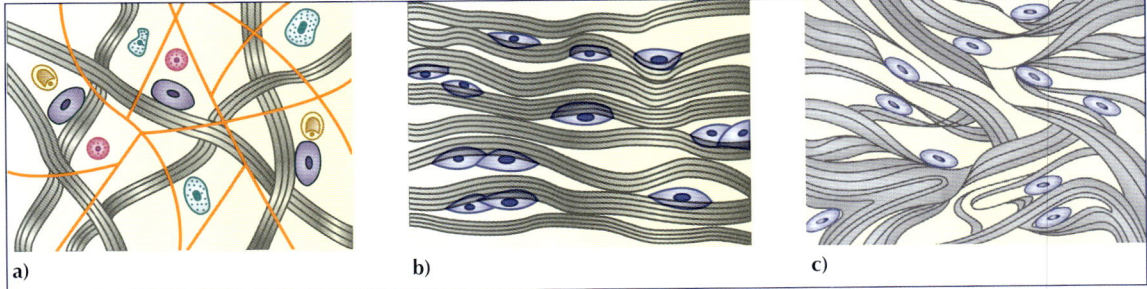

Figure 2.22. The structure of connective tissue: (a) loose connective tissue (e.g., areolar); (b) dense regular connective tissue; (c) dense irregular connective tissue.

ECM
The ECM of areolar tissue consists of a gel-like substance called ground substance, which contains a loose arrangement of collagen, elastic fibers, and reticular fibers.

Appearance
Under the microscope, areolar tissue appears as a loose, open network of cells and fibers with abundant ground substance filling the spaces between.

Function
Areolar tissue provides support and elasticity to organs and serves as a medium for the exchange of nutrients and waste products between blood vessels and surrounding tissues. It also plays a role in immune defense and inflammation.

Dense Regular Connective Tissue

Cellular Composition
The cells in dense regular connective tissue are primarily of fibroblasts, which are elongated cells responsible for producing collagen fibers.

ECM
The ECM of dense regular connective tissue is densely packed with collagen fibers, which are parallel to one another.

Appearance
Under the microscope, dense regular connective tissue appears as densely packed collagen fibers with few visible cells and minimal ground substance.

Organization
Collagen fibers in dense regular connective tissue are arranged in parallel bundles, providing high tensile strength in one direction.

Location
Dense regular connective tissue is typically found in structures that require strong, unidirectional tensile strength, such as tendons and ligaments.

Dense Irregular Connective Tissue

Cellular Composition
Dense irregular connective tissue contains fibroblasts and other cells, similar to loose and dense regular connective tissues.

ECM
The ECM of dense irregular connective tissue is composed of densely packed collagen fibers that are irregularly arranged in multiple directions.

Appearance
Under the microscope, dense irregular connective tissue appears as densely packed collagen fibers arranged in a random, mesh-like pattern with scattered fibroblasts and other cells.

Function   Dense irregular connective tissue provides strength, support, and resistance to tensile forces in multiple directions. It is found in areas where strength and support are needed but where tension may occur from different directions, such as the dermis of the skin, capsules of organs, and the outer layers of some organ walls.

Piezoelectric Activity

At the molecular level, the myofascial system exhibits a configuration akin to organic crystalline structures, endowing it with the capacity to both generate and conduct electrical fields. The optimal hydration of tissues plays a pivotal role in enhancing the efficacy of electromagnetic functions within this intricate system, encompassing processes such as ionic bonding, nutrient and waste transfer, and the transmission of neural signals. James Oschman, a notable cellular biologist, has extensively explored the interplay between the myofascial system and its electromagnetic properties.

The manipulation of the ECM by techniques employed by fascia-focused therapists serves to draw fluid into the matrix. This orchestrated influx of fluid facilitates the proficient execution of cellular electrical functions. This helps preserve the critical fiber distance, allowing an unrestricted range of motion. Notably, interventions such as pressing on the tissue can help cells perform more optimally, mitigating the potential

for micro-injuries associated with overuse stress. Failure to address such injuries may trigger the cumulative injury cycle, which typically starts with repetive stress (or strain), leading to a cycle of microtrauma, inflammation, and tissue repair, resulting in the formation of inelastic, fibrous adhesions, which detrimentally impact both mechanical function and tissue extensibility.

From the muscular perspective, connective tissue enwraps the muscle tissue and its contractile fibers, with white and yellow fibrous tissues being the main types. White fibrous tissue, characterized by its strength and inelastic nature, has fibers consisting predominantly of types I, II, III, and IV collagen. In contrast, yellow fibrous tissue, with fibers of elastin, exhibits elasticity. This specialized tissue demonstrates significant deformability, while possessing the capacity to revert to its original shape, epitomizing the characteristic resilience of elastic tissues—a concept elucidated by my friend and colleague, cellular biologist and biophysicist James Oschman, within the broader framework of fascia tissue dynamics. I recommend his book *Energy Medicine* (2nd ed., New York: Elsevier, 2016) for a deeper understanding of this topic.

Functions of Fascia as a Connective Tissue

Connective tissue generally, and fascia specifically, has six main functions:

- It acts as a structural support framework, or scaffolding, for all the internal organs and tissues of the human body, providing a highway for transportation and immune defense. It has been described as a spider's web, interwoven throughout the organism and providing an elastic rigid structure for the body.

- It functions in metabolism—nutrients pass from the capillaries through the connective tissue into cells, while by-products of energy production move into the capillaries and lymphatic system.
- It has a role in fighting infection—the removal of dead cells and foreign proteins is facilitated by the connective tissue in repair and regeneration.
- It functions in tissue repair—fibroblastic activity leads to the deposition of collagenous fibers in damaged tissue to form a scar.
- It acts as a nutrient reservoir—excessive water, dietary protein, carbohydrates, and lipids are all stored in the connective tissue. As fat is stored in the connective tissue, this provides vital heat insulation for normal physiological activities.
- Fascia contains an abundance of sensory receptors, including interoceptors, nociceptors, baroreceptors, chemoreceptors, mechanoreceptors, and proprioceptors. These receptors contribute to the body's awareness of its position in space (*proprioception*) and play a vital role in sensing dynamical changes, such as pressure and stretch. The influence of interoception on emotion is multifaceted and involves complex neural pathways. The brain receives signals from these receptors and integrates them with emotional and cognitive processes. The insula, a brain region involved in interoceptive processing, is particularly important in

this regard. Interoception contributes to emotional awareness by providing information about the physiological state of the body. For example, increased heart rate or shallow breathing may be associated with emotions such as anxiety or fear. The brain uses interoceptive signals to regulate emotional responses. Being aware of internal bodily sensations allows individuals to recognize and manage their emotional states. Mindfulness and other practices that enhance interoceptive awareness can be effective in emotion regulation. Interoception can directly contribute to the subjective experience of emotion. Changes in visceral sensations, such as those associated with autonomic nervous system responses, are linked to emotional experiences.

Differentiated connective tissue in the skeletal system includes cartilage, periosteum, ligaments, blood, and bone marrow.

Overview of the Nervous System

The nervous system allows us to react and respond to stimuli and comprises two main divisions (figure 2.23):

- The CNS, which consists of the brain and spinal cord
- The peripheral nervous system, which consists of all nerve tissue outside of the spinal cord

The peripheral nervous system is subdivided into the *somatic* (voluntary) nervous system and the *autonomic* (involuntary) nervous

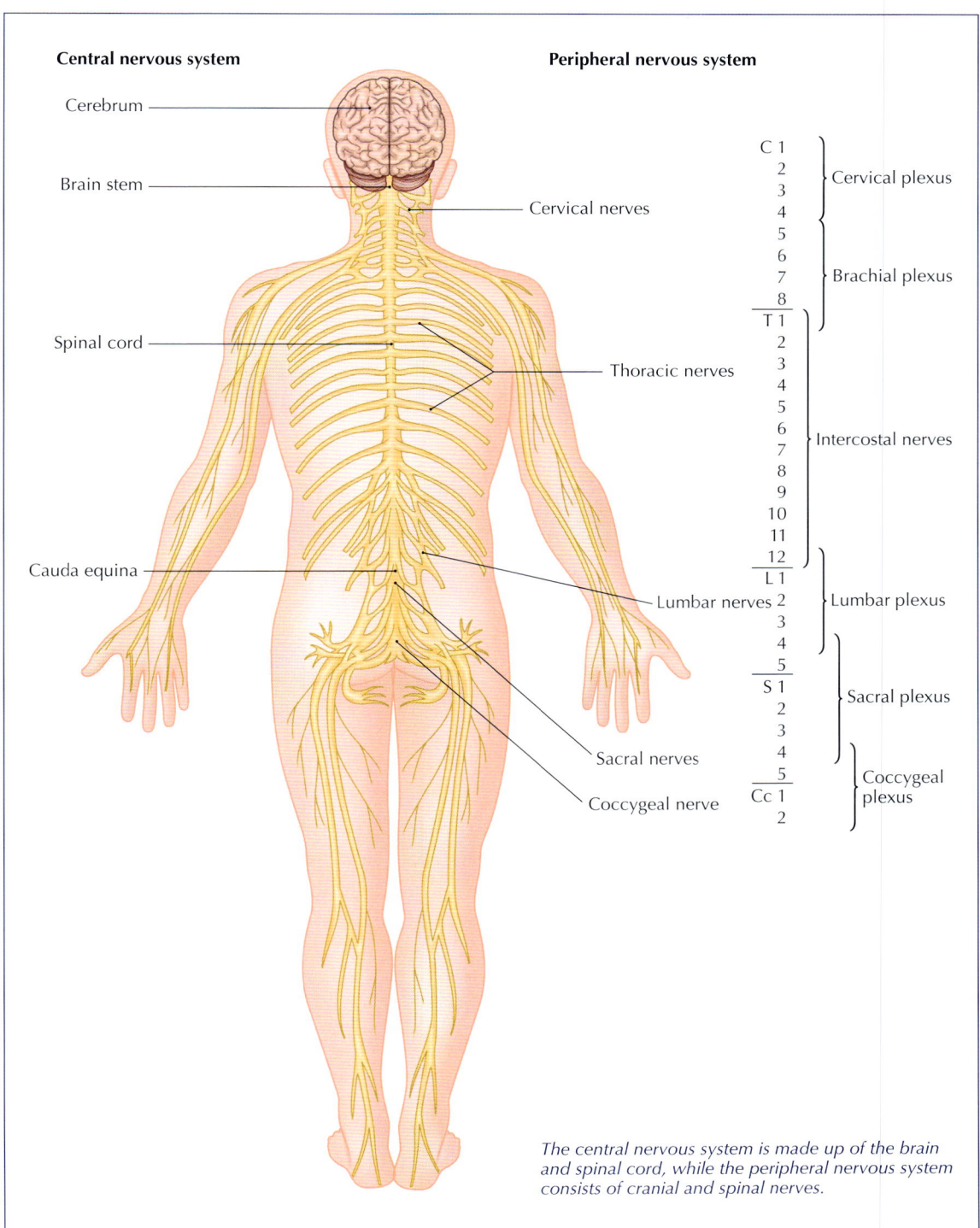

Central nervous system

Cerebrum

Brain stem

Spinal cord

Cauda equina

Peripheral nervous system

Cervical nerves

Thoracic nerves

Lumbar nerves

Sacral nerves

Coccygeal nerve

C 1
2
3
4
5
6
7
8
T 1
2
3
4
5
6
7
8
9
10
11
12
L 1
2
3
4
5
S 1
2
3
4
5
Cc 1
2

Cervical plexus

Brachial plexus

Intercostal nerves

Lumbar plexus

Sacral plexus

Coccygeal plexus

The central nervous system is made up of the brain and spinal cord, while the peripheral nervous system consists of cranial and spinal nerves.

Figure 2.23. An overview of the central and peripheral nervous systems.

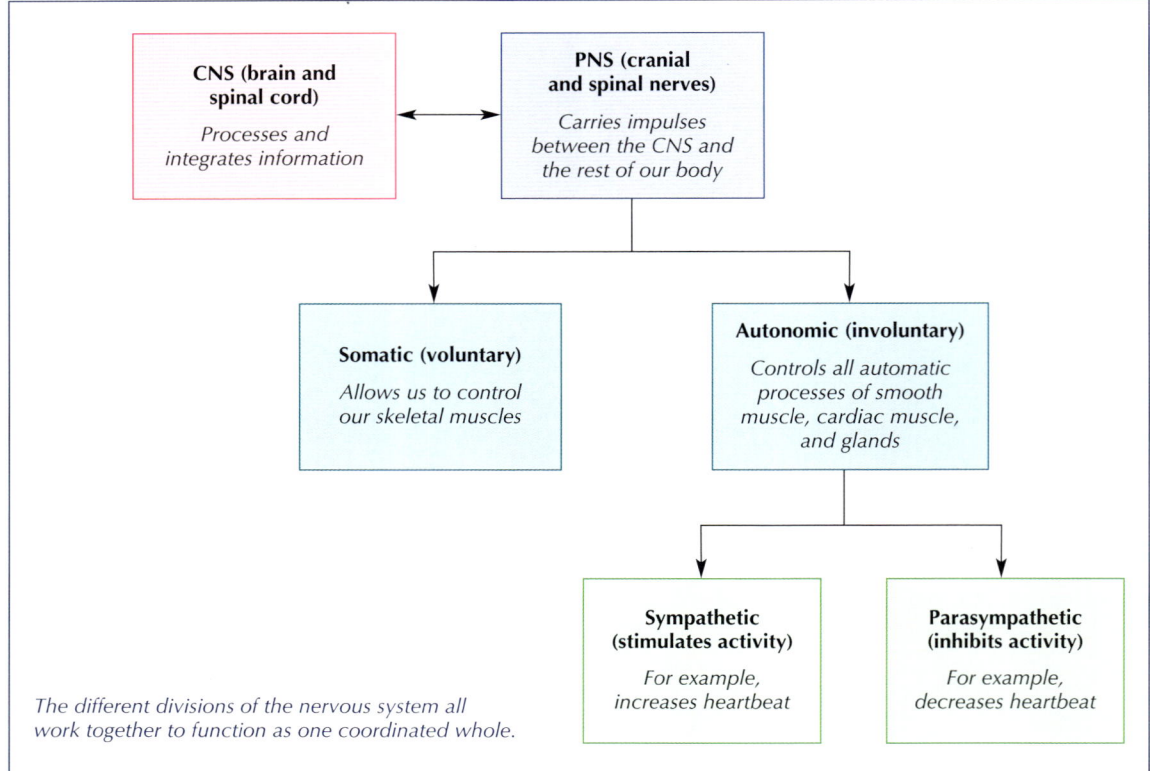

The different divisions of the nervous system all work together to function as one coordinated whole.

Figure 2.24. Divisions of the nervous system.

system, which is further subdivided into the *sympathetic* and *parasympathetic* nervous systems (figure 2.24).

Nervous tissue is composed of *neurons*, which transmit nerve impulses (figure 2.25), and neuroglial cells. A neuron is made up an axon, a cell body, and dendrites, with the axon resembling a long thin wire that arises from the cell body conducts nerve impulses away from it, and the dendrites being short, protruding fibers that convey impulses toward the cell body.

The axon may have an outer covering called a *myelin sheath*. This fatty covering is constricted at intervals along its length; these

locations where the myelin is absent are called *nodes of Ranvier*. Axons that have this outer covering are known as *myelinated* nerve fibers, while those without it are called *unmyelinated*. Such fibers are found mostly in the autonomic nervous system. All axons outside the CNS have an outer covering called the *neurolemma*.

The nervous system sends signals to all the body's trillions of cells twenty-four hours a day. Neurons that connect the spinal cord (which typically ends between your first and second lumbar vertebrae) to the toes can be 20 inches (50 cm) or more in length. Nerves can be as thick as your little finger or as thin as a fine thread—in fact, they can be microscopic.

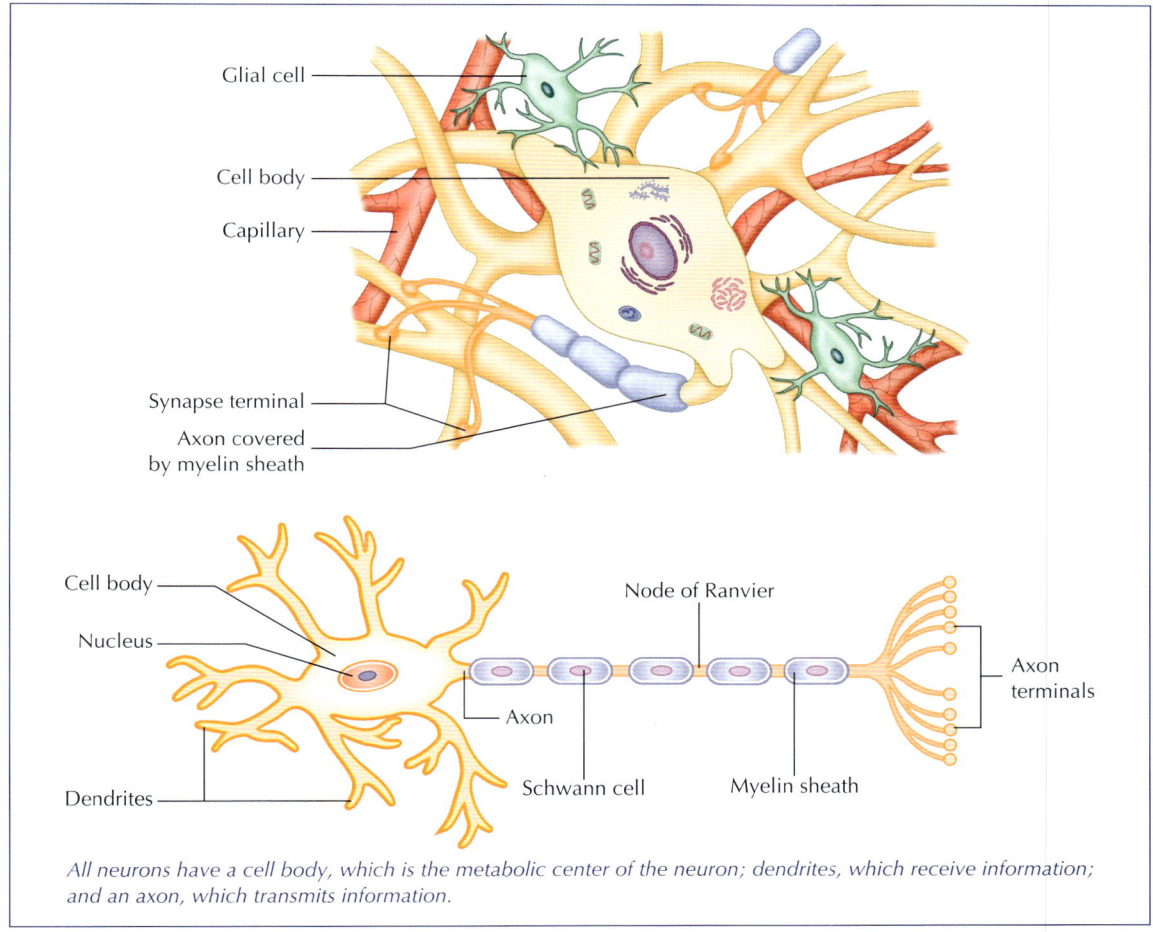

All neurons have a cell body, which is the metabolic center of the neuron; dendrites, which receive information; and an axon, which transmits information.

Figure 2.25. Nervous tissue and nerve cells.

In addition to the obvious roles of nerves and blood vessels, neurovascular bundles provide an important structural component to our connective tissue. Fascia-focused dissections conducted in the University of Dundee, Scotland, have highlighted the decussated anatomical arrangement of these structures. This latticed, chiral, crisscrossing arrangement of neurovascular tissues provides additional structural integrity, lending strength, stability, and resilience (see figure 1.7).

Overview of the Cardiorespiratory System

The term *cardiorespiratory* encapsulates the intricate interplay of two essential systems within the body, even as all bodily systems harmonize as a unified whole. Envisioning someone enduring a prolonged treadmill run while deliberately holding their breath underscores the indispensability of both systems. In such a scenario, the imperative to breathe becomes apparent, to allow the vital taking in of oxygen and expulsion of carbon dioxide. The growing deficit of oxygen and accumulation of carbon dioxide in sustained breath-holding builds a powerful feeling of the need to inhale.

The relationship between the respiratory and circulatory systems is pivotal (figure 2.26). These systems are not isolated but interdependent partners; any lapse or inefficiency in one system invariably reverberates through the other. Thus, optimal functioning of both systems is indispensable for the seamless orchestration of physiological processes, especially during activities demanding heightened cardiovascular and respiratory efforts.

Blood (a connective tissue and a liquid fascia) circulates throughout the body in an enclosed, one-way system. It is made up of both solid and liquid portions (figure 2.27). The solid portion comprises the formed elements: *erythrocytes* (red blood cells), *leukocytes* (white blood cells), and *thrombocytes* (platelets). Blood is a thick, bright red liquid whose color depends on the quantity of oxygen that it contains. Of course, blood always contains *some* oxygen. It is never actually blue as some diagrams suggest, but is darker when it contains less oxygen, almost rust colored. Normally the pH of blood is slightly alkaline. Oxygenated blood is carried away from the heart in arteries, and deoxygenated blood is returned to the heart by veins.

Blood volume in the adult male is approximately 10 pints (5.68 l). Blood in veins will always move toward the heart—no matter in which direction a therapist may apply compression, such as compressive effleurage—because of *valves*, which allow the blood to

move in only one direction. As a clinical anatomist, I call on the international massage community to collectively agree on removing the guideline that massage must always be applied toward the heart.

The three main functions of blood are:

- **Transportation.** Respiratory gases and nutrients, waste products, hormones, antibodies, and more are moved from one place to another.
- **Protection.** White blood cells and antibodies provide protection against pathogens, while platelets provide protection against blood loss through hemorrhage.
- **Regulation.** Our body temperature constantly remains close to homeostasis. Blood transfers heat throughout the body to where it is needed. When we are producing more heat than required, blood will dissipate the excess by vasodilating blood vessels just beneath the skin.

I want to mention the heart and the unique system in place for providing blood to the coronary arteries. The heart is a spiraled muscular structure containing four chambers, which receive and release blood at least once every second at rest. This is known as the *cardiac cycle*. Normal resting heart rates are sixty to one hundred beats per minute.

The Cardiac Cycle

The cardiac cycle occurs at least once every second and involves an active and a passive phase, with variability in each phase. The heart wall (*myocardium*) is the muscular part of the heart and comprises involuntary and

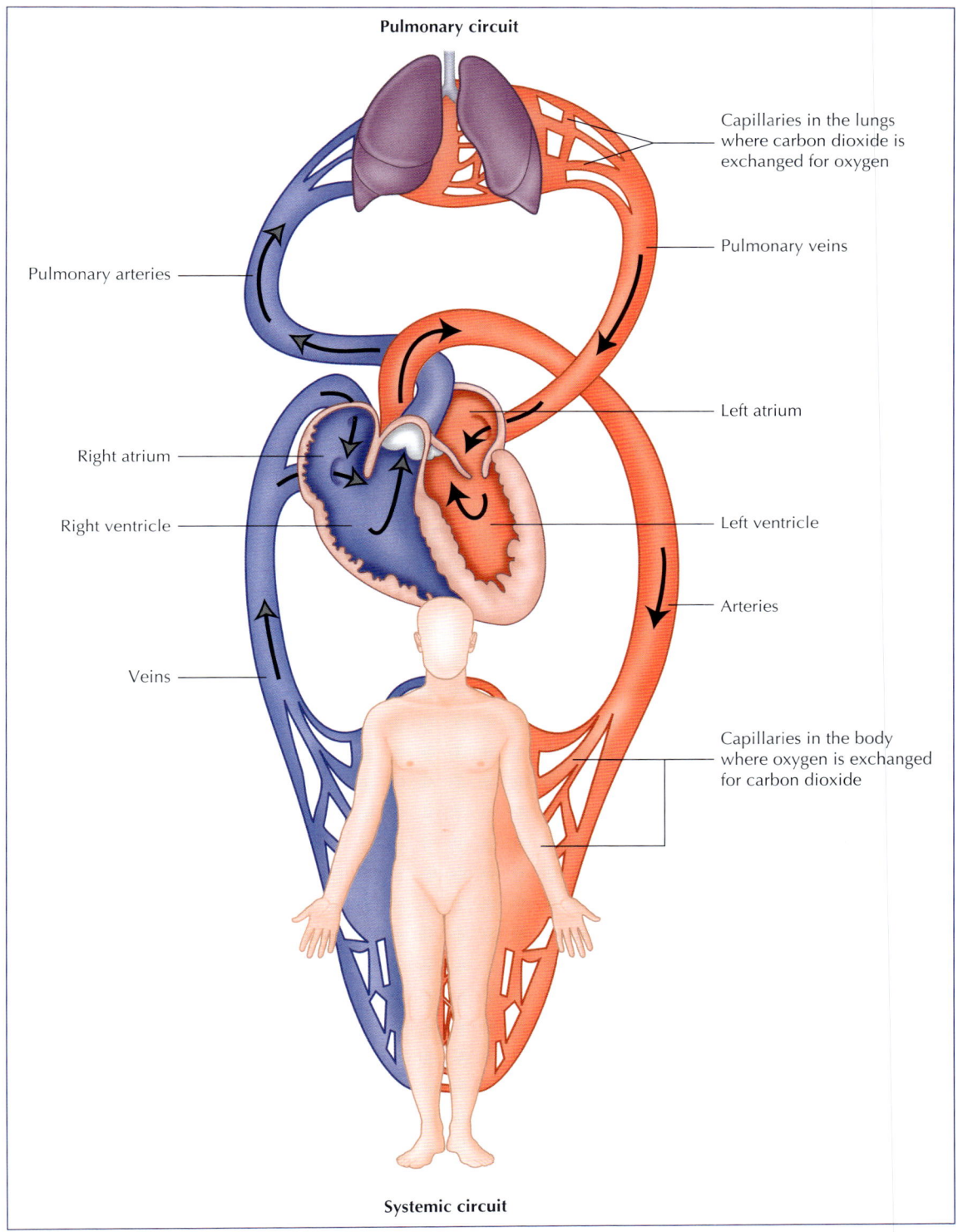

Figure 2.26. Pulmonary and systemic circulation.

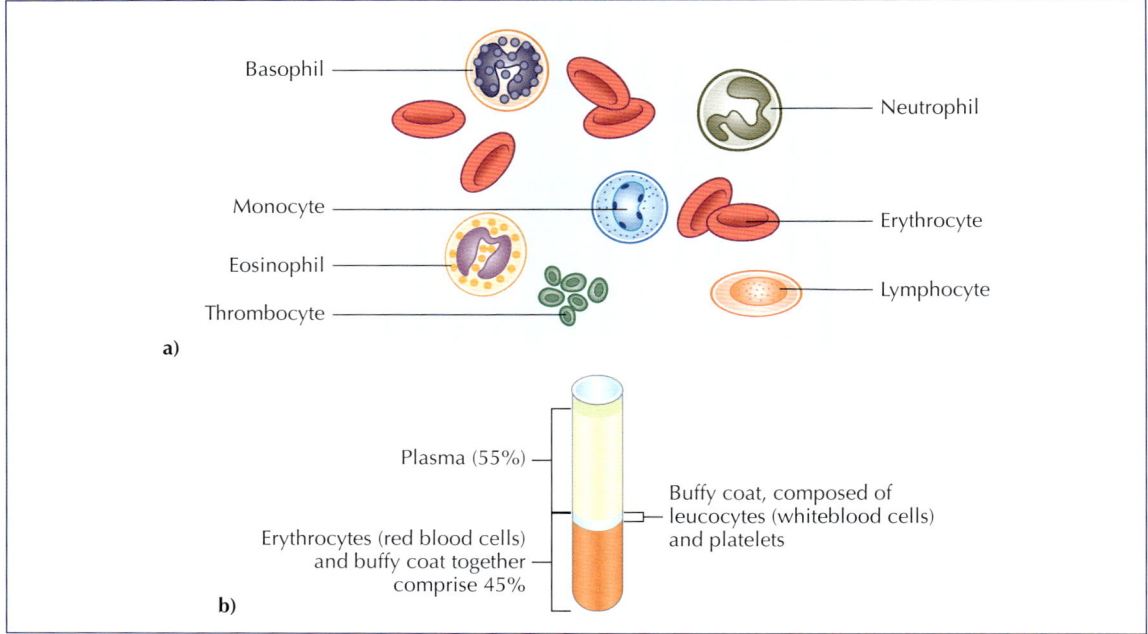

Figure 2.27. The anatomy of blood: (a) its structure; (b) its components.

striated muscle (figure 2.28). The myocardium requires a supply of nutrient-rich blood. The active phase of the cycle involves the spiraling contraction of the myocardium to create a vortex, which ejects the blood up and out of the chambers; this is *systole*. In between beats, the heart muscle relaxes for a fraction of a second. This is the passive phase, *diastole*, when the pressure within the heart chambers drops and blood flows back into the heart.

Blood vessels, the conduits in our circulatory system, are intricately continuous with the heart. The aorta, a key player in this cardiovascular symphony, emerges from the left ventricle and drives blood upward, toward the head and upper spinal cord. Remarkably, the aortic arch then gracefully curves downward, leading to the systemic

blood supply that nourishes the entire body. Intriguingly, a fraction of the blood undergoes retrograde flow back into the aorta, a phenomenon observed during the passive phase of the cardiac cycle. The aorta's sophisticated valve system, strategically positioned to prevent the backflow, simultaneously facilitates blood pooling, ensuring a portion enriches the coronary arteries and sustains the myocardium. How this is achieved is remarkable.

Our knowledge of the heart's profound intricacies owes much to the groundbreaking work of the late Spanish cardiologist Francisco ("Paco") Torrent-Guasp, whose unfortunate demise in 2005 marked the end of an era. Guasp's revolutionary insights debunked the simplistic notion of the heart as a mere pump,

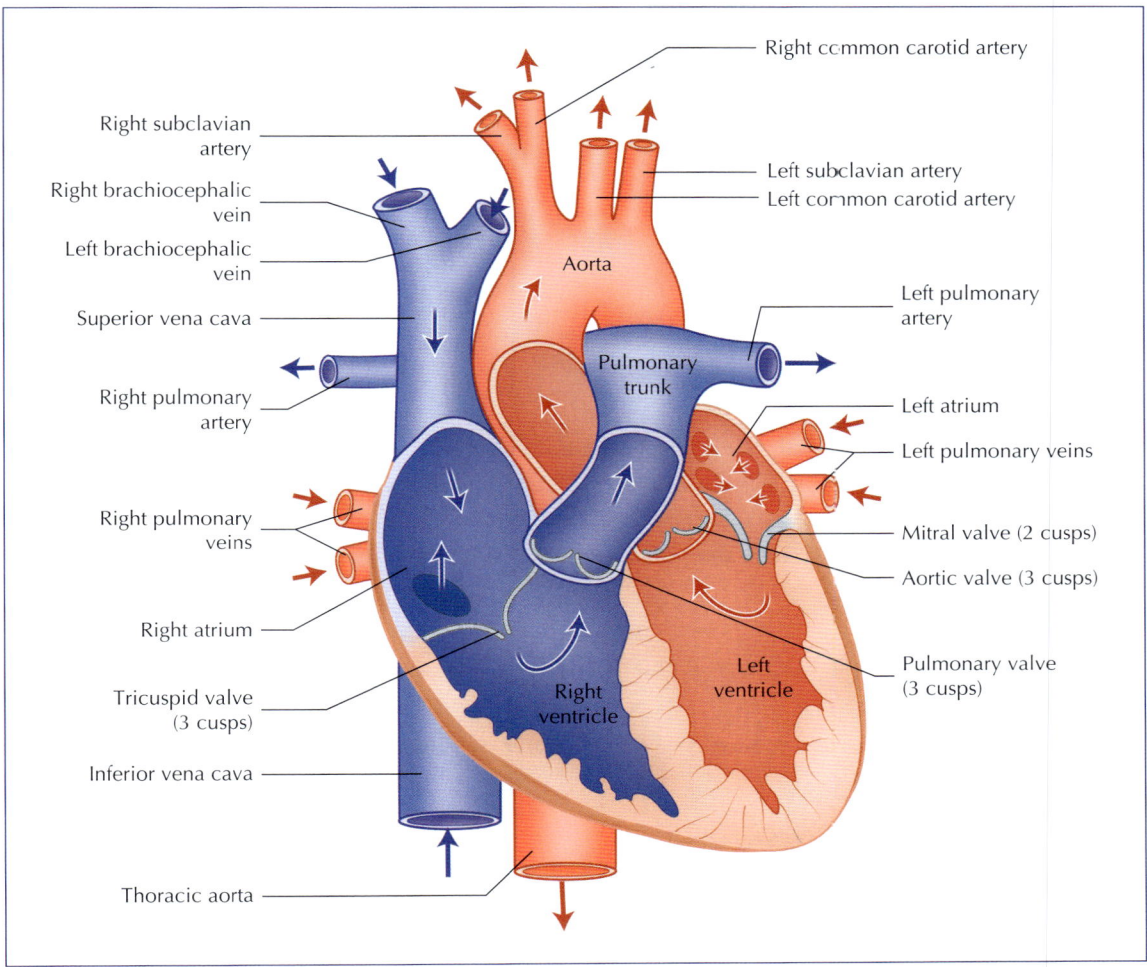

Figure 2.28. The heart and the cardiac cycle.

revealing a myocardial loop that orchestrates a vortex-like motion, efficiently propelling or sucking blood throughout the body. This paradigm shift challenges conventional perspectives, shedding light on the seemingly enigmatic passive phase of the cardiac cycle and elevating our understanding of cardiovascular physiology.

The profound implications of this knowledge extend beyond the realm of theoretical understanding. It underscores the importance of a gradual warm-up before engaging in physical activity, allowing the body the necessary time to adapt. Abrupt shocks to the system induce an accelerated heart rate and vasoconstriction in the coronary arteries, reducing the passive phase of the cardiac cycle (figure 2.29). Thus, this information becomes not just an exploration of the heart's complexity but a practical guide for optimizing cardiovascular health and performance.

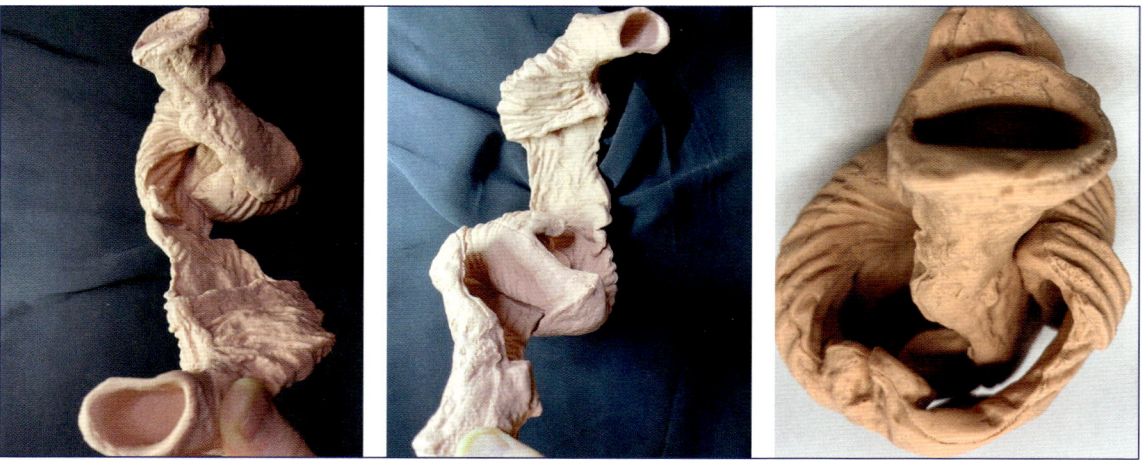

Figure 2.29. Francisco Torrent-Guasp's anatomical dissection revealed the helical ventricular myocardial band, a result of spiral folding. Many great anatomists have attempted to unravel the secrets of the heart—Erasistratus, Leonardo da Vinci, Galen, and others—but did not discover its true helical nature, a feat deserving of the Nobel Prize.

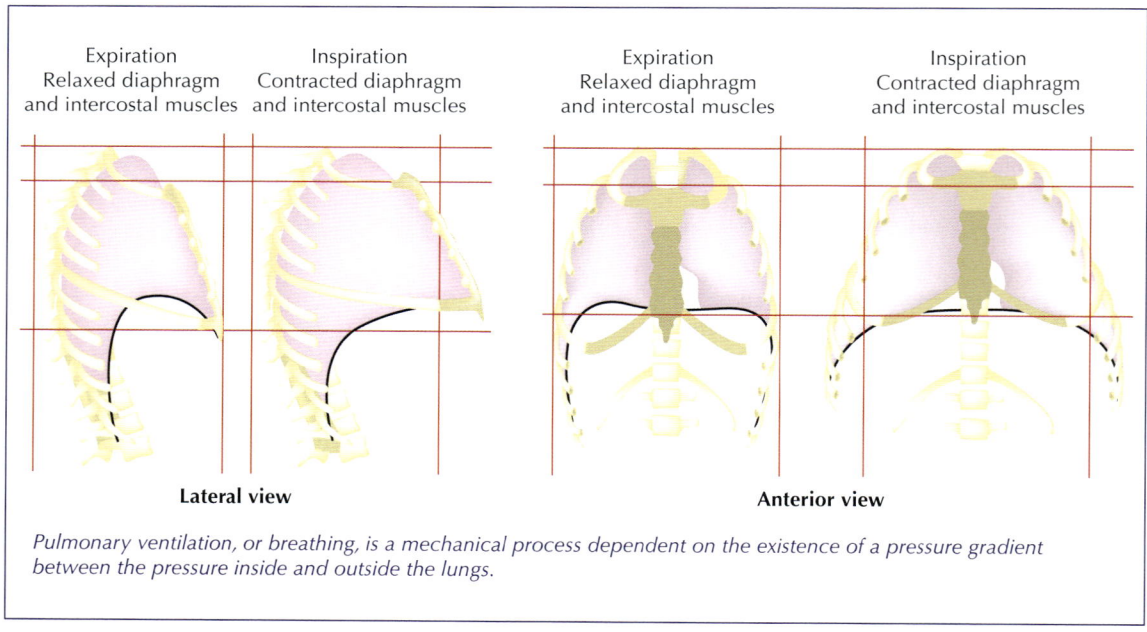

Figure 2.30. Changes in the thoracic cavity during breathing.

The combined efforts of the heart and the circulatory and respiratory systems maintain the state of allostasis required for an efficient kinetic system. Allostasis involves providing the necessary oxygen for cellular activity while ensuring the delivery of appropriate nutrients and removal of metabolic by-products in a homeostatic environment.

Ventilation involves inhaling and exhaling. The chest wall expands and compresses through muscular and fascial activity, including the diaphragm, external intercostals, and pleural membranes (figure 2.30). The internal intercostal muscles are not involved in quiet normal breathing (this is a passive action based on recoiling of the connective tissues). Only during exertion do accessory muscles take part, to increase the thoracic volume and increase the speed at which air is expelled.

Oxygen is necessary to aerobically create enough ATP for the body's needs. This is the combined function of the circulatory and respiratory systems. Failure to provide the internal environment with the correct balance of oxygen and CO_2 results in fatigue, retarded circulation, disturbed sleep, heightened feelings of anxiety, inability to think clearly, headaches, and painful muscles.

Useful Terms

Blood pressure   Force exerted on the walls of the vessels that contain blood

Cardiac output   Effective volume of blood expelled by either ventricle of the heart per unit of time (usually volume per minute); equal to the stroke volume multiplied by the number of beats per minute (heart rate)

Stroke volume   Volume of blood ejected from a ventricle with each heartbeat, equal to the difference between the end-diastolic volume and the end-systolic volume

Vasoconstriction   Reduction in the diameter of blood vessels

Vasodilation   Increase in the diameter of blood vessels

Muscles, Tensegrity, Fascia, and the Kinetic System

To advance knowledge about safe, effective, and appropriate physical activities, one must first appreciate the classification of myofascial structures and understand each of the integrated anatomical, physiological, and neurological facilities.

There are three types of muscle (figure 3.1):

- **Skeletal muscles**—also known as striated or voluntary—are under direct nervous control. They fatigue easily but can be strengthened, and are capable of powerful, rapid contractions, but also longer, sustained contractions. The contractile body (the muscle proper) is usually attached to two bony points. Attachments may be by tendon, by aponeurosis, or by raphe (see figure 3.3).
- **Cardiac muscle** is also striated but is under involuntary nervous control. It is confined to the heart.
- **Smooth muscle**—also known as visceral—is similar to cardiac muscle

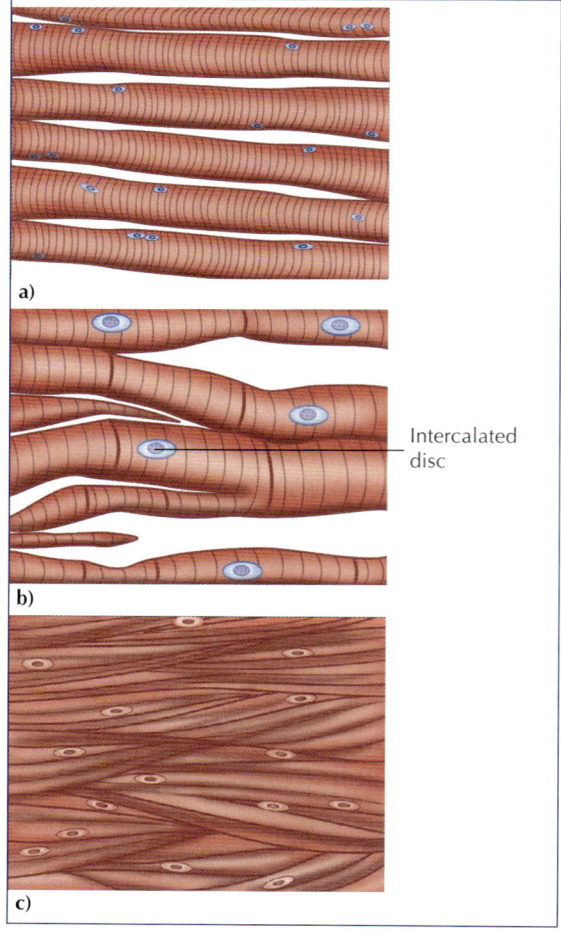

Intercalated disc

Figure 3.1. Structure of muscle: (a) skeletal muscle; (b) cardiac muscle; (c) smooth muscle.

in being under involuntary nervous control. Found in the walls of the alimentary tract, blood vessels, and stomach, it provides a slow and sustained contraction. Smooth muscle is usually seen in flat sheets, sometimes wrapped around an internal organ such as the gut in circular and longitudinal layers or arranged as a sphincter to close off a tube (as in the opening to the stomach).

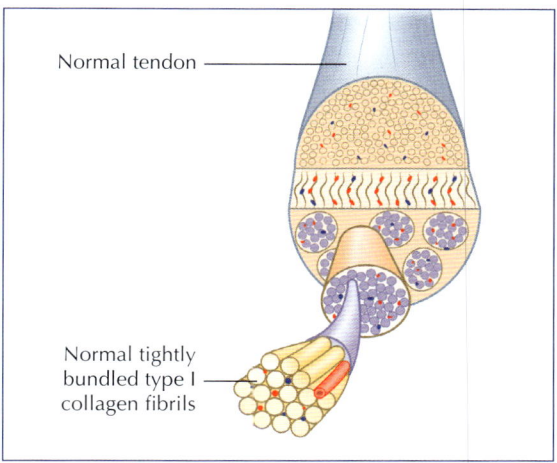

Figure 3.2. Normal tendon structure.

Skeletal Muscles

Skeletal muscles make up approximately 40 percent of total human body weight. They pull but cannot push, which means that you use the same muscles to pick up your shopping bags as you do to put them down again.

If you imagine a person sitting in a pec deck exercise machine, although they push the pads away from their body, it is in fact the pulling action of the pectoralis and associated muscles that provides the "pulling" force to overcome the resistance. Muscles can provide forces only in the direction that their muscle fibers are running. This is known as *directional force* or *line of pull*; however, one must remember the forces are also shared via the associated fascia in an omnidirectional manner.

Tendons are an integral part and continuation of muscle. The tendon is a fibrous band of tissue that is flexible enough to bend around bones and joints (figures 3.2 and 3.3a). It is less vascular than muscle and therefore appears white in color and heals slower than muscle fiber.

Tendons take the form of cords or strips, in cross section circular, oval, or flattened.

They are made up of bundles (*fascicles*) of collagen fibers, mostly parallel.

Where tendons have to move independently of other tissues, various friction-eradicating strategies are used. The tendon may run over cartilage or over a sesamoid bone, such as the patella, or a bursa may be interposed. This bursa may be elongated and folded around the tendon to form a sheath. A flattened tendon is an *aponeurosis* (figure 3.3b).

A *raphe* attachment is a fleshy continuity of muscle and bone without the intervention of a collagenous tendon or aponeurosis (figure 3.3c). The collagen is still there, however, among the muscle fibers or forming a very short tendon.

Origins and Insertions

In classical anatomy, muscles are said to have an *origin* at one end and an *insertion* at the other (figure 3.4). The origin (the one that moves least on contraction) is often proximal, with the insertion distal.

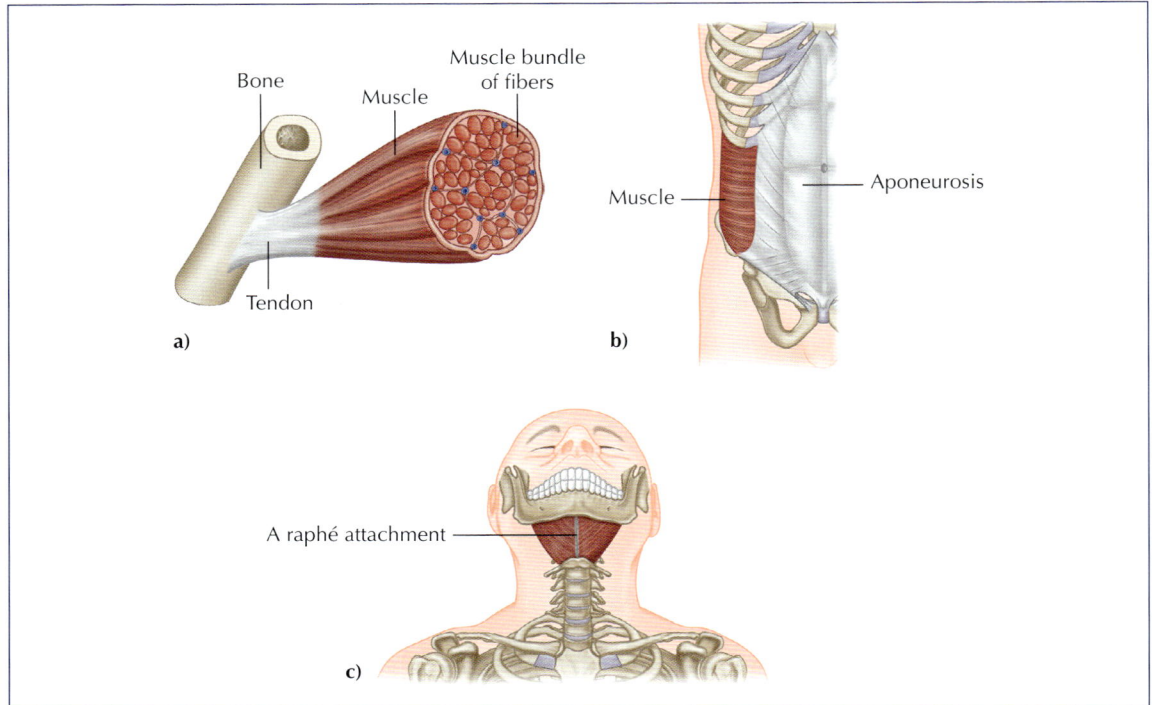

Figure 3.3. Muscle attachments: (a) by tendon; (b) by aponeurosis; (c) by mylohyoid raphe.

Origins and insertions can change their role, depending on the body's position relative to gravity. As this is the case, we can also refer to muscle attachments as opposed to origins and insertions. Often a muscle originates from more than one place, and it is then said to have two heads (e.g., biceps brachii) or three heads (e.g., triceps brachii).

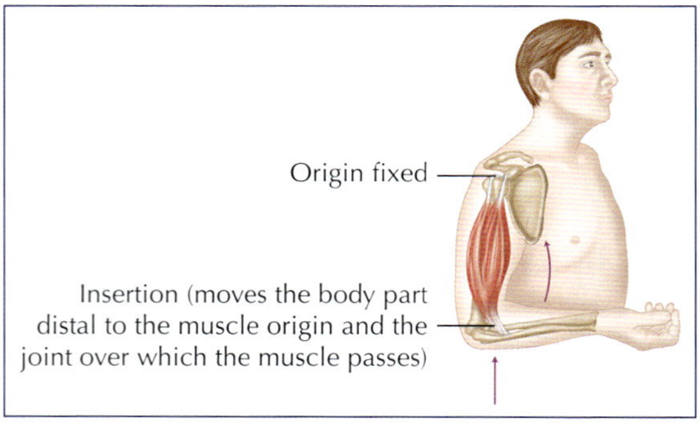

Forms of Muscles

Muscles vary widely in size and shape, according to the task they are required to perform. Skeletal muscles are made of bundles of fascicles, which are bundles of muscle fibers, with each muscle fiber being a single cell. Muscle fibers vary in size from 0.004 inches (0.10 mm) to 12 inches (30 cm) in length. To put the diameter of a muscle fiber into context, consider that a fiber is typically ten times smaller than a human hair. The diameter, length, and arrangement of fascicles also varies from muscle to muscle, with fine bundles in precision muscles, coarse ones in power muscles. Fascicles may be parallel,

Figure 3.4. Muscle working with origin fixed and insertion moving.

oblique, or spiral, according to the position of attachments.

Variations (Shapes) and Explanations

There are seven different muscle shapes: circular, unipennate, bipennate, multipennate, strap (parallel), convergent, and fusiform (figure 3.5).

The simplest is the strap muscle, which has a fleshy, wide attachment at each end.

It can be long and narrow, so long as the maximum length of the muscle fiber is not exceeded. If it is, there will need to be fibers in parallel, with tendinous insertions between groups. The range of contraction of a muscle depends on its length, but its local "tuning peg" power depends on how many fibers it contains.

Strap muscles have a good range but low "tuning peg" power. For greater power, the muscle needs to become fusiform (spindle shaped)—that is, thicker and more

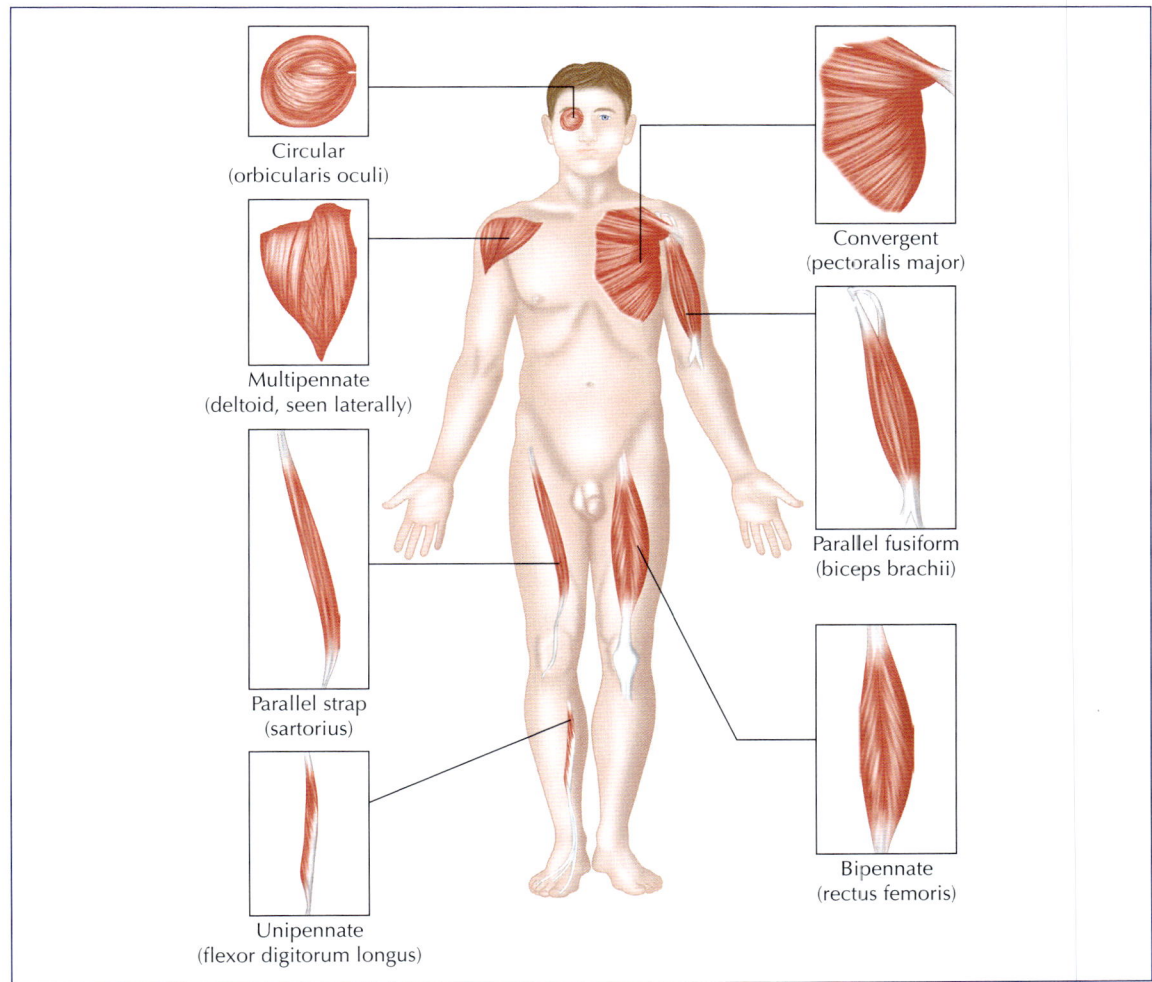

Figure 3.5. Muscle shapes.

three-dimensional. This tends to make the attachment into the tendon less flat and more circular in cross section. Many muscles have their fibers concentrated at one end in a single belly, but digastric (i.e., with two bellies) muscles work just as well. Another way to increase power is for a muscle to have more heads—so in effect, two or three or four muscles are pulling the same tendon.

Having more than one head results in muscle fibers pulling obliquely on the tendon, while dissipating forces through the epimysium that wraps around the muscle in an omnidirectional manner. This can often balance out, but in a unipennate muscle, where fibers insert all along one side of a tendon, the resultant force is the combination of multiple vectors. Multipennate muscles are common compound muscles with a short range but with lots of power.

All muscles are spiralized. Muscles not only pull their associated fascia when they contract but also attempt to untwist or unwind as they accelerate or decelerate a motion. A similar twisting or winding can be further facilitated by wrapping the course of a muscle around a bone. Good examples are levator scapulae and psoas major.

Action of Muscles

Muscles do not suddenly jump from a state of relaxation to one of contraction, they are always "on." At any given time, some functional units (motor units, groups of fibers of various sizes) will be contracting, some inhibiting, and some in stasis, providing either muscle tone or a state of readiness. If the proportions doing each stay constant, so too

will muscle tone, although individual motor units will cycle.

When an individual fiber contracts, it tends to approximate its ends by a spiraling motion, but whether or not this results in movement depends on the force generated and the forces opposing the contraction. The net result for the whole muscle may be contraction, inhibition, or stasis.

A muscle trying to initiate contraction is opposed by:

- passive internal resistance of muscle,
- passive internal resistance of articular tissues,
- opposing muscles (inhibition),
- stiffening of opposing soft tissues,
- inertia of whatever it is trying to move,
- load,
- gravity and ground reaction.

If the force generated exceeds the sum of the above, the limb is accelerated from rest—once moving, a smaller force will keep it moving. A muscle doing this is referred to as the *prime mover*, or *agonist*. *Antagonists* can slow or stop the movement. When both groups act together, nothing moves, or the movement is moderated or controlled. If the movement is prevented, the real result is that the joint across which the muscles act will be stabilized. This cannot be done exclusively by close packing or gravity.

Movement is always opposed or aided by gravity, and this is used wherever possible. The action of a prime mover often exerts a little unwanted movement. For example, the flexion of the fingers by long flexors also flexes the wrists, which is opposed by wrist extensors.

It is easy to see that inhibited muscles cannot provide the decelerating force needed to avoid excessive end ROM resulting in microtrauma. In a simple arrangement of two bones joined by a synergy of muscles, the pull of the muscles can be resolved into:

- **swing**, tending to move the mobile bone;
- **shunt**, compressing the joint;
- **spin**, rotating the mobile bone.

Moving the attachments of the muscles varies the relative size of each component. The largest swing is best for initiating movement—spurt muscle. A large shunt will allow a mobile bone to be loaded by compressing the joint, and a large spin can be used for prime movement or as a synergistic "soaker-up" of unwanted rotation.

Levers

A lever typically involves a rigid bar moving about a fixed point, known as the *fulcrum*. In the absence of physical levers in the human body, I use this popular conceptual framework for ease of understanding.

In the language of levers, *effort* is the force applied to the lever in a specific direction, capable of inducing movement if unopposed. The *resistance* is the force acting against the applied effort force. The fulcrum, though not a tangible pivot point in the human body, is the theoretical support around which the lever would pivot.

Levers are traditionally categorized based on the relative positions of the fulcrum, resistance (load), and effort. These classifications give rise to first-, second-, and third-class levers (see figures 3.6–3.8).

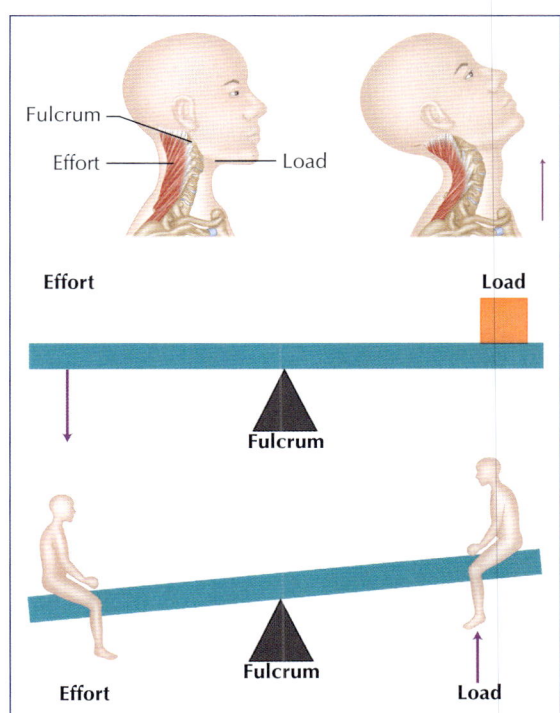

Figure 3.6. First-class lever (EFR): the effort (E) and resistance (R) are located on opposite sides of the fulcrum (F). Examples include animal jaws, seesaws, and crowbars.

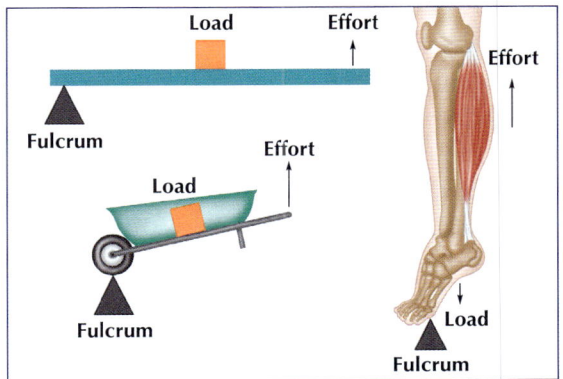

Figure 3.7. Second-class lever (FRE): the effort (E) and resistance (R) are located on the same side of the fulcrum (F), with the resistance between the fulcrum and the effort. An example is a wheelbarrow.

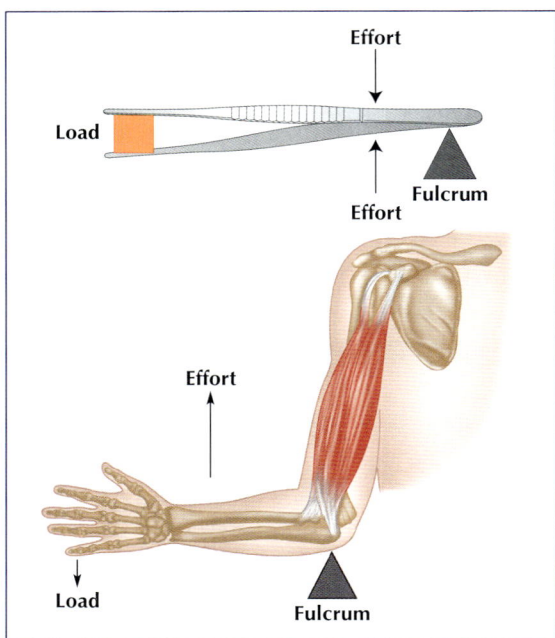

Figure 3.8. Third-class lever (FER): the effort (E) and resistance (R) are located on the same side of the fulcrum (F), but the effort acts between the fulcrum and the resistance. Examples include tweezers. A large effort gains speed of motion in this type of lever. It is the most common lever type in the human body.

It's important when using the lever analogy in the context of the human body that we acknowledge the absence of pin joints and actual mechanical constructs resembling levers. If, hypothetically, we were to consider the relationship between the distal end of the femur and the proximal end of the tibia as a lever, a deep squat might result in the femur figuratively shooting off the tibial plateau. This highlights the theoretical nature of the lever analogy in describing biomechanical interactions within the human body.

Muscle Kinematics

Classification of Muscle Kinetics

Agonist	A muscle that is shortening to perform an action (also known as the *prime mover*) or maintain a posture
Antagonist	A muscle anatomically opposite to the agonist that can stop or reduce the speed (acceleration) of the agonist
Neutralizer	A muscle that counteracts unwanted actions of secondary or tertiary muscles
Stabilizer	Also known as a *fixator*, this type of muscle contracts to offer tension as support to stabilize a body part while a more distal part is moved
Synergist	A muscle that assists the agonist or prime mover to fine-tune a functional movement but is not capable of producing the movement efficiently by itself

Muscles function together synergistically in "force couples" to generate finely-tuned forces, decrease forces, and fixate the kinetic system. A good example is thoracolumbar fascia gain.

In figure 3.9, the transversus abdominis (TA), a muscle on the side and front (deep) of the body, contracts to pull the abdominal wall inward. Acting in a synergistic fashion, the internal oblique (IO) contracts to exert a force on the thoracolumbar fascia. This tension affects the second and third lumbar

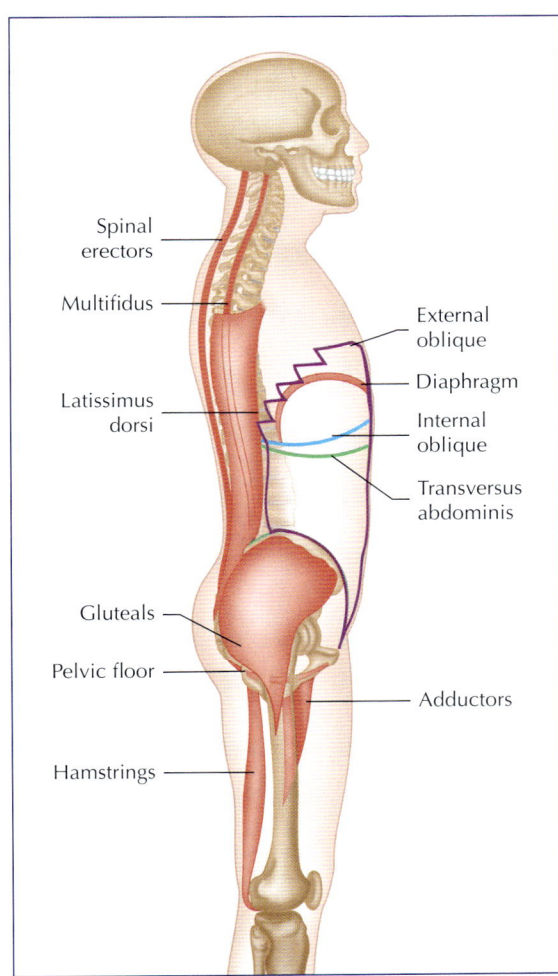

Figure 3.9. Schematic diagram of core stability (inner unit) muscles, and the global (outer unit) muscles.

vertebrae, causing a lift or extension, releasing compression from the fourth and fifth lumbar vertebrae and sacral base. In response to this tension, the deep so-called "fourth layer" muscles—including the multifidus and erector spinae—contract to offer decelerating forces to trunk flexion, thereby neutralizing the forces of forward flexion. Failure of these muscle synergies, such as in the case of poor core neuromuscular efficiency, leads to increased

lumbar compression, and an increased risk of prolapsed or herniated discs.

The muscles to target first are those spastic muscles inhibiting the IO and TA tuning pegs. Significant factors that influence arthrokinematics include: muscle spindles, force couple relationships, reciprocal inhibition, synergistic dominance, neuromuscular efficiency, leverage, muscle fiber arrangement (fasciculi arrangement), and fascia migration.

Stretching

In this new edition of the book I would like to invest more words on the topic of stretching specific to human tissues: fascia, osseofascia, muscle fibers, nerves, blood vessels, lymphatics, and more. I describe myself as a critical friend of stretching, if stretching means taking tissues through their normal anatomical range of motion.

The word *stretch* represents one small battle in a larger war of words, where, in most cases, the opposing army views the body as a machine (figure 3.10) Materialism and reductionism are essential components of a flat-space Euclidean view of a mechanical universe based on a finite number of mathematical shapes. This model resulted in attempts to describe entirely biological phenomena using mechanical descriptions and laws. The ensuing battle is an attack on the true nature of reality. Autonomous, self-formed, self-generated, self-developed, self-aware human forms can self-regenerate and self-heal (within reason), something man-made constructs cannot do.

Advocates for the principles of continuity, connectedness, wholeness, and rationality

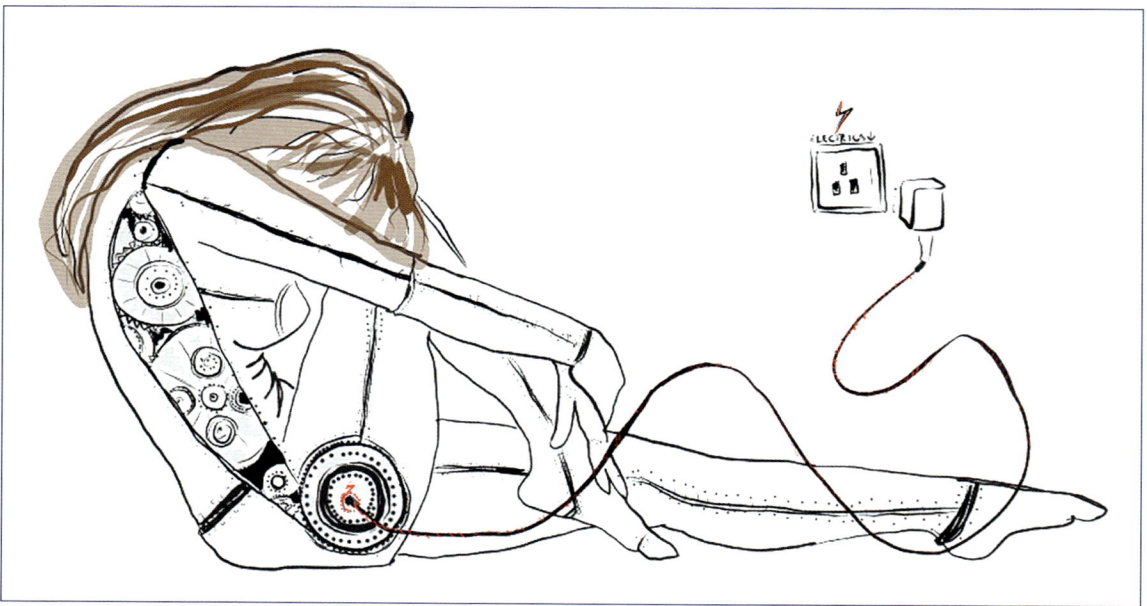

Figure 3.10. For centuries anatomists have viewed the body as a mechanical construct. (Image: commissioned by John Sharkey and drawn by J. Avison, 2021).

often find themselves utilizing the same language as their mechanistic counterparts, often resorting to imprecise or, at times, misleading definitions. This has resulted in the unclear use of words, with many meanings becoming lost in translation, all in an endeavor to uphold a vision that may not fully honor our nervous system. My worry is that many people, myself included, may have developed an inability to see alternative perspectives, because of the influence of models and explanations from our upbringing. These models, relying on evidence better suited to mechanical devices, automobiles, skyscrapers, elevators, and watches, assert strong positions on cause and effect, and have inadvertently limited our openness to more accurate and nonmechanistic viewpoints.

I am seldom satisfied with my current resource of vocabulary, and I feel I have never truly had an *esprit de l'escalier* moment where I came up with the most fitting words to support my argument. (That pursuit is a continuous journey of discovery.)

The discussion is made all the more difficult, in part, by the numerous definitions that exist for *stretch* or *stretching*. Here are a few examples of dictionary definitions:

- To extend or lengthen something beyond the normal length (*Vocabulary.com Dictionary*, Vocabulary.com, https://www.vocabulary.com/dictionary/stretch, accessed February 22, 2024)
- To cause something to reach, often as far as possible, in a particular direction (*Cambridge Dictionary*, Dictionary, https://dictionary.cambridge.org/dictionary/english/stretch, accessed March 27, 2024)
- To pull something to make it longer or wider or to change the length of something

(Macmillan English Dictionary app, last updated January 3, 2024)
- To be able to be made longer or wider without tearing or breaking (*Oxford English Dictionary*, https://www.oed.com/dictionary/stretch_n?tab=meaning_and_use, accessed March 27, 2024)

The term *stretch* has its roots in the 1550s, denoting the action of enlarging beyond proper limits, a manifestation of exaggeration. From an anatomical perspective, *stretch* has been intertwined with the concept of *tension*, leading to the emergence of the term *tendon*. Specifically, the tensor veli palatine, a distinctive muscle situated in the palate, played a crucial role in this context. It engaged in tensing the soft palate, providing the necessary tension for the expansion of the Eustachian tube. This specialized tube, integral in equalizing pressure within the internal auditory mechanism, becomes notably relevant during experiences such as the constriction felt during high-altitude flights.

Fascia-focused therapists have not merely embraced but actively incorporated the term *stretch* into their lexicon. We've not just borrowed it; we've drawn inspiration, derived meaning, appropriated, and absorbed it from the realm of scientific mechanics and hard-matter physics. This word has become an integral part of our ideological framework, serving as a foundational presupposition in explaining and characterizing our practices in manual and movement therapies.

In our approach, there's an underlying assumption that the principles applied to metals and rubber can yield analogous results and outcomes for the intricate web of fascia within the human body. However, this analogy must carry a cautionary note, echoing the criticism often leveled at doctors who, it is said, address symptoms rather than the true root of a patient's ailment. In a parallel vein, some therapists have been criticized for merely "stretching the symptoms," neglecting the deeper complexities of fascial dynamics.

As Ida Rolf, founder of structural integration, is famously reported to have said, "Where you think it is, it ain't." That said, what most people refer to as stretching is not stretching at all but is, in fact, taking tissue through its normal physiological ROM, and that is to be welcomed. So why is there an issue? In essence there are two problematic questions that need to be answered:

- What is occurring during a typical statically held stretch? These static poses have been popular with manual and movement therapists, exercise specialists, dancers, gymnasts, martial artists, and athletes from long before we considered fascia, nerves, blood vessels, and lymphatics.
- Why would stretching (in the true sense of the word) not cause changes to the plasticity of our hard to soft specialized fascia in a harmful way, and most often in a manner that is irreversible (i.e., entropy; and think, *stretch marks*)? I diverge from the numerous accommodationists who promote stretching as harmonious tuning that is congruent with living connective tissues. I view statically held stretching as inappropriate in most cases, harmful and out of tune with the reality of our soft matter, fluidic, electromagnetically vibrant matrix.

My experience over the past forty-two years is that when I ask people *what* they are stretching, the most common, almost exclusive, response is "my muscle." When asked *why*, the most common responses include "My muscle feels tight or stiff," and "I want to make my muscle longer."

I suspect that this underscores the widespread undervaluation or misunderstanding of the profound continuity in the human form and our limited comprehension of the intricacies of nervous fascia. There is a pressing need for a process of de-education. In the first edition of this book, I opted for the term *stretch* because of its pervasive use in various practices. But boldly advocating for the avoidance of stretching, I believe, might have caused more confusion than enlightenment, given the concise nature and word constraints of the book.

While I persist in using the term *lengthen*, it is crucial to clarify that the entire anatomical structure cannot inherently shorten or lengthen (unless affected by dislocation or subluxation). Rather, a transformative shape change occurs, visually resembling a shortening or lengthening, akin to the intricate folding and spiraling of an origami.

It's noteworthy that early anatomists chose the term *contract*, synonymous with *shrink*, to depict the shape change in muscles. Consider the analogy of a backscratcher (figure 3.11). Each module of the backscratcher extends relative to the module within which it is contained, allowing the entire backscratcher to elongate without any individual component altering its length. A more precise syntax is essential to fully grasp the nuances of this intricate subject.

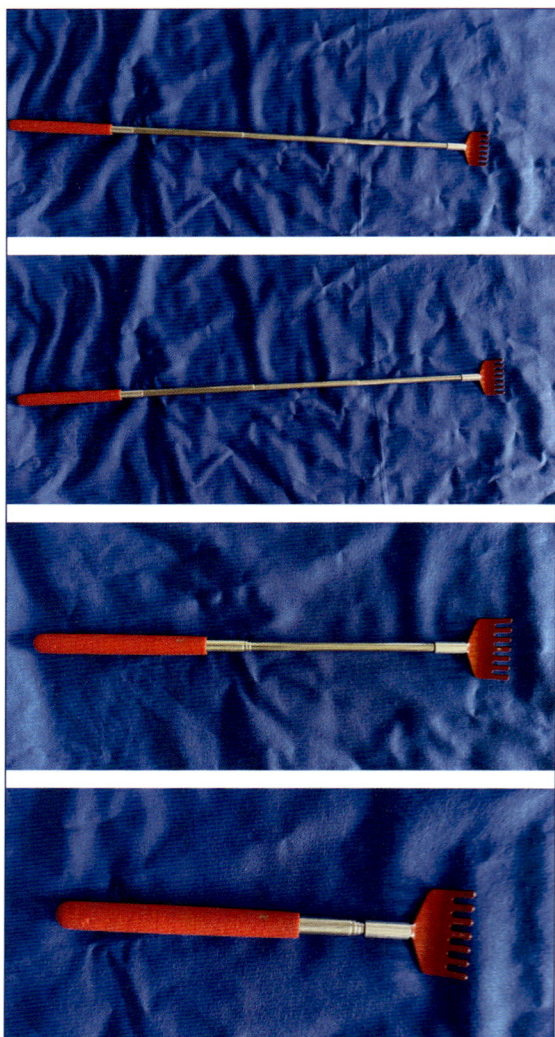

Figure 3.11. Backscratcher 1, 2, and 3. Each module of the backscratcher extends relative to the module within which it is contained, allowing the entire backscratcher to elongate without any individual component altering its length.

A stimulus applied to the surface of a cell can instigate movement, either away from or toward the source of the stimulus. The coordination of our everyday movements involves specialized cells known as sensory (afferent) and motor (efferent) cells. In the realm of fascia-focused therapy, crucial sensory organs include muscle spindles, Golgi tendon organs (GTOs), and receptors that provide information on pressure, pain, temperature, and position, while also being attuned to changes in muscle shape. This information is essential for enabling our muscles to accelerate, decelerate, or initiate reflexive inhibitory responses as protective or facilitating actions.

For instance, to perform a function requiring flexion at the elbow, the triceps brachii must be inhibited to allow the biceps brachii to engage. Simultaneous contraction of both muscles would impede movement at the elbow joint unless cocontractions are specifically required for a particular movement. In such cases, the elbow joint remains fixed, and movement occurs at the shoulder (glenohumeral) joint.

Muscle spindles play a pivotal role in monitoring the speed at which a muscle changes shape, particularly when lengthening. As a muscle accelerates its lengthening, the muscle spindles relay this information to the spinal cord, signaling the nervous system to facilitate appropriate responses. During our daily activities, such as walking, climbing stairs, or sitting, muscles constantly receive neural input from spindles, maintaining a state of readiness or tone—essentially, muscles are always engaged.

One often-misunderstood aspect of muscle spindle activity is its static component. Even when seemingly stationary, we are in motion. When a muscle is isometrically held or elongated eccentrically, it maintains a contractile response. This phenomenon is known as the *muscle stretch reflex*, or *monosynaptic reflex arc* (figure 3.12). The static aspect represents a tonic component, while the dynamic or accelerated aspect is the phasic component.

Muscle spindles remain stimulated as long as the "stretch" is held. The extent of stretch imposed on a muscle correlates with the level of spindle irritation and activation, prompting a neurological resistance to lengthening. This situation essentially manifests as an isometrically held eccentric contraction.

Muscle spindle activity also involves inhibition. This involves a neural response resulting in the release of chemicals that inhibit the antagonist muscle to that being stretched. The patellar tendon stretch (or knee jerk test) is an excellent example of the stretch reflex (figure 3.13).

My understanding of these myotactic reflexes has led me to avoid recommending static and ballistic stretching in most situations of physical activity over the past forty-two years. As static poses are an integral part of some sports, such as the start of a run or swim, we should not rule out static poses for athletes. However, I refer to this as "static dynamic."

The judicious application of static stretching, when administered by a knowledgeable and well-trained therapist, can indeed yield therapeutic benefits. However, it is crucial to recognize that static stretching, if not carefully implemented, has the potential to induce architectural damage and compromise the structural integrity of connective tissues. The decision to employ static stretching as an intervention requires meticulous consideration.

Contrary to the notion that increasing ROM with every stretch is a universal goal, I advocate for caution. Subjecting muscles to prolonged static stretches may contribute

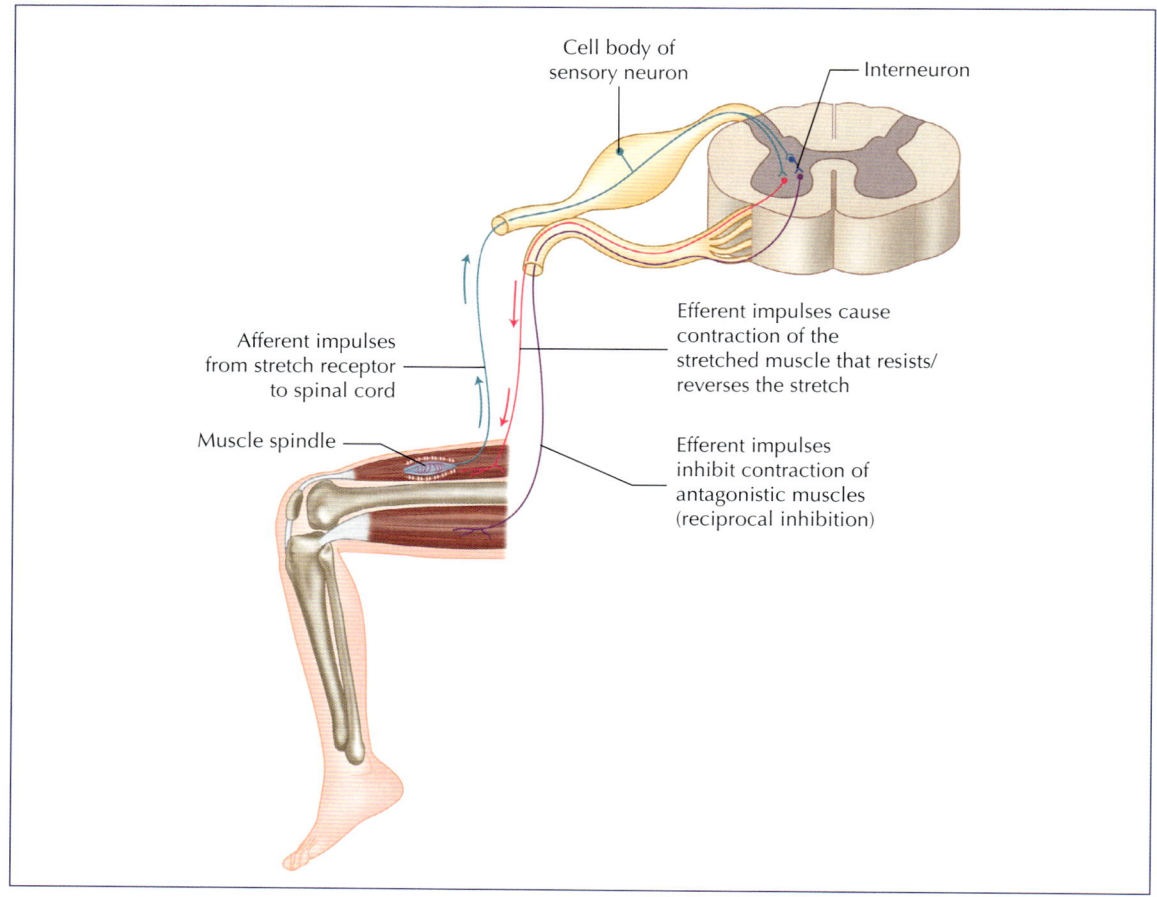

Figure 3.12. The muscle stretch reflex, or monosynaptic reflex arc.

to elevated muscle tension, diminished neuromuscular efficiency, and a decline in relative strength. In the pursuit of elongating muscle fibers, an unintended consequence may be the temporary reduction in reaction times due to the lengthening of nerve tissue. Additionally, the disassociation of actin/myosin proteins during muscle fiber elongation could compromise both strength and neuromuscular efficiency.

I posit that inappropriate static stretching has the potential to exert forces pulling individual sarcomeres (see later this chapter) in opposite directions, leading to the disassociation of contractile proteins and potential reduction in force output. This, over time, may contribute to increased or sustained hypertonicity in the muscle. The resulting tension impedes blood and nerve tissue circulation, fostering tissue hypoxia and additional tension, potentially laying the groundwork for myofascial trigger point (MTrP) activity.

Many individuals feel compelled to incorporate static stretching into their warm-up routines, often just minutes into the session. It's crucial to remember that

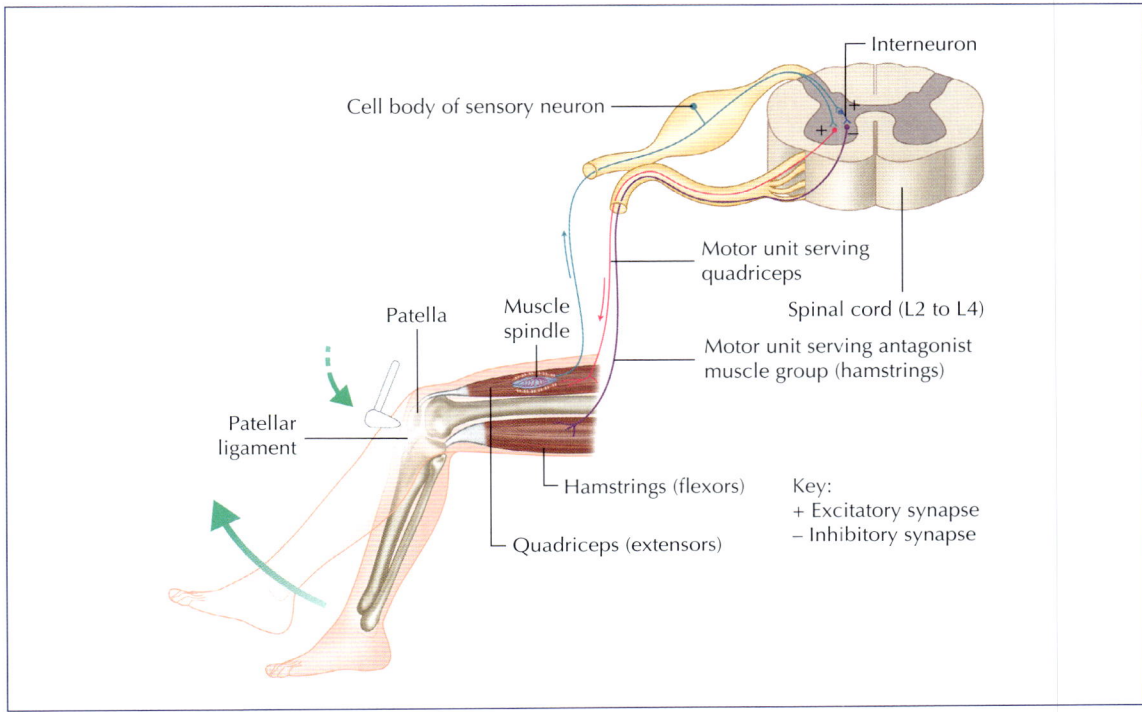

Figure 3.13. Patellar tendon stretch.

warm-up activities should be low in intensity, gradually elevating body temperature from core to extremities. Beginning with small movements, these warm-ups increase body temperature from the core to the extremities, enhance blood flow, reduce fluid viscosity, and render muscles and fascia more pliable. Elevated temperature promotes neural activity and improves diffusion. Exercises appropriate for warm-ups do not induce muscle tightness. If one does, a reassessment of exercise intensity and/or impact is warranted.

Interrupting the warm-up phase to engage in static stretching can reverse the physiological benefits gained. During static stretching, heart rate and body temperature drop, fluid and tissue viscosity increase, and respiratory benefits diminish. Nerve augmentation is

also reversed, emphasizing the importance of maintaining a warm, pliable state for muscles before escalating activity demands in terms of intensity, ROM, and duration.

Fascia-focused therapy promotes neuro-muscular efficiency or dynamic ROM as well as active cold therapy spray (using a safe cold spray), as opposed to classical static stretching. It is my recommendation that static stretching has little place in medical exercise, or athletic or recreational training.

Static stretching may have a therapeutic role in injury rehabilitation—however, the therapist or trainer, as previously mentioned, must understand how to use static stretching in an appropriate and effective manner. Many fitness experts have promoted static stretching as an effective means of reducing injuries, yet time and time again this notion is not supported by research. Many other unsupported claims regarding the benefits of static stretching have also been made; for example, with the toe touch or sit and reach test.

These standardized tests are widely acknowledged for evaluating hamstring flexibility. If an individual is identified as having limited ROM or flexibility in the hamstrings, a common manifestation is bending at the knees (figure 3.14). However, it is essential to consider that the tension within the posterior kinetic system, residing in the associated fascia either above or below the hamstrings, might be the actual origin of excessive neurologically driven tension, adhesion, inhibition, or densification.

Addressing the interconnected fascial components, such as releasing tension in the plantar fascia of the feet or the thoracolumbar

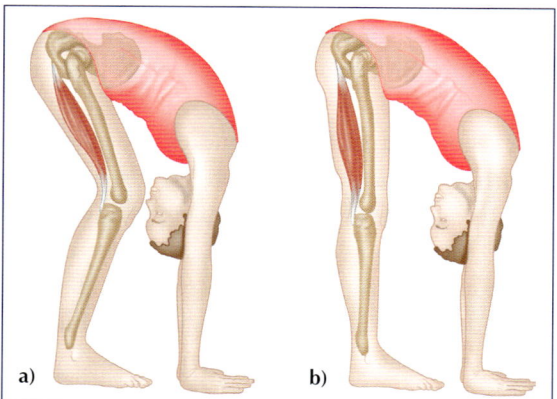

Figure 3.14. (a) Having to bend the knees to touch the toes is interpreted by many as passive insufficiency of the hamstrings; (b) being able to touch the toes with the knees straight would mean there is much less passive insufficiency of the hamstrings.

and cervical fascia, often leads to notable enhancements in hamstring flexibility test scores. Recognizing and addressing tension in these broader fascial networks can provide a more comprehensive approach to improving overall flexibility and mitigating issues attributed to neurologically based tension, perceived or felt by the patient as "stiffness."

It is my recommendation to all personal trainers and all manual and physical therapists, including physiotherapists, osteopaths, chiropractors, sports therapists, and others, to encourage appropriate warm-ups and cool-downs, incorporating gradual increases in ROM with control. Control involves decelerating toward the end ROM.

As mentioned before, recent studies have shown that static stretching has a negative effect on neuromuscular efficiency, including agility and power, as well as reduced force production in the stretched muscles. In fact, studies have demonstrated that making a fast, dynamic movement following a static stretch increases the risk of injury to that muscle. I want to point out that this is very different to pre-stretching a muscle under load and then immediately following it with a concentric contraction, as you would during weight training following an appropriate warm-up. Such a pre-stretch is by its very nature dynamic and causes the stretch reflex, thereby increasing force output.

It is worth noting that recent research regarding proprioceptive neuromuscular facilitation stretching (PNF) has identified increases in electrical activity in the stretched muscles, while there is also an increase in muscle stiffness during the stretch. It appears that PNF techniques have a pronounced short-term analgesic effect on the target muscles. This would not be a desired effect for athletes about to engage in high-risk, high-intensity eccentric actions.

Critical reviews of scientific literature highlight that, similar to weight training, both force and power decrease immediately after static stretching. The decreases are mild and range from 2 to 5 percent. This difference may not be clinically significant for a normal individual with a healthy lifestyle, but to the elite athlete it may be the difference between first and first loser, also known as second. Of course, the debate on stretching must continue and we must be ready to change our views if quality evidence is produced.

Force Couple Relationships

Imagine for a moment you are throwing a ball (figure 3.15). As the ball leaves your right hand, your left leg/foot has remained firmly on the ground. Now, like watching a movie, let's freeze that image. A tensional relationship now exists between the opposite lower and upper limbs moving in opposite directions, causing a rotation in the vertebral column; this is one example of a force couple.

Current research supports the benefits of moderate exercise or physical activity in maintaining the health of the myofascial system. There needs to be a full body kinetic system postural assessment before an individualized medical exercise or physical activity program can be prescribed.

For example, imagine a client presenting with hypertonic spastic psoas muscles. Such a scenario would create an inhibition to the gluteus maximus. As gluteus maximus offers a force couple to the sacroiliac (SI) joint, in conjunction with latissimus dorsi, it is easy to see how the hamstrings will have to offer additional force, as compensation, to maintain the necessary tension to assist in force closure of the SI joint.

In walking, as the left leg is propelled forward, the left ilium rotates backward in relation to the sacrum, producing an increase in tension through the sacrotuberous and interosseous ligaments. This helps to provide turgor, which in turn supports the SI joint, in preparation for heel strike. The ipsilateral hamstrings are activated.

When considering joint biomechanics (arthrokinematics), it is helpful to understand the diversity in degrees of ROM available at various joints. Familiarity with joint ROM will play an important role in evaluating a client, including the kinetic system postural assessment and the medical exercise prescription.

The following are useful examples of normal ROM at the shoulder complex.

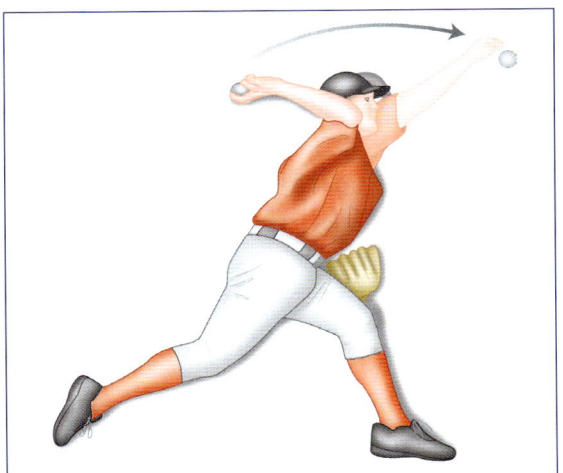

Figure 3.15. Force couple relationship.

Flexion (anteversion)	0 to 180 degrees
Extension (retroversion)	0 to 50 degrees
Adduction	0 to 45 degrees
Abduction	0 to 90 degrees
Elevation	90 to 180 degrees
Lateral (external) rotation	0 to 80 degrees
Medial (internal) rotation	0 to 100 degrees
Horizontal extension	0 to 40 degrees
Horizontal flexion	0 to 140 degrees

Joint Biomechanical Terms

Acceleration	Rate of change of velocity with time
Compression	Force that compacts an object
Displacement	Location of one point in relation to another
Energy	Capacity to work, produce motion, overcome resistance, or effect physical change
Fluid	Composed of elements or particles that freely change their relative positions without separating
Force	Push or pull resulting from physical contact between two objects
Hydrostatic pressure	Intensity of loading within a fluid

Mass	Amount of matter composing an object and the resistance of that object to being moved with speed—i.e., acceleration
Momentum	Mass of an object multiplied by velocity
Shear	Deforms a structure without compacting or stretching it
Strain	Amount of deformity when an object has force applied to it
Stress	Intensity of load, equal to the force exerted divided by the area over which it is applied
Tensile	Force that pulls apart
Velocity	Rate of change of displacement with time
Weight	The force acting on an object due to gravitational pull; force + mass × acceleration, Newton's law

Two Members of the Movement Club

For movement to take place, two members—compression and tension—act together to translate generated forces produced by the muscle fibers into orderly, synchronized, adaptable, efficient, and precise movement—i.e., mechanotransduction (figure 3.16). The skeletal (osseofascial) system, with its joints, provides compression by "pushing out" while the skin and soft tissues are tensioned, activating muscle spindle activity, in turn providing constantly required tension "pulling in."

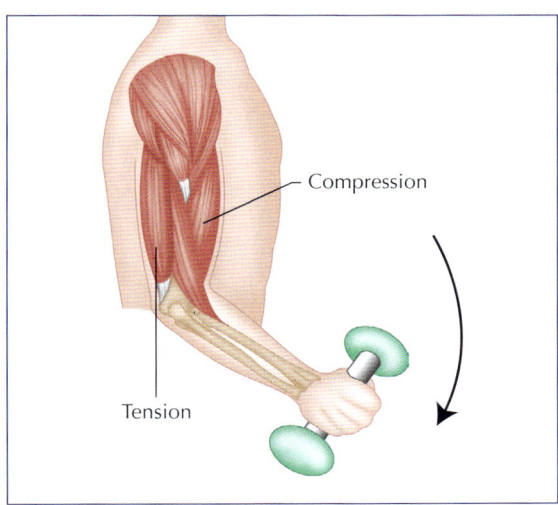

Figure 3.16. Two members of the movement club: (a) compression; (b) tension.

As muscles are integrated into the osseofascial tissue through the periosteum, their pulling forces generate a tensile stress providing the necessary force to produce tension at a joint. This tension is generated to facilitate movement. For movement to occur in a manner that is compatible with the structure of the body, one should avoid creating muscles that dominate inappropriately within a global myofascial system. Training a muscle in a manner that is sagittal-plane dominant while focusing on developing strength through large force output is commonplace within the gym setting. This approach to training does little to reduce risk of injury (in fact, it may increase such risk) as a significant number of injuries occur during eccentric movement in the transverse plane.

Reciprocal Inhibition

Reciprocal inhibition (RI) is the automatic inhibition of a muscle when its antagonist contracts, also known as Sherrington's law. Under special circumstances, both the agonist and antagonist can contract together, known as a cocontraction.

Inhibition is a central theme in fascia-focused therapy. Let me use eye movement in one direction—say, rotated to the right—as an example to describe RI. The number of motor units and their discharge rates increase in the contracting muscles, while there must be an invariant corresponding decrease in contraction resulting from an increase in chemical neuroinhibitors—for example, gamma-aminobutyric acid, glycine, phosphates, lactates, and serotonin—in the opposing, but synergistic, muscles.

This does not mean that the muscle relaxes or that it is not being innervated—that would be a misrepresentation of the complexity of muscle synergies. While the opposing muscle still receives the neurochemical stimulus to contract, it also receives twice as much of a neural inhibitor chemical, stopping the muscle from contracting—in other words, it becomes inhibited.

When flexing at the elbow, the synergistic roles refer to the coordinated action of muscles working together to achieve a specific movement. In the context of inhibition rather than relaxing, this means that certain muscles are actively preventing excessive movement or contraction by inhibiting their activity. Inhibition, in this case, suggests a controlled suppression of muscle activity to a level that supports and maintains stability or control during the fixation at the elbow. This mechanism helps to stabilize the joint and prevent unwanted or excessive motions. As in figure 3.17, when fixing at the elbow, several muscles work synergistically to stabilize the joint.

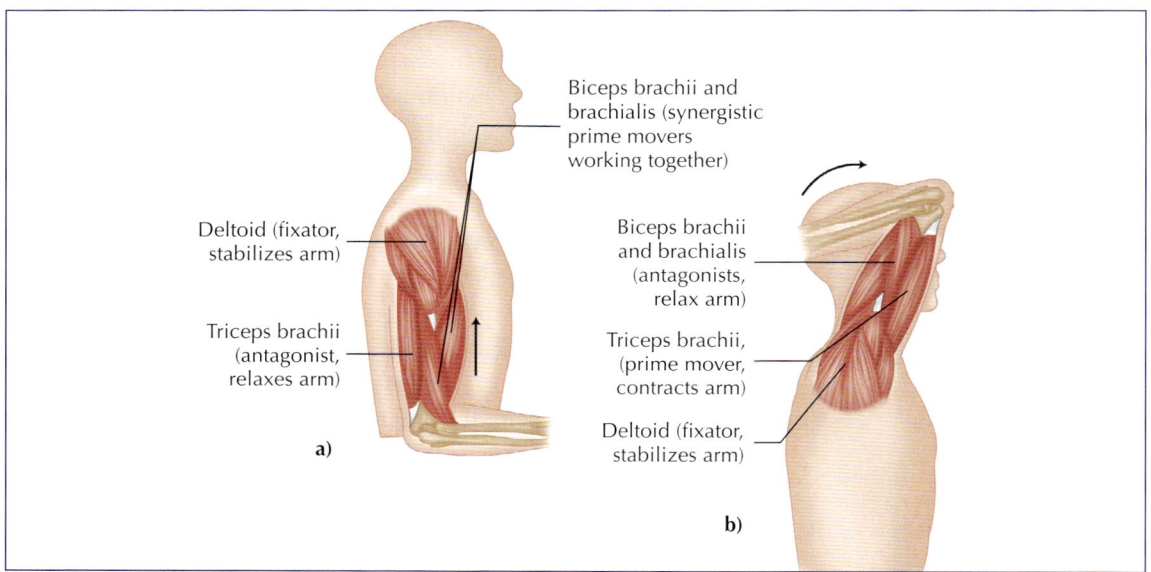

Figure 3.17. Group action of muscles: (a) flexing the arm at the elbow; (b) extending the arm at the elbow (showing reversed roles of prime mover and antagonist).

Let's consider the flexors and extensors:

- **Flexors:**
    - **Biceps brachii** flexes the elbow and plays a role in supination of the forearm.
    - **Brachialis** is a prime flexor of the elbow and assists the biceps brachii.
    - **Brachioradialis** also aids in elbow flexion and is particularly active when the forearm is in a mid-position between pronation and supination.
- **Extensors:**
    - **Triceps brachii** is the primary extensor of the elbow; it helps in straightening the upper limb at the elbow.
    - **Anconeus** is a small muscle that assists the triceps in extending the elbow.

In terms of inhibition, these muscles would be actively controlled to prevent excessive contraction or inhibition, maintaining a balanced and stable position at the elbow joint. For example, while the flexors are active in bending the elbow, there is simultaneous inhibition of the extensors to prevent the joint from straightening too much. This coordinated activity ensures precise control of movement and stability during tasks involving fixation at the elbow.

It is crucial to reiterate that when a muscle is inhibited, the term *relaxed*, while commonly used, is somewhat misleading. The muscle is not truly relaxing; rather, it receives a neural impulse to contract but refrains from doing so because of a greater influx of neurochemical substances that actively "inhibit" the amplitude of contraction. These inhibitory substances include phosphates and lactic acid, which exert a significant influence on decision-making concerning the prescription of physical activities for rehabilitation or promoting balance in synergies. The initial phase of rehabilitation should focus on treatment reducing tone in the hypertonic muscles that are creating inhibition in synergistic muscles.

Understanding the neural dynamics of inhibition underscores the impracticality of instructing a patient to "strengthen" a muscle already under inhibition. In the early stages of therapeutic intervention, therapists should steer clear of strengthening exercises. Instead, the focus should be on establishing synergistic balance and enhancing neuromuscular efficiency. Furthermore, a specialized emphasis on fascia rehabilitation is imperative, necessitating the incorporation of physical activities specifically designed for the fascial system (see p. 131).

Synergistic Dominance

The role of synergists is to assist prime movers to perform functional movements. Owing to poor exercise practices, inappropriate posture, and repetitive strain on muscles, fascia, and joints the neural aspects of kinesiology will adapt and change. A kinetic reaction both up and down, anterior to posterior, and lateral to medial, will occur. If an individual has learned to perform an exercise incorrectly, they will always perform that exercise incorrectly. To address this they need to learn correct static and dynamic posture during physical activity.

Minute alterations occur in muscle recruitment, stabilization, proprioception and motor skills, strength, and joint positioning. Over time, this leads to faulty recruitment of muscles within kinetics and inhibition of prime movers. When gluteus maximus is inhibited, the synergistic hamstrings and lumbar erectors will inappropriately provide movement of hip extension. Such synergistic dominance could, in time, lead to pain and injury.

Neuromuscular Efficiency

This concerns the capacity of the neuromuscular system to provide safe, effective, and appropriate forces in a synergistic fashion, involving agonists, antagonists, synergists, stabilizers, and neutralizers, while stabilizing the kinetic system in all planes of motion.

Neuromuscular efficiency takes into account the global effect of movement and the integrated relationship of local muscles (a link) within any given synergy of muscles (a chain)—the integrated functional unit. As mentioned on page 126, a more precise term would be "kinetic system" to describe the dynamic interconnectedness within the human body. Unlike a chain where a single broken link would render it useless, our biological systems possess remarkable adaptability, allowing for continuous function despite disruptions. Neuromuscular retardation—or reduced efficiency—leads to postural adaptations and increased risk of injury. For example, retardation of the reaction time response would increase risk of sprains and strains.

Biophysical Dynamics as an Alternative to *Biomechanics* (Arthrokinematics)

Understanding human movement is an essential prerequisite for safe, effective, and suitable fascia-focused therapy and medical exercise. Aristotle could be seen as a pioneer of biomechanics, because of his seminal work *De motu animalium* (Movement of animals). This foundational text explores the intricacies of animal motion.

In the intellectual landscape of ancient Greece, Aristotle—alongside luminaries like Socrates and Plato—laid the groundwork for our most fundamental scientific tools: deductive and mathematical reasoning. Their collective insights not only laid the philosophical groundwork for subsequent generations but also provided the conceptual underpinning for the development of biomechanics. Aristotle's exploration of animal movement in *De motu animalium* provides a foundation for understanding the mechanical principles governing the human body. His observations and analyses of anatomical structures, coupled with his keen philosophical mind, set the stage for a discipline that would later become indispensable in the realms of therapy and medical exercise.

The evolution of biomechanics owes much to the enduring relevance of Aristotle's contributions. The essence of deductive and mathematical reasoning, identified by Aristotle, remains integral to contemporary biomechanics. In this book, the study of human movement is expanded beyond Aristotle's foundational work, incorporating tensegrity architecture and fascia research, advanced technologies, sophisticated methodologies, and a deeper understanding of the intricate interplay between our myofascial structures.

Today, practitioners in fascia-focused therapy and medical exercise should draw upon the rich legacy of Aristotle's insights but integrate contemporary advancements and move away from the view of man as a machine. We need to replace the term *biomechanics* with *biophysical dynamics*, to reflect this dynamic and evolving discipline to promote safe, effective, and tailored approaches to enhancing human movement and well-being.

Care is needed when choosing the vocabulary to describe the research supporting fascia

Theories and Proof

Theories

In the realm of science, a plethora of theories abound, each representing someone's best attempt to elucidate the intricate workings of the universe. Among these, significant examples are the theory of evolution by natural selection, conceived by Charles Darwin; Albert Einstein's theory of relativity; Copernicus's heliocentric model, positing Earth's orbit around the sun; and atomic theory, asserting the existence of atoms. Each has undergone rigorous scrutiny through observation and experimentation, earning them the status of accepted facts.

In 1916, climatologist and geologist Alfred Wegener boldly proposed that continents floated across the Earth's surface. He suggested that West Africa and the East Coast of South America once interlocked like a jigsaw puzzle and subsequently drifted apart owing to tectonic movements. Wegener faced ridicule for his audacious theory, but by the late 1950s it had transformed from outrageous to accepted and accurate science, taught in schools.

Delving into the intricacies of muscle physiology theories lays the groundwork for comprehending the diverse techniques employed in fascia-focused therapies and their

Theories and Proof *(Continued)*

therapeutic efficacy. While acknowledging established theories, it's crucial to remain vigilant about emerging academic research, ready to adapt our perspectives and challenge ingrained beliefs.

One such theory, the *sliding filament theory*, presents a viewpoint that I find flawed. The notion of "sliding" implies friction, potentially leading to inflammation and swelling. Nevertheless, the theory contributes a plausible account of how electromagnetic activity generates forces culminating in muscle contraction. Acknowledging its strengths and weaknesses fosters a nuanced understanding of the complex dynamics underlying muscle physiology.

Proof

Newspaper and magazine articles frequently employ attention-seeking headlines, replete with catchphrases like "dramatic proof." But if one reads further and investigates, it often becomes evident that such an assertion lacks substantiation, and it turns out that it is neither dramatic or proof. The term *proof* has been wielded to discredit therapeutic approaches perceived as less "academic." Many proponents of therapeutic modalities assert that they have been unequivocally "proven" effective. However, it is imperative to realize that having been shown to be efficacious, or exhibiting positive therapeutic outcomes, is distinct from having been incontrovertibly proved. To give reliable results, academic research must be very carefully designed, and there is much "bad science" published. Despite the wealth of evidence supporting

the role of cigarette smoking in promoting lung cancer, the tobacco industry has been able to find research that apparently "proved" that smoking mitigated the risk of specific medical conditions. Over time, evidence builds up that supports or doesn't support one theory or another, and a widely accepted consensus may be achieved, although that must always remain subject to change if new evidence arises.

While emphasizing the imperative for science-based foundations for fascia-focused therapies, a word of caution is extended to therapists against invoking the term *proven*. Instead, employing more tempered expressions such as *research supports* or *research has demonstrated* is advised.

The quality of a research study needs to be assessed in terms of its nature and methodology; whether it adopts a quantitative or qualitative paradigm; the size and recruitment methodology of the study cohort; and other factors that contribute to the reliability and validity of its findings. Empirical research, where data are collected, summarized, and analyzed, is reliant on the quality of those data for its conclusions and recommendations. If the instruments employed for data collection lack robustness, the resulting data may be rendered inherently inaccurate. As an accumulating body of data substantiates the therapeutic efficacy of fascia-focused therapies and various NMTq, vigilance is required to avoid using the "proof" criterion as a weapon against less academically endorsed therapeutic modalities.

therapy. Avoid the words *proven* and *proved*. Not even Darwin could prove anything 100 percent.

Titin and the So-Called Sliding Filament Theory

In 1954, H. E. Huxley and J. Hanson proposed the *sliding filament theory* of muscle contraction (figure 3.18). The structural unit of muscles, the sarcomere, had been understood to consist of two interdigitating filament systems, which slide past each other when a muscle shortens. Special proteins were identified as forming one thin and one thick protein filament. This description is the most widely used in medical and exercise science texts to this day.

Credit must be given to Huxley and Hanson all those years ago when they noted that removing the actin and myosin protein filaments did not lead to a collapse of the sarcomere. The presence of some third protein filament was proposed, but its size and proximity to the other filaments made firm conclusions regarding its disposition and function difficult to reach. Over the years many terms have been used to describe the function of these filaments, including *S filaments*, *gap filaments*, *T filaments*, and *core filaments*.

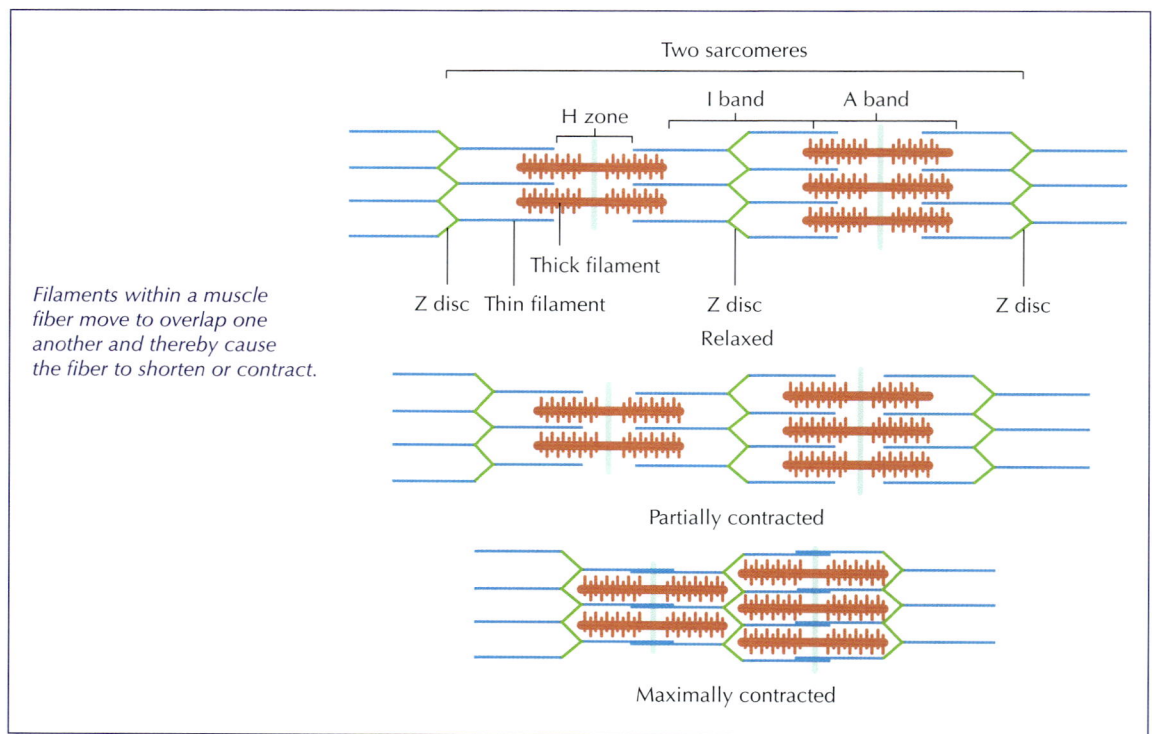

Filaments within a muscle fiber move to overlap one another and thereby cause the fiber to shorten or contract.

Figure 3.18. The sliding filament mechanism.

In 1977 a new myofibrillar protein was identified, and later in 1999 it was given the name *titin*. It appears that titin is the third-most-abundant protein in striated muscle, accounting for about 11 percent of its combined protein content.

I mention this because it is important to recognize that we are still learning about the architecture of sarcomeres and how muscles contract. Of course, that is why we still say the sliding filament "theory," because it is the best theory we have to explain how muscles go about their business.

But there is no sliding in the human body unless there is pathology, and so there cannot be a "sliding filament" at play. Heat production in the human body comes from the production of energy through the splitting of ATP. Sliding would cause friction, and that would not be a valuable component of muscle activity (figure 3.19).

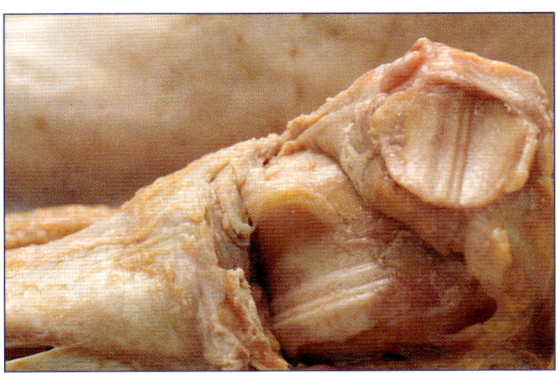

Figure 3.19. This image of the posterior surface of the patella (kneecap) and anterior surface of the femoral condyles is a perfect example of pathology caused by friction. Bones should never touch, but through inappropriate synergistic activity or inhibition because of spastic hypertonic tissues, excessive compression can result.

Muscle Anatomy—Only One Muscle in the Human Body

This section is of the utmost importance in providing essential science related to the structure and workings of muscle fibers. Without this knowledge it is not possible to understand and appreciate the anatomy of MTrPs. The following explanations are offered in a simplified science-based language yet offer a fresh view on the topic of anatomy. This view is one of continuity, a unified body, one muscle with possibly 670 individual fascial bags or compartments.

The one-muscle concept was first introduced at the World of Fitness conference held in 1992, organized by Jan Field and Roger Byrne. The presentation, called "The Never-Ending Story," was an attempt to encourage personal trainers and aerobics instructors to view connective tissue (CT) as a continuous insulation of muscle bellies condensed into tendons and ligaments with no beginning and no end.

Skeletal muscle is continuous with *periosteum*, the outer covering of bone (figure 3.20). Skeletal muscle is squeezed by the fascia into individual muscle tubes. These fascial tubes contain the central part of the muscle, called the *gaster* or *belly*, where the tube is dilated, and the more condensed portions either end are called the *tendon*. This in effect means there is only one muscle in the human body. One continuous muscle with its associated fascia. This fascia rises and falls as it waves throughout the body, embracing the sandy shores of the osseofascial tissue with its more solid component, the periosteum. Muscle tissue spirals and twists as it makes its way from origin to insertion. Muscle fibers are not arranged in straight lines but rather in spiral

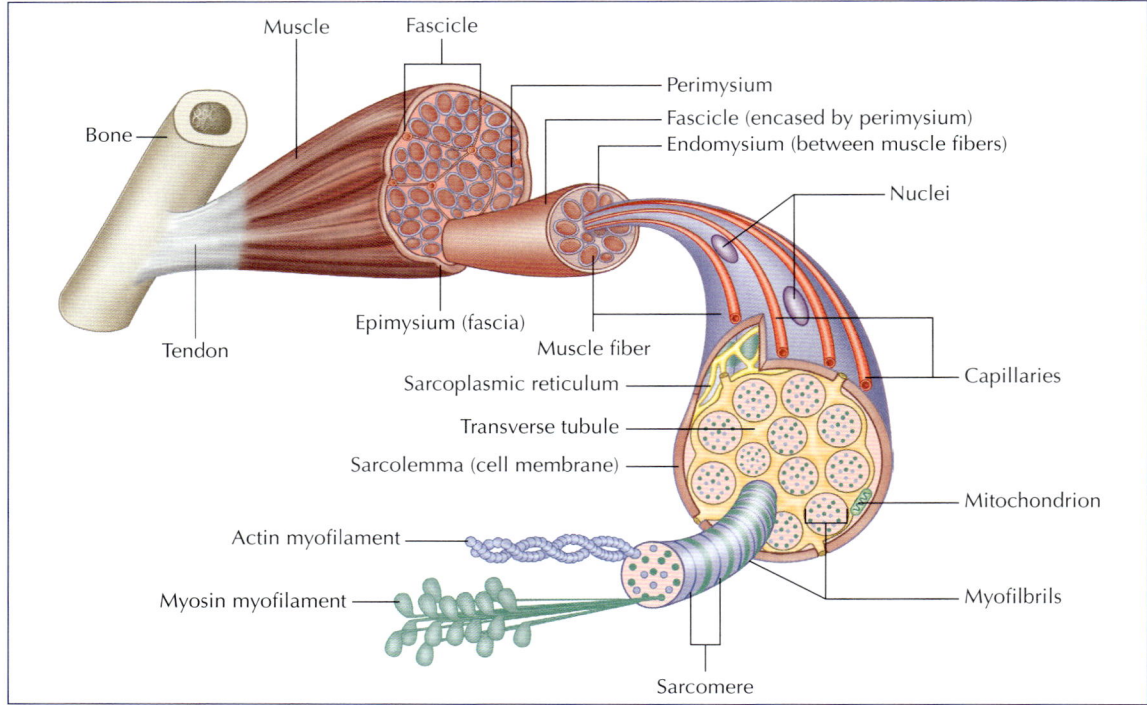

Figure 3.20. The structure of skeletal muscle.

and diagonal patterns. There are no straight lines to be found in the human body.

Muscles may have anatomical individuality, but they have no functional individuality. The one muscle of the human body is continuous from superior to inferior, anterior to posterior, side to side, birth to death. Muscle makes up about 35 percent of human body weight, and 85 percent of body heat is produced by muscles.

The fascia wraps and covers the muscles, viscera, and skeleton. The fascial coverings wrapping your organs and viscera are called the *subserous fascia*. The skeletal fascia is the *periosteum*. The fascia beneath your skin is called the *superficial fascia* (subcutaneous). This is one continuous system of connective tissue throughout the body, linking distant body parts to one another. From embryonic development, a system of interconnecting tubes, including your arterial system and the alimentary system, combines with an interlocking system of fascial planes, including the crural fascia, around the legs, merging at the inguinal ligament, with the transversal fascia surrounding the peritoneal cavity and continuing up to connect to the diaphragmatic fascia. It continues, integrating with the parietal pleura surrounding the lungs and goes on to merge with the cervical fascia from the neck up to and into the head.

The idea of compartmentalizing muscle function has led to the invention of machine-based exercises. I want to encourage a shift in perspective from trying to isolate and improve strength in one muscle to improving multidirectional, multidimensional neuromuscular efficiency (the firing patterns throughout the entire kinetic system). It is essential to recognize that the body does not contract only one muscle when performing a task but several muscles in a specific sequence or in concert. As muscles contract to accelerate, decelerate, stabilize, and neutralize, the forces generated are facilitated along the continuously formed continuities of myofascial tissue. A global view of human movement is required.

Not all tendons are thick, cord-like structures; some are flat, thin and/or thick tissues called *aponeuroses*. A good example of an aponeurosis is the thick tendon and fascia of the lower back known as the *thoracolumbar fascia*. The outer covering of muscle is the *epimysium*, a tissue that encapsulates the entire muscle. Each muscle contains subunits or bundles known as *fascicles*. Fascicles are, in turn, surrounded and separated by a connective tissue called *perimysium*.

Fascicles come in various shapes and sizes. Each fascicle contains numerous individual muscle fibers, or cells. Each individual muscle cell is separated from its neighbor by a connective tissue called *endomysium*. The virtual space between muscle fibers is called the *critical fiber distance*, and should be maintained for normal, healthy muscle function. When muscles are injured or dehydrated, this space can become compromised. The distance between the fibers reduces and the fibers become adhered. This virtual space is occupied by a special lubricating glycosaminoglycan called *hyaluronan*.

Each individual muscle fiber has an outer covering or membrane called the *sarcolemma*. It is important to note that the sarcolemma maintains a membrane potential, allowing impulses to travel along the muscle cell in a similar way to how impulses are propagated in nerves.

Of course, the main function of impulses in muscles is to generate or inhibit contractions. A muscle never relaxes. A typical muscle fiber is about one-tenth the diameter of a human hair, yet it can support a thousand times its own weight. Muscle names sometimes provide us with essential information regarding the muscle's own individual features. Muscles have been named for many different reasons, such as:

Size	Gluteus maximus (largest), gluteus minimus (smallest)
Position	Tibialis anterior (in front [of the tibia]), tibialis posterior (behind [the tibia])
Shape	Deltoid (shaped like a triangle)
Number of tendons	Biceps brachii (two-headed), triceps brachii (three-headed)
Fiber direction	Rectus abdominis (rectus means straight)
Action	Extensor digitorum (extends)

Examining the structure of the muscle cell will provide you with the necessary technical information to grasp how a muscle contracts and provide the foundation for understanding MTrP etiology.

Structure of a Muscle Cell

Muscle cells contain long protein strings called *myofibrils* (figure 3.21). Each myofibril runs the length of a fiber. If a fiber is 4 inches (10 cm) long, then the protein myofibrils making up that fiber will also be 4 inches long.

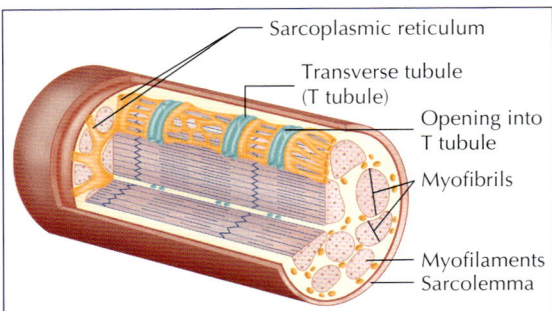

Figure 3.21. The structure of a muscle cell.

Contained within each myofibril are protein molecules called *myofilaments*. Each myofibril contains special protein molecules within small room-like structures called *sarcomeres* where contractions take place. The special relationship between the various molecules contained within these sarcomeres causes a shortening, pulling the walls of each sarcomere closer together, what the early anatomists called "shrinking."

The outer covering of individual muscle cells, the *sarcolemma*, has special holes and openings in it. These holes lead to tubes known as *transverse tubules*, or *T tubules*. Similar in some ways to microscopic blood vessels, these specialized tubes cover the myofibrils. T tubules function to conduct impulses originating on the surface of the sarcolemma into the muscle cell, specifically to the *sarcoplasmic reticulum* (SR).

The Theory of Sliding (or Gliding) Filaments—Essential Information for Understanding the Formation of MTrPs

The sliding filament theory is currently internationally accepted as the basic mechanism of muscle contraction.

The hollow SR functions to store calcium ions, which are constantly being pumped into the SR from the cytoplasm (*sarcoplasm*) of the cell. When muscle fibers are not contracted, a high concentration of calcium is located in the SR and low concentrations exist within the sarcoplasm. Special calcium gates remain closed, blocking calcium from escaping into the sarcoplasm. When an impulse travels along the membrane of the SR, these calcium gates open, allowing a flood of calcium ions to rush out of the SR and into the sarcoplasm of the sarcomere, where the myofilaments are located. This is a key step in the normal sequence leading to muscle contraction.

The sarcomere is the basic functional unit of the myofibril. When viewed under a microscope, the ends of a sarcomere appear lighter than the center. This is because the thick myofilaments are situated in the center, while the thin myofilaments are located toward the ends. The name *striated muscle* was used for this reason. Sarcomeres appear as dark A bands, with a narrow H zone in the center divided by an M line, and light I bands. Near the center of the I band is a thin, dark line known as the Z line, or Z disc. The Z line is where sarcomeres come together, and the thin myofilaments of adjacent sarcomeres overlap slightly.

Myofibrils are composed of three types of myofilaments: *myosin* in the thick filaments, *actin* in the thin filaments; and *titin*, which is sticky, associated with the thick filaments. The myofilaments are arranged in a very precise pattern. The thick myofilaments are surrounded by six thin myofilaments, while the titin acts as tails to anchor the myosin to

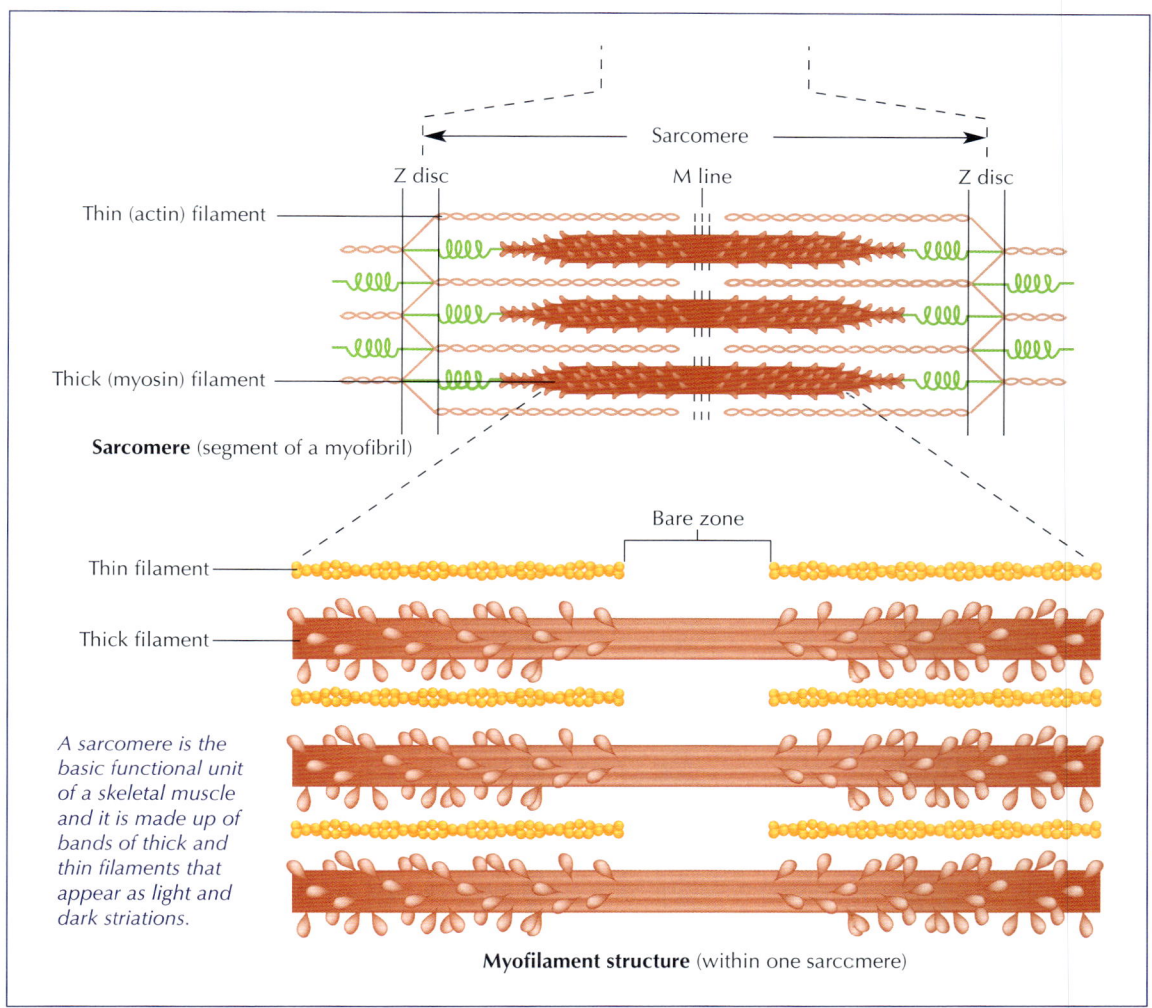

Figure 3.22. The structure of a sarcomere.

the Z disc. The thin actin myofilaments can be seen above and below each thick myofilament (figure 3.22). In reality, they spiral around the thick proteins in a snake-like chiral fashion.

The A bands are composed mainly of thick filaments, with only a few thin filaments. The H zone contains only thick filaments. the M line is protein molecules that hold the thick filaments together. The I bands are made of up thin filaments only.

Within each sarcomere, the myofilaments overlap in a way similar to placing the bristles of two yard brushes into each other.

The thick myosin myofilament, made up of two protein strands wrapping around each other, has a core, or body, with heads that project out like the head of a golf club (two heads, actually). These are called *myosin cross-bridges* (or cross-heads) and they have numerous important facilities including:

- ATP-binding sites,
- Actin-binding sites,
- a hinge allowing a swiveling action, so that the head can move the thin proteins. resulting in a contraction.

Note the helical shape of the long chain of actin molecules (also called G actins). The thin actin filament is constructed of two chains spiraling around each other. A smaller associated protein called *tropomyosin* in turn coils around the actin. Another protein called *troponin* attaches itself at specific intervals to the tropomyosin. As the troponin and tropomyosin are connected to each other, when the troponin moves it will pull the attached tropomyosin with it.

Here is the important point. Tropomyosin covers the myosin-binding sites on actin, and when it is pulled away by the movement of troponin, the sites become free for the cross-bridges of the myosin to attach to and pull. This is how a muscle contracts.

Contractions: Pulling it all Together

Understanding the sequence of events leading to a muscle contraction will provide you with a simple step-by-step picture of how a muscle fiber contracts. So far, I have discussed the structure of muscle and described some of the key players. Now we must look at the chemical neurophysiology. I will keep it simple, but at the same time I want to challenge you and advance your understanding. This will hopefully change the way you think about muscles (figure 3.23).

When muscles are working normally, a nerve impulse (an action potential) is the very first (or last) step leading to a contraction. This nerve impulse will travel along the sarcolemma and into the T tubules. From there, the it will travel to the SR, leading to the active opening of calcium gates, allowing calcium to diffuse into the sarcomere where the myofilaments are located.

Calcium now binds to the troponin molecule, altering the shape of the protein and causing it to move, thereby moving the attached tropomyosin. After the tropomyosin has moved, the myosin-binding sites on actin become free, permitting the myosin heads to attach to and pull the actin. As the myosin heads contact the actin, the myosin cross-bridges hinge and swivel, pulling the actin myofilament, similar to a team in a tug-of-war. The pulling action occurs in a synchronized manner, some myosin heads attaching while others disassociate, and the collective effort leads to a *concentric contraction*. Should the pulling action be overcome by an external force, or when a person consciously allows the muscle to be overcome, this leads to a lengthening of the muscle while it is pulling on the myofilaments, which is known as an *eccentric contraction*. (Remember, muscles can only pull, they cannot push.)

For muscles to work effectively energy is required, and this is supplied by the breakdown of ATP. As long as calcium remains in the presence of the myofilaments, the sarcomeres will remain shortened. Under normal circumstances, when the nerve impulse stops, the membrane of the sarcoplasmic reticulum is no longer permeable

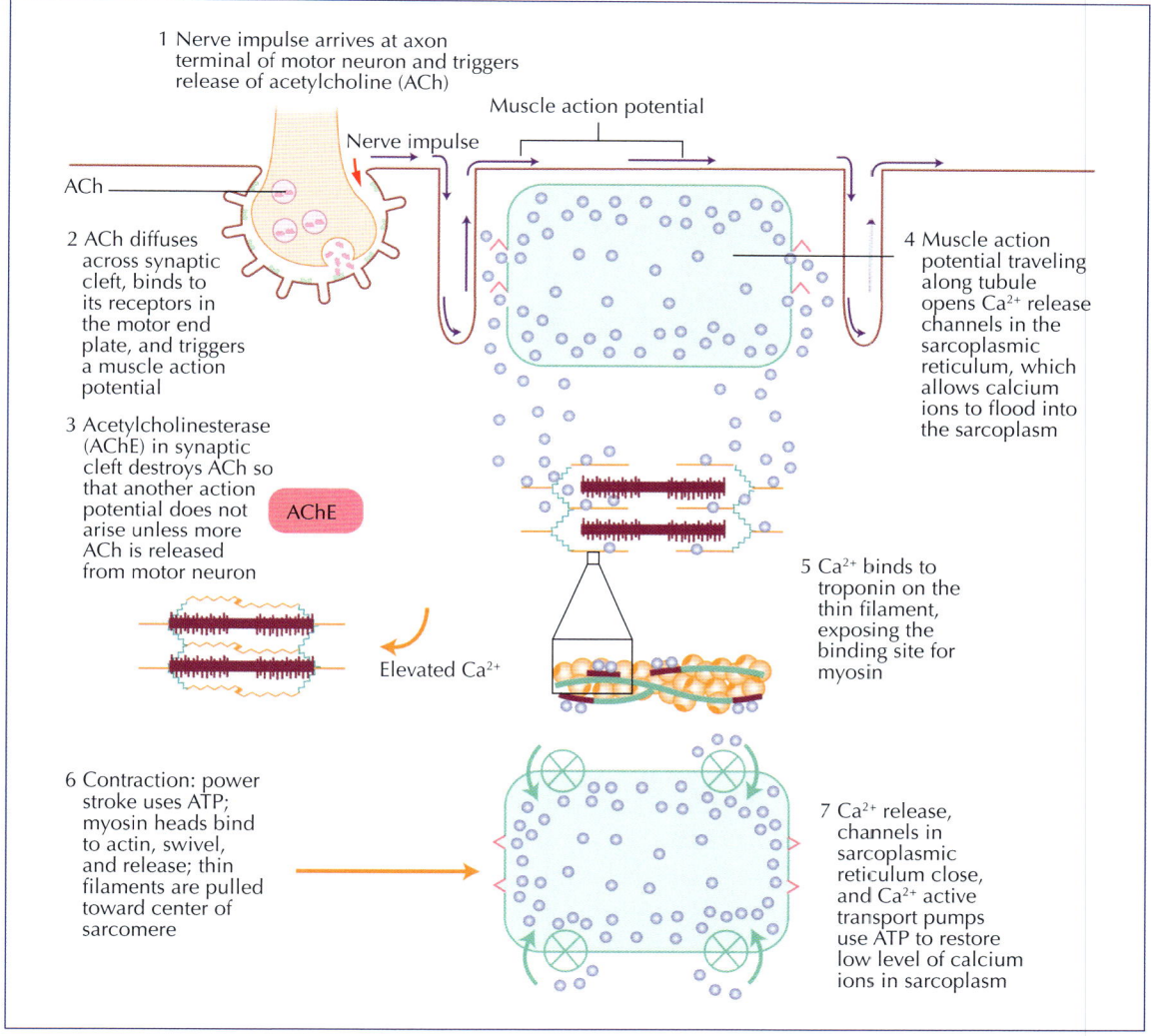

Figure 3.23. The seven steps of muscle contraction.

to calcium and the calcium gates now act in reverse, allowing the calcium to move from the sarcomere back into the SR. As the calcium disassociates from the troponin, it pulls the tropomyosin back into its resting place covering the myosin binding sites. Tropomyosin now, once more, blocks the cross-bridges from touching the thin actin filament, inhibiting a contraction from taking place (i.e., phase change).

From this description of muscle contraction, you can see that calcium is the key that "turns on" a contraction, or, for that matter, turns it off. If for some reason calcium ions cannot escape from the sarcomere, the myofilaments will remain shortened. Sometimes, it may require more energy to rectify this situation than to maintain it, and so the muscle fiber remains short, thereby increasing tension (i.e., a contracture).

The seven steps of cross-bridge cycling are:

1. the influx of calcium, triggering the exposure of binding sites on actin;
2. the binding of myosin to actin;
3. the *power stroke* of the cross-bridges, which causes the sliding or gliding of the thin filaments;
4. the binding of ATP to the cross-bridges, which results in the cross-bridges disconnecting from actin;
5. the hydrolysis of ATP, which leads to the reenergizing and repositioning of the cross-bridge;
6. the transportation of calcium ions back into the sarcoplasmic reticulum;
7. the provision of an action potential (this could be step 1 or 7).

Imagine you are witnessing the players in the dynamic action potential that will lead to a muscle contraction. A spark ignites, nerve impulses crackle down the axon terminal, coaxing the release of acetylcholine (ACh) into the synaptic space. ACh whips across the synaptic cleft, finding its partners in the motor end plate, triggering a resonance of the muscle action potential. Acetylcholinesterase (AChE) tiptoes into the synaptic cleft, erasing the ACh signal, ensuring the stage remains clear for the next act (unless summoned again by the motor neuron). Gates of calcium swing open. The muscle action potential, a wave of energy, surges along the tubule, unlocking the gates of the sarcoplasmic reticulum, flooding the stage with calcium ions. Calcium ions alight upon troponin, pulling free the binding site for myosin, ushering in the grand performance of contraction. Myosin heads, fuelled by ATP, grasp hands with actin, spiralling and releasing in a rhythmic cadence, pulling the thin filaments closer to the center of sarcomere. The channels sealing the sarcoplasmic reticulum shut, and the calcium ions, spent from their performance, are escorted back to their chambers by the ATP-powered pumps, leaving the stage set for the act to begin anew.

Exercise Science—Energy and ATP

Energy is not created or destroyed but, whatever it is, converted from one form to another. It takes different forms, such as light, heat, electrical, magnetic, and chemical energy, and much as we know it allows work to be done we still do not know what energy actually is.

Animals from the lowly worm to humans all convert chemical energy from the food we eat to mechanical energy for work. When we do this we also produce by-products, including carbon dioxide, water, and heat. In fact, of the energy we gain from food, only 20 percent results in work or movement, with the remaining 80 percent being released as heat.

For both humans and animals, the main chemical energy source to provide the energy to run, walk, jump, digest food, or have a thought is adenosine triphosphate (ATP), which has to be produced and stored in all cells of the body. ATP consists of adenine attached to ribose and three inorganic phosphates. Ribose is a sugar that is a building block of the backbone chains in nucleic acids, and is classified as a monosaccharide. Adenine is one of the four bases of DNA. Only a small amount of ATP can be stored in cells. When muscle cells contract, ATP is broken down into adenosine diphosphate (ADP) and phosphate.

Muscle Fatigue

As ATP supplies begin to diminish—as they will if muscles are used either over an extended period or for short time of high intensity—myosin heads remain bound to actin and can no longer swivel. If calcium cannot escape from the sarcomere, the fiber may remain in a short state even though no nerve impulse is being received. This can lead to muscle spasm—or, at the micro-level,to tight muscle fibers. As muscles produce energy for high-intensity activity through anaerobic metabolic pathways, this results in the production of lactates and inorganic phosphate.

Lactic acid is often described as a waste product, which is not the case. As lactic acid builds up in the muscle, being produced faster than it can be removed, this offers a feedback mechanism whereby the innervation of muscles diminishes, and contractions can no longer be sustained. Eventually, the individual will have to stop and catch their breath. If this important feedback mechanism did not exist, the person might continue beyond their limits in the high-intensity activity, resulting in a strain or even a heart attack.

An additional and perhaps a more potent source of inhibition is the build-up of inorganic phosphate from the breakdown of ATP to ADP.

Equine and feline physiology take advantage of adenosine diphosphates in a unique way. As ATP breaks down to ADP, one ADP can give up one of its two phosphates to another ADP, thereby making an ATP and an adenosine monophosphate.

Motor Units

A *motor unit* is the combination of a motor nerve and all the muscle fibers to which it connects or that it innervates (figure 3.24). When a nerve impulse travels the length of a nerve cell along its axon, all the muscle fibers attached to that nerve contract. A motor unit can have as few as three muscle cells or many thousands. This large variety in motor units allows muscles to perform precise or coarse muscle control. It also allows muscles to recruit increased numbers of fibers when needed, depending on the required effort, known as *gradual increments of contraction*. It takes fewer motor units (and therefore fewer muscle fibers) to lift an 11 pound weight than a 33 pound weight.

If we contracted all the fibers we have in a muscle every time we contracted that muscle, we would not be able to distinguish between the effort required to lift a pencil compared to the effort needed to lift a telephone.

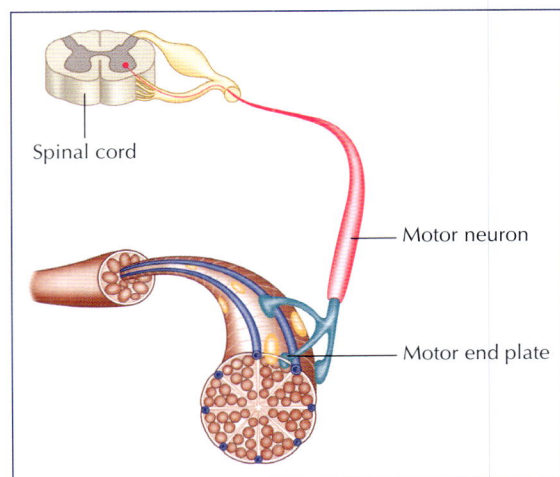

Figure 3.24. A motor unit of a skeletal muscle.

Muscular Tone

Muscular tone refers to the basic and constant ongoing contraction or muscular activity in the muscles—a state of readiness or preparedness. It can be understood as a baseline or background level of innervation. It is what helps to keep us upright or to give us "lift."

Tone may be normal, too low, or too high. When muscular tone is too high (*hypertonic*), muscles can appear somewhat stiff and do not move in a smooth and natural way. Identifying a basic muscle tone that is too low or too high is one of the key motor skills of therapists. We need to be able to recognize and identify any hypertonic muscles and their inhibited (and therefore *hypotonic*) antagonists.

Gross Motor Skills

Gross motor skills are those that require large muscles or groups of muscles. Muscles or groups of muscles should act in a coordinated fashion to accomplish a movement or a series of movements. Examples of gross motor tasks are walking, running, throwing, and jumping.

Posture is a very important element to consider in assessing gross motor skills. Adequate posture may make all the difference between being able or unable to execute a movement.

Fine or Precise Motor Skills

Fine or *precise motor skill*s consist of movements of small muscles that act in an organized and subtle fashion to accomplish more difficult and delicate tasks—e.g., the hands, feet, and muscles of the head (as in the tongue, lips, and facial muscles).

Precise motor skills are the basis of coordination, which begins when we learn to transfer things from one hand to the other across the midline at about six months. Examples of fine motor activities are writing, sewing, drawing, imitating subtle facial gestures, pronouncing words (coordination of soft palate, tongue, lips), blowing bubbles, and kissing. Many individuals, particularly children, who have difficulties in their fine or precise motor skills also have difficulties in the articulation of sounds or words.

Muscles Do Not Work in Isolation

Any muscle performing an action is providing a portion (or all) of its available muscle fibers, while the arrangement allows it to provide a "line of pull" (resulting in omnidirectional forces) to offer a given movement at a given joint. For example, muscles with fibers running vertically on the anterior side of the knee joints are agonists of extension. Conversely, muscles with a portion of their fibers running vertically on the posterior side of the knee are agonists of flexion. It is important to remember that muscles fibers are localized, while the fascia (in this case the deep fascia) is unbroken and continuous. If one muscle involved in making up the synergy fails to engage effectively (is inhibited) or is hypertonic, the tonus of the fascia will be compromised, leading to a disruption in the coordinated effort required for efficient joint movement. This breakdown can result in an imbalance of forces within the fascial plane, inhibiting the smooth transmission of tension across the interconnected myofascial synergies. Consequently, even though the fascia remains uninterrupted, the absence or inefficiency of one muscle can alter the distribution of tension, affecting the optimal functioning of the entire kinetic system. In essence, the interdependence of muscles within the fascial system underscores the significance of each muscle's contribution as a "tuning peg" to maintain harmony and facilitate seamless movement patterns.

In the context of so-called musculoskeletal physiology, the term *antagonist* is commonly employed to delineate a muscular entity that opposes a specific physiological action. To illustrate, when an individual concentrically contracts their biceps brachii (agonist), the triceps brachii undergoes a shape-changing process (it lengthens) with concurrent inhibition, facilitating the flexion of the elbow (antagonist). Rather than characterizing this dynamic as strictly antagonistic, it is more aptly construed as a symbiotic partnership marked by mutual agreement on a global level. This intricately balanced partnership affords seamless movement, ensuring controlled acceleration and deceleration across the full range of motion (ROM). Such coordination serves to safeguard both muscles and joints, preserving optimal joint space. Noteworthy are instances where specialized movements necessitate the simultaneous contraction of both an agonist and its antagonist, a phenomenon referred to as *cocontraction*.

Agonists, antagonists, synergists, stabilizers, and neutralizers must work effectively and synergistically to provide neuromuscular efficiency.

Many soft-tissue and musculoskeletal injuries concerning the spine and extremities are caused or perpetuated by muscle imbalances and inhibition in the core musculature. People with a weak, inhibited core substitute primary muscles to compensate during dynamic functional movements. Popular machine-based exercise may be a significant contributing factor leading to overuse injuries.

The core system is ultimately a system of stabilization. If it is not functioning optimally the result is neuromuscular substitution—utilizing the strength, power, and neuromuscular control in the rest of the body. Unfortunately, many individuals use exercise to develop strength and neuromuscular control in their prime movers and neglect core stabilization, or even worse, establish ineffective kinetic system patterns that prove stressful and lead to pain and injury. Understanding the kinetic system will assist you in connecting pain in the head or neck, for example, to possible tension or spasm in muscles or fascia some distance away, even in the feet. By appreciating these relationships, you can carry out visual, structural, neuromuscular assessments to identify those tissues that are short, tight, adhered, and spastic (possibly housing MTrPs). Treating those structures first and providing a fascial release will provide the foundation for the possibility of a return to homeostasis or allostasis and the introduction of functional movement challenges.

Stabilization

Analysis of movement will usually focus on the moving bone or segment, but focus must also be on the muscle forces that produce movement in that segment. Equal force is exerted on the "stable" part (or bone), known as the "origin." When the biceps brachii exerts force on the radius, an equal force is also placed on the muscle's attachment to the scapula (coracoid process and glenoid fossa). In this example, the scapula does not move because of a stabilizing force offered by the muscles attaching to it.

When your quadriceps exert force on your tibial tuberosity, your tibia will move. The stabilizing force in this example is gravity: the weight of your body would be too much for the muscles to move. When you perform a sit-up (on the floor), the abdominal muscles will pull the rib cage toward your pelvis. An equal and opposite force is pulling on your pelvis, yet it does not go into posterior pelvic tilt. Why? The pelvis will not posteriorly tilt because of forces generated by the hip flexors.

Now think of what force will help to stabilize the lower extremities to which the hip flexors attach. All this time, what forces are acting on the vertebrae (think kinetic), all the way up to the base of the occiput?

Planes of Motion

In NMTq, when we speak of the *kinetic system*, we are referring to all the body systems, as they form an unbroken, ubiquitous, continuous network. This text will focus on the relationships of the skeletal, muscular, and nervous systems as one interconnected system generating, absorbing, and dissipating forces, resulting via mechanotransduction into metabolism, physiology, and human movement.

All human movement takes place on three planes of motion throughout the kinetic system (figure 3.25). The kinetic system must adapt in a synergistic, body-wide manner to

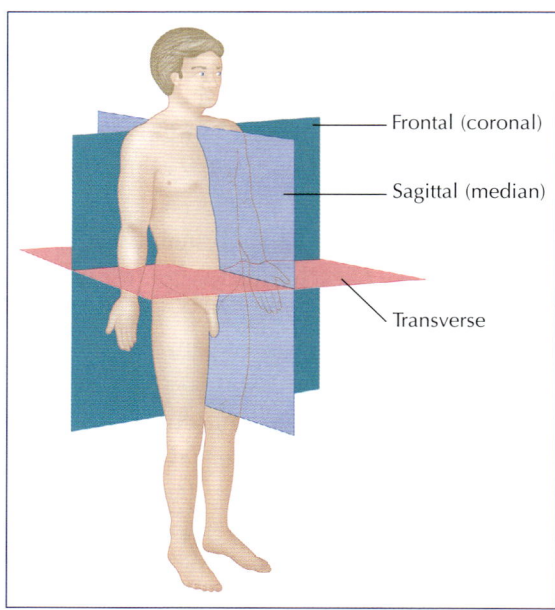

Figure 3.25. Planes of motion.

accept and accommodate the dynamics of functional movement. As the base of support constantly changes, the body makes subtle arthrokinematic changes to maintain dynamic balance. Within each plane, a single axis can be identified in association with a joint or joints around which movement takes place.

The Sagittal Plane

The *sagittal plane*, also known as the *midsagittal* or *median* plane, is an imaginary line running vertically through the body moving along an anterior to posterior plane, cutting the body into equal right and left sides.

A sagittal slice or section that is not on the median plane is also referred to as a *parasagittal* section. Any plane running parallel to this line is known as a parasagittal plane.

The Frontal Plane

The *frontal plane*, also known as the *coronal* plane, passes through the body from top to bottom at right angles (perpendicular) to the sagittal plane. This plane divides the body into front (anterior) and back (posterior). The term *posterior* refers to the back half of the body, behind the coronal plane, and *anterior* refers to anything in front of this plane.

The Transverse Plane

The *transverse plane*, also known as the *horizontal* plane, is perpendicular to both of these planes and divides the body into an upper and a lower half. Positions above the transverse plane are called *superior*, and positions below the transverse plane are called *inferior*.

Planes in between these three and formed at a 45-degree angle are known as *oblique* planes.

However, there are several cases where the meaning of these planes is slightly different. This is apparent in the foot, the tongue, the hand, the brain, and sometimes the perineum.

Foot and Hand

As the foot is discontinuous with the coronal plane, it is described by analogy, and with embryological considerations, to the hand.

The palm (adj. *palmar*) of the hand corresponds to the sole (adj. *plantar*) of the foot, and the *dorsum* (back) of the hand corresponds to the dorsum (top) of the foot. *Dorsiflexion* means to flex upward (true flexion), and *plantar flexion* to extend

downward (true extension). The term *volar*, used mainly in orthopedics, is synonymous with palmar and plantar.

The foot is also capable of movement along another axis, owing to the flexibility of the ankle joint: *eversion*, which is movement of the sole of the foot away from the median plane, and *inversion*, which is movement of the sole toward the median plane.

The position of the hand in the anatomical position is considered supine. Rotation of the hand—so that the palm faces backward—is called *pronation*, and the reverse action, *supination*.

What Is Tensegrity?

There is no better model than the human body to represent and explain living tensegrity.

A tensegrity icosahedron is typically made up of two types of component: *isolated compression* members and *infinite tensional* members. As everything is connected to everything in human tensegrity, there is, and can only be, one member providing both tension and compression as required in the moment. To build a biological organism on the principles of tensegrity, the tensegrity truss must reflect continuity within a hierarchical construction, starting at the infinitely small subcellular component. Importantly, it must have the potential to build itself and provide self-stability.

The structure would be one integrated tensegrity that includes an integrated series of *trusses* (a truss is a structure composed of interconnected triangles), which evolved from infinitely smaller trusses that could be both

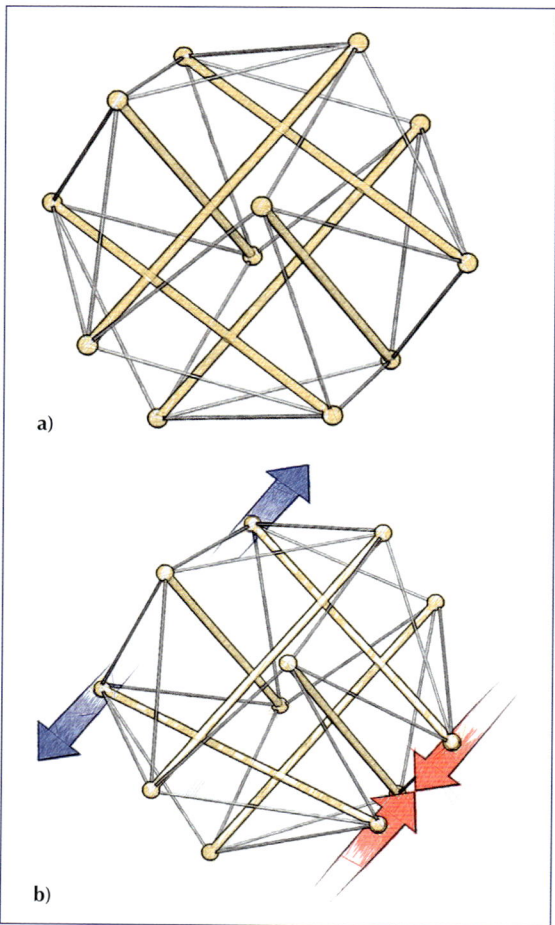

a)

b)

Figure 3.26. Tensegrity model. (From Movement Integration: The Systemic Approach to Human Movement by Martin Lundgren and Linus Johansson (Chichester: Lotus, 2019).)

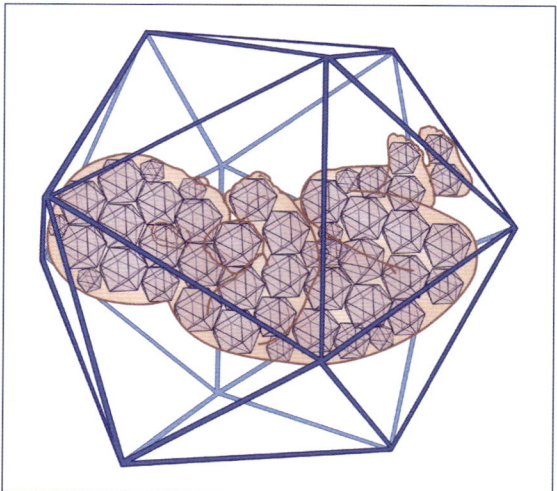

Figure 3.27. The icosahedron baby reflects the premise that we are scale-free icosahedra from micro to macro.

structurally independent and interdependent at the same time (figure 3.26). The triangulated arrangement of a truss offers stability without movement, and for movement to be facilitated, we need one or more additional three-bar trusses, essentially constrained by the lengths of the links and the angles between them. Therefore, living tensegrities consist of multiple-bar, closed kinematic systems of trusses (figure 3.27).

We can use "anatomy for the twenty-first century" to appreciate self-constructed living forms and provide us with a different paradigm to inform appropriate therapeutic interventions and movement modalities, as we attempt to support people in our communities to move with greater ease and with less or no pain.

Based on the principle of uncertainty, science has grown to a level of maturity and sophistication that allows us to feel confident about topics including evolution, embryology, ontology, phylogeny, biomechanics, and how we experience our own reality. Right? Quite the contrary. That process is still ongoing.

This book does not require the reader to be the intellectual equivalent of Einstein to comprehend or appreciate the new anatomical narrative of human form and function. In its most unabridged form, this book wishes to make it abundantly clear that humans are not machines. Brains, muscles, nerves, lymphatics, and blood vessels are not mechanical nor mechanistic. The habit in medicine and anatomy of defining and describing humans, and all life on earth, as mechanical constructs has led us down the wrong epistemological path. This has resulted, at best, in inaccurate descriptions and models of human form and function, and at worst set us back years from achieving an understanding closer to truth.

Grounded on a seventeenth-century vision, we currently see the body as made up of disconnected parts, pin joints, and levers, through the lens of hard-matter physics and, most worryingly, using linear explanations for a complex, nonlinear, unified system. Put simply, there are no straight lines in the human body and everything is connected and in continuity.

Muscle-associated fascia has morphologically different manifestations (figure 3.28). The muscles of the limbs—both upper and lower—contain predominantly cord-like tendons, while those of the torso—for example, the rectus abdominis—present with flat tendons referred to as *aponeuroses*. Fascia aponeurosis allows for omnidirectional transmission of forces—for example, from muscle-generated force in the lower limbs to the upper limb via the thoracolumbar aponeurosis, finely tuned by associated fascia tuning pegs, including deep pelvic myofascial units.

Muscle forces are never linear, no matter how tempting it is to suggest it is so; however, the forces are not always shared equally in every direction because of normal dampening or pathological adhesions, arrangement, and the number of skin ligaments tasked with coordinating the forces and translating them

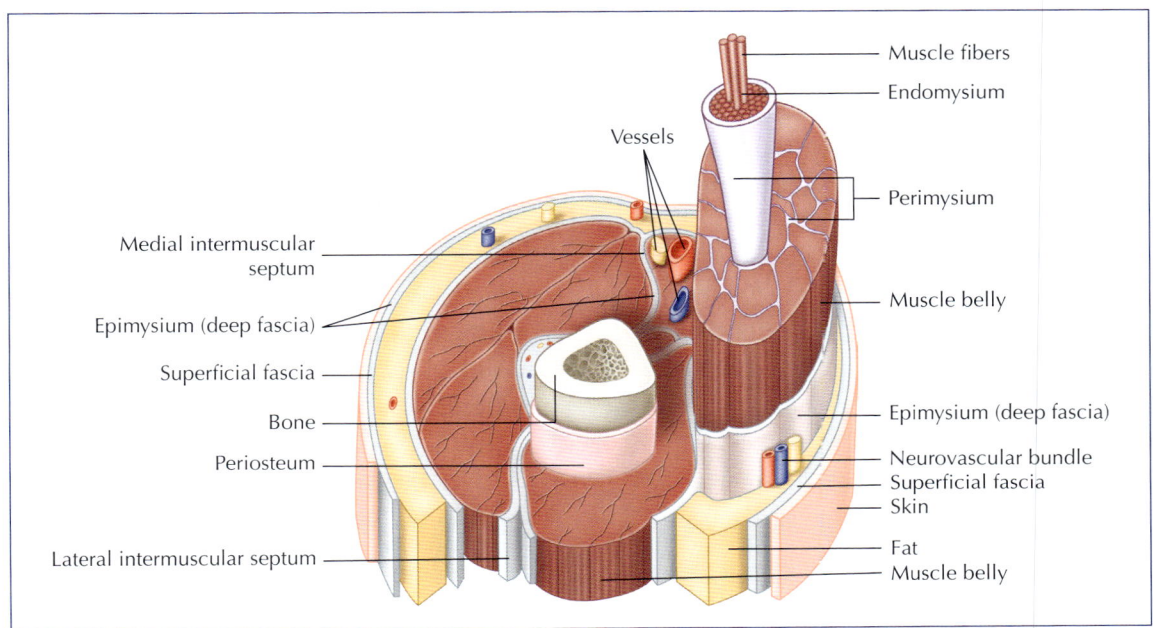

Figure 3.28. A cross-section through the skin, showing the fascial layers—superficial and deep fascia.

into appropriate metabolism, physiology, and motion.

Deep to the superficial fascia, fascia tuning pegs include quadratus femoris, piriformis, obturators internus and externus, superior and inferior gemelli, as well as paraspinal myofascial units such as the spinalis, longissimus, iliocostalis, multifidus, and serratus posterior inferior. Neuromuscular-associated fascia and muscle epimysium, perimysium, and endomysium translate forces without friction (unless there is pathology that would lead to friction, excess heat, and subsequent inflammation, nerve insult, and pain). This frictionless motion is facilitated by the gliding of a deeper tissue relative to a more superficially or laterally placed tissue in continuity. This fascia does not contain high levels of fat and has a chiral arrangement of collagen fibers, providing structural integrity (figure 3.29).

The relationship of force exchange, or *mechanotransduction*, facilitated by the superficial fascia through the associated retinacula cutis and the fascia profunda is poorly understood. Extramuscular force pathways include the neurovascular tracts, lymphatics, and the interstitium. These forces provide an expansive or reductive hydraulic effect on fascia locally or at distance, as demonstrated in fascia-focused dissections carried out at the University of Dundee by this author.

The morphology and histology of fascia are location-specific, and reflect the local operating forces and epigenetic influences informing its formation. Fascia-focused Thiel dissections have provided unique insights to fascial anatomy, resulting in

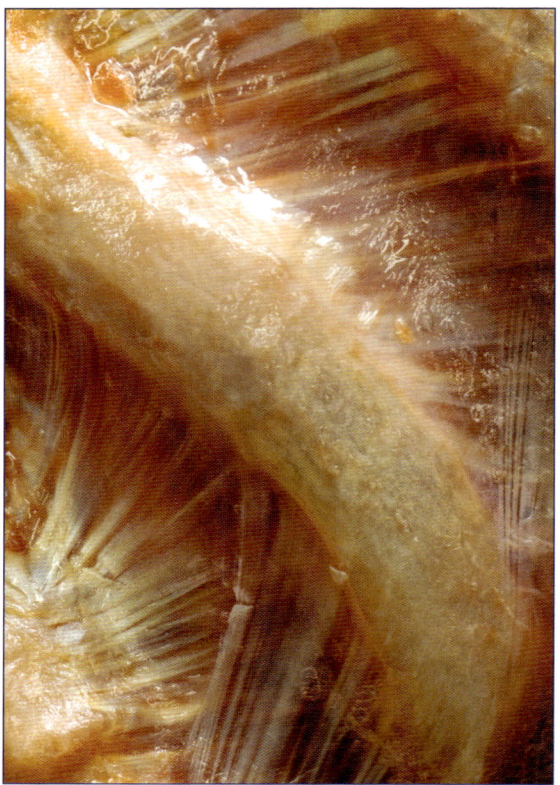

Figure 3.29. Ribs and chirality. Note the lattice-based decussation of the collagenous fibers running at angles over the red protein we call muscle and continuing to cross each rib. This beautiful image is a two-dimensional representation of what is a three-dimensional process, omnipresent in the entire soma.

a new classification based on functional hierarchical categories, which include gliding, restraining, containing, force-transductive, communicating, septal, invaginating, and osseous.

In the first edition of this book, I referred to the *kinetic chain* as an analogy. I have mostly dropped this term in the intervening years, as the analogy does not work well for living constructs. If one link in a chain were to break it would render the chain useless. This is not the case in the living body, as if one so-called link in the body's continuity was damaged or broken the body would adapt. In this updated edition I will refer to the *kinetic system*.

In the 1970s, Doctor Steven Levin proposed a model for the structure of organic tissue accounting for many of its physical and clinical characteristics. Levin suggested that all organic tissue must be composed of a type of truss, and that the essential building material for all tissues was constructed on the tension icosahedron and Buckminster Fuller's tensegrity model. This is the soft scaffold of the myoskeletal system and forms the basis of the four-bar, closed myokinetic system. The complexities and body-wide continuity of the fascia are global. Fascia is an organ of communication.

> Fascia offers a unifying medium, a structure which literally "ties everything together", from the soles of the feet to the meninges which surround the brain. This ubiquitous material offers support, separation, and structure to all other soft tissues and because of this produces distant effects whenever dysfunction occurs in it.
> —*Chaitow (2015, 171)*

In 1957 D. L. Stillwell confirmed the abundant sensory innervation of fascia. He estimated that there are as many as ten times more sensory receptors in fascial tissues compared with muscle. In 2016, Martin Grunwald in his book *Homo hapticus* estimated that there are a hundred million receptors in the body-wide fascial system. More recent estimates by Doctor Robert Schleip and other fascia researchers have suggested a significantly larger number, and fascia has been identified as the body's richest sensory organ, profusely innervated with proprietors and nociceptors far exceeding Grunwald's proposed number.

Doctor Donald Ingber of Boston proposed a model of developmental control based on tensegrity architecture, in which tissue pattern formation in the embryo is controlled through mechanical interactions between cells and extracellular matrix (ECM) that place the tissue in a state of isometric tension (prestress). Ingber hypothesized that local changes in the mechanical compliance of the ECM—for example, due to regional variations in basement membrane degradation beneath growing epithelium—may result in local shape changes in the ECM and associated adherent cells, similar to a "run in stocking." Experiments have established a firm correlation between basement membrane thinning, cell tension generation, and new bud and branch formation during tissue morphogenesis, and that this process can be inhibited or accelerated by dissipating or enhancing cytoskeletal tension, respectively. This work confirms that mechanical forces generated in the cytoskeleton of individual cells and exerted on the ECM scaffolds play a critical role in the sculpting of the embryo.

Presently, embryogenesis (how tissues and organs are formed in the developing embryo) is explained in terms of genes, hormones, and chemical gradients. This is one part of the story. What is important for the professional fascia-focused therapist to appreciate is that while biochemistry and molecular biology have found the power switches that turn on or off different embryological programs by means of specific genes, identification of the light switch on the factory floor does not explain how a finely crafted car is constructed.

It is the micromechanical perspective of the cytoskeleton—how cells sense mechanical forces and convert that information into changes in intercellular biochemistry and finally in the tissues, the fascia, our posture, joint positioning, and tissue status—that is fascinating. Of course, these changes are not exclusive to embryogenesis but continue throughout our life. Due to repetitive daily tasks or habits—for example, sitting, typing, and exercising—these forces we place on our tissues, the fascia, form and shape the myokinetic fascial system, which responds to the tension placed upon it. The result is your posture—your fascial outline—which friends can recognize even at a distance.

Fascia and Tensegrity—A Fasciategrity Perspective

As discussed, fasciategrity speaks about the distribution of tensional and compressional force relationships, of balance and integrity within a unified fascial system or body-wide fascial net (figure 3.30). All living and nonliving forms and constructs on this planet—be they beehives, the interlocking basalt columns of Giant's Causeway, trees, animals of all kinds—are tensegrity constructs.

Embryologically, we emerge from the fundamental embryonic soup contained within the oocyte and morph into one multifunctional original fabric we call fascia.

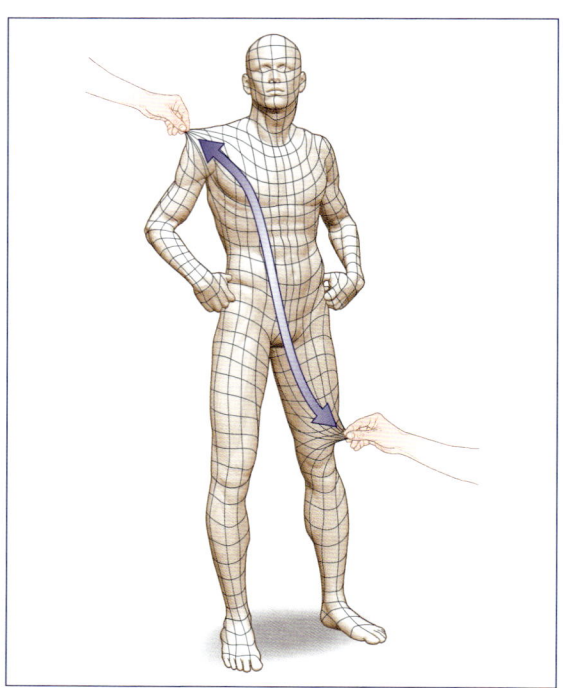

Figure 3.30. The distribution of tensional and compressional force relationships within a body-wide fascial net. Courtesy of Handspring Publishing.

The embryological process of genetic and epigenetic self-assembly organizes its way through a series of complex developmental shape changes, twisting, permeating, wringing, folding, spiraling, invaginating—ultimately expressing itself as a variety of specialist thinner and thicker tissues on a spectrum from hardness to softness.

Joanne Avison and myself employ an innovative approach in teaching clinical anatomy to elucidate the intricacies of the fascial net and other first principles of tensegrity, such as pretension and mechanotransduction. We orchestrate learning in a dynamic experiential exercise,

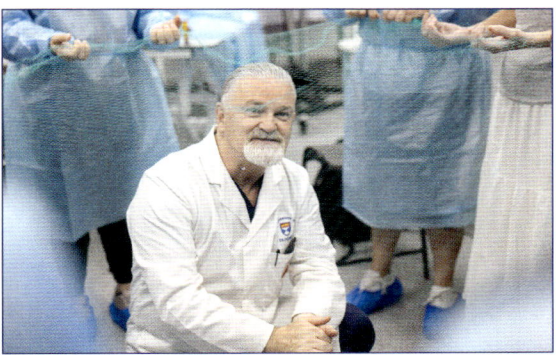

Figure 3.31. The net was first introduced as an analogy of the fascia net. Students standing in a circle can pull on the net, and everyone feels the expression of shared forces. Creating a hole in the net allows learners to appreciate how surgical intervention, or scars and other fascial insults, can impact the normal transfer of forces. With students pulling gently on the garden net one can immediately appreciate the concept of pretension.

using a garden net to represent the fascial net (figure 3.31).

We direct students to exert force upon the net, creating a state of pretension within the fascial system. This serves as a palpable metaphor for the physiological dynamics inherent in living tissue. Subsequently, we guide our students to manipulate the net, rolling it into a configuration that mimics the increased density reminiscent of tendons and ligaments. This illustrates the transformation of a pliant network into a structured and resilient matrix, vividly exemplifying the biomechanical nuances of connective tissues.

Not content with a unidimensional demonstration, we introduce further complexity by folding the net to illustrate the concept of invagination within the fascial continuum. The folds serve as a tangible representation of the intricate layers and sheaths inherent in the fascial architecture, showing the dynamic interplay between structure and function.

As a denouement, we further embellish this didactic exposition by elucidating the spiraling nature of the fascial net, using the net as a metaphorical canvas, articulating the sinuous trajectories and interconnectedness characteristic of the fascial matrix.

In this odyssey through the anatomical realm, our use of a humble garden net transcends the mundane, transforming the pedagogical landscape into an arena of intellectual and tactile discovery. Through the lens of this captivating narrative, students are beckoned to embark on a journey of enlightenment, exploring the profound tapestry of the fascial net with what we hope is a newfound sense of awe and understanding.

Fascia comes on a continuum of rigor, or flexibility, including soft, hard, stiff, fluidic, turgid, and all the in between. Bone—or osseofascial tissue—is located at one end of the spectrum and our leptomeninges, for example, could reflect the opposite end. Time is a key component, as self-organization occurs in a hierarchical, time-dependent sequence of events. Tendons, aponeuroses, epineuria, muscle fibers, retinacula, ligaments, cartilage, and bodily fluids all occupy the "in between" of harder to softer matter.

Bodily fluids—including lymph, blood, mucus, cerebrospinal fluid, and synovial fluid—are all liquid crystal matrices, with viscosities along a spectrum that could be compared to thick paint (e.g., emulsions or colloids). Importantly, the ground substance of these liquid crystalline matrices is bound water. A crucial point to consider is that connective tissue naturally expresses nonlinear behavior; in other words, forces are shared in an omnidirectional manner.

In the light of overwhelming evidence to the contrary, explaining human beings and all living constructs as mechanical is simply unsatisfactory, false, out of tune, and inharmonious. Elegant mechanistic theories have been put forward, but under scrutiny, they do not make the problems go away. Fascia-focused dissections in the world famous Trecchi Human, under the auspices of the Department of Clinical-Surgical, Diagnostic and Paediatric Sciences of the University of Pavia in Cremona, Italy and directed by clinical anatomist John Sharkey, have provided clear evidence to the contrary (figure 3.32a). The observations of historical figures such as Vesalius, Descartes, Newton, and Borelli of the natural world generally, and of anatomy specifically, did much to add to the perception of all living forms as mechanical constructs. For hundreds of years, we have applauded the biomechanical insights gained from describing bodies in terms of pin-joints, lever systems, bone to bone origin-insertions, and individual "parts," elucidated and compounded by hard-matter physics.

Our understanding of the "body as a machine" has evolved from the fifteenth-century Renaissance period to the modern era, and medical specialists are now able to replace body parts with acrylic resin, silicone,

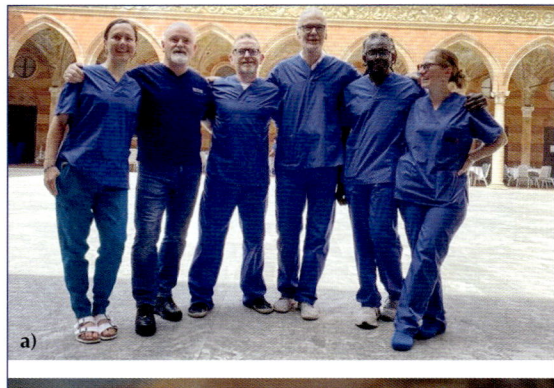

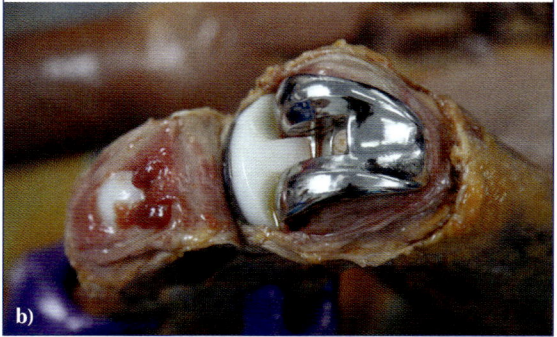

Figure 3.32. (a) Left-to-right: Karen Kirkness, John Sharkey, Mark Flannigan, Robert Schleip, Wilbour Kelsick, and Carla Stecco. (b) Knee replacement using modern technology.

aluminum, titanium, copper, magnesium, iron, stainless steel, super glue, screws, metal plates, and my favorite, cement. These, it would seem, are perfectly suitable replacement materials for a self-constructed life form (figure 3.32b).

As the world's population ages, demand for knee and hip replacements continues to rise. With a tensegrity-focused approach to developing soft-matter materials, we can reduce our dependence on traditional replacements made from hard-matter materials such as metal or ceramic. These materials are subject to wear and tear over time and create an imbalance in the body's natural tensional forces, leading to further complications and necessitating remedial surgeries. New soft-matter materials have been developed that are promising alternatives, owing to their superior ability to mimic natural tissue. Such materials include hydrogels, which are highly absorbent and can retain water. These properties make them ideal for mimicking the natural lubrication found in joints. Additionally, hydrogels have a similar stiffness to cartilage and so can provide a more natural feel than traditional replacements. Other soft-matter materials such as elastomers, polymers, and fibrous composites have also shown promising results in preclinical studies.

I advocate for using tensegrity principles to guide the design of soft-matter replacements. By designing replacements that adhere to tensegrity principles, the body's natural and appropriate tensional-compressional forces can be maintained, reducing the risk of complications and improving outcomes.

Kinetic System Anatomy

In the body there is an interlocking of fascial planes that connect one muscle group with another. Due to this interconnectedness of the fascial system, restriction in one area will result in reduced ROM in another local or distant area. The crural fascia covering the anatomical leg merges at the inguinal ligament with the transversalis fascia wrapping the peritoneal cavity. The transversalis fascia merges with the fascia of the diaphragm and continues on to merge with the parietal pleura

surrounding the lungs. The parietal fascia merges with the cervical fascia, and on up to the galea aponeurotica. In this way, the fascia represents the largest organ system in the human body.

The lumbo-pelvic-hip (LPH) complex musculature produces dynamic forces and stabilizes the spine and pelvis during functional movements. Many of these deep pelvic muscles provide support to the pelvic viscera and help to maintain intra-abdominal pressure.

No less than thirty-six muscles attach to the pelvis unilaterally. They are the rectus femoris, hamstrings (× 3), iliopsoas (iliacus and psoas major with the possibility of a psoas minor) (× 3), rectus abdominis, internal and external obliques (× 2), transversus abdominis, pyramidalis, quadratus lumborum, quadratus femoris, sartorius, obturators internus and externus (× 2), gemelli superior and inferior (× 2), gluteus maximus, medius, and minimus, adductors (including adductor longus, brevis, and magnus, gracilis and pectineus), tensor fasciae latae, erector spinae (iliocostalis, longissimus, spinalis), latissimus dorsi, multifidus, piriformis, levator ani, iliococcygeus, puboccygeus, pubococcygeus, and coccygeus.

The "core" typically refers to the group of muscles in the torso region that are responsible for stabilizing the spine, pelvis, and shoulders, and for generating power and force during movement. While there isn't a strict consensus on which muscles exactly constitute the core, it generally includes a number of muscles from the previous list, including the rectus abdominis, transversus abdominis, internal and external obliques, multifidus, erector spinae, quadratus lumborum, and pelvic floor muscles (including levator ani and coccygeus). The primary function of the core's myofascial structures, including fascia and ligaments, is to provide postural control by keeping the center of gravity over our base of support during dynamic movements. One can consider these myofascial structures as *fascia tuning pegs*, providing specific notes contributing to a symphony of movement.

Myokinetic System and Subsystems: The Evolution from Linear Chains to Omnidirectional Dynamics

The concept of *chains of movement* has long been foundational in manual and movement therapies, as well as in the study of human and animal anatomy. This idea underscores the interconnectedness and interdependence of muscles and tissues in producing movement, tracing back to several pioneering figures who have significantly contributed over many decades.

One of the earliest proponents of this concept was Françoise Mézières (1909–91), a renowned French therapist and anatomy instructor. In the 1940s, Mézières developed innovative techniques focusing on the role of what she called "muscular chains" in maintaining posture and facilitating movement. Her groundbreaking work emphasized the importance of viewing the body as an integrated whole, rather than as isolated parts, in therapeutic practices. Mézières's insights were revolutionary, laying the groundwork for a more holistic understanding of the body's movement dynamics.

Following in Mézières's footsteps, Doctor Serge Gracovetsky, author of the groundbreaking book *The Spinal Engine*, introduced the idea of "transmission chains" in 1987. Gracovetsky's research delved into the complex pathways through which so-called "mechanical forces" are transmitted across the body. Gracovetsky's work provided a deeper understanding of how different regions of the musculoskeletal system interact during movement. This pioneering research offered invaluable insights into the dynamics of human motion, setting the stage for further advancements in rehabilitation and manual therapies.

Credit is also due to Doctor Raymond Dart, an Australian-born South African anatomist and anthropologist. Dart's images and descriptions of his double-spiral arrangement of voluntary musculature significantly influenced my own journey into anatomy and also profoundly impacted Tom Myers, the author of *Anatomy Trains*. Inspired by Dart's description of the double-spiral arrangement in the anterior abdominal wall, Myers expanded the concept to encompass the entire body, leading to his comprehensive model of myofascial meridians. Dart recognized the fundamental and interconnected nature of spirals and cyclical patterns in physiology, embryology, anatomy, and cosmology, even relating these phenomena to local and global climate change and human migration. He observed that everything moves in a spiral pattern and all growth follows a helical structure.

Another key figure who has likely been influenced by such pioneers is Luigi Stecco, a distinguished manual therapist from Italy. Stecco expanded upon foundational ideas with his concept of "myofascial sequences." His work highlighted the critical role of fascia in coordinating and facilitating movement. By mapping out these myofascial continuities, Stecco provided manual and movement therapists with a practical framework for diagnosing and treating a variety of myofascial disorders. His contributions further enriched our understanding of functional anatomy.

In the spirit of ongoing development and new insights influenced by up-to-date research, we move from *chains* to *whole-body systems* and *whole-body strategies*. The contributions of Mézières, Gracovetsky, Dart, Myers, and Stecco illustrate the evolution of the *chains of movement* concept to the more modern understanding of a self-developed continuity, rather than isolated parts. Their collective insights underscore the necessity for a holistic approach to fascia-focused manual and movement therapy, acknowledging the intricate interplay of muscles, the omnidirectionality of fascia, and the continuity of differentiated tissues in optimal movement and function.

While not discarding the foundational principles, we must now recognize the genesis of spirality and the cyclical nature of forces within the human body, considering the omnidirectionality of the ubiquitous fascia. Fascia pervades every part of the body, providing structural support and transmitting mechanical forces in all directions.

This understanding moves us beyond the linear and segmented view of movement chains, embracing a more comprehensive perspective that sees the body as a dynamic and integrated system of processes.

This holistic approach acknowledges that forces within the body are not linear but omnidirectional, meaning that they can be transmitted and absorbed in multiple directions simultaneously. This is crucial for understanding how the body maintains balance, adapts to different stresses, and recovers from injuries. The fascia's ability to distribute forces omnidirectionally is essential for efficient movement and the prevention of injuries.

We can now appreciate the evolution from linear chains of movement to a more comprehensive understanding of omnidirectional dynamics within the myofascial system, giving due consideration to the role of shared forces in synergistic fascial planes.

Primary neuromuscular strategies exist that coordinate muscular contraction in whole-body stability and orientation. All body systems and structures work together to establish continuities that are ultimately interdependent to form a functional kinetic system.

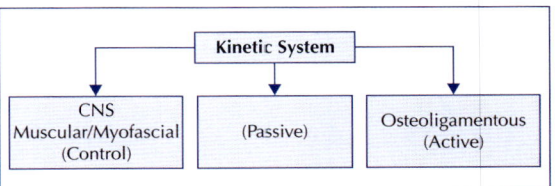

Within fascia-focused therapies, these strategies are known as the *spiral/oblique*, *lateral*, *posterior sagittal*, and *anterior sagittal*. Several other secondary links also exist, both deep and superficial. These continuities exist as one continuous facility through which forces are translated and dealt with omnidirectionally through the periosteum and out into the ubiquitous softer fascia, and vice versa, linking toes to head and head to toes.

The Spiral (Oblique) System

The spiral (oblique) system (figure 3.33) includes the external oblique, internal oblique (contralateral), adductors, iliotibial tract, tibialis anterior, and fibularis longus and brevis. This system can also include the following myofascial structures:

serratus anterior, ipsilateral rhomboids, and contralateral splenius capitis.

The Lateral System

The lateral system (figure 3.34) includes the fibulares, iliotibial tract, tensor fasciae latae, the gluteals, obliques, ipsilateral adductors, and quadratus lumborum (contralateral). The lateral system may include the following links: intercostals, sternocleidomastoid (SCM), splenius capitis/cervicis, and the scalenes).

The Posterior Sagittal System

The posterior sagittal system (figure 3.35) includes occipitofrontalis, erector spinae, thoracolumbar fascia, multifidus,

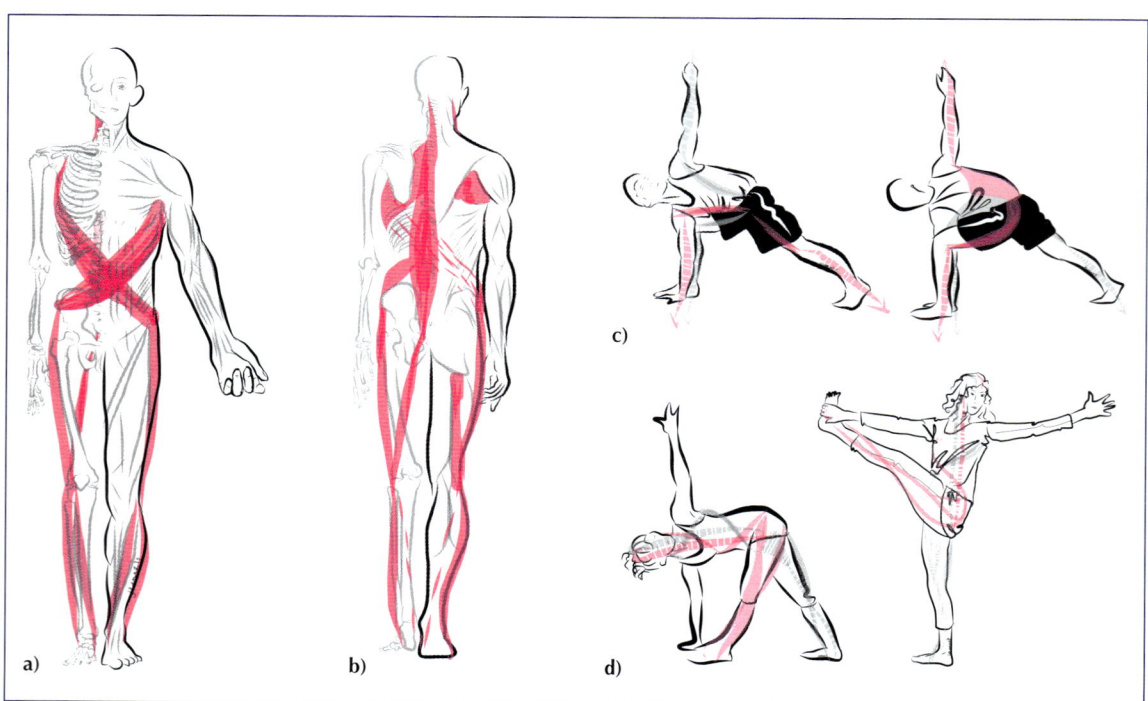

Figure 3.33. The spiral (oblique) system: (a) anterior view; (b) posterior view; (c and d) in motion. (Images: Joanne Avison, 2021).

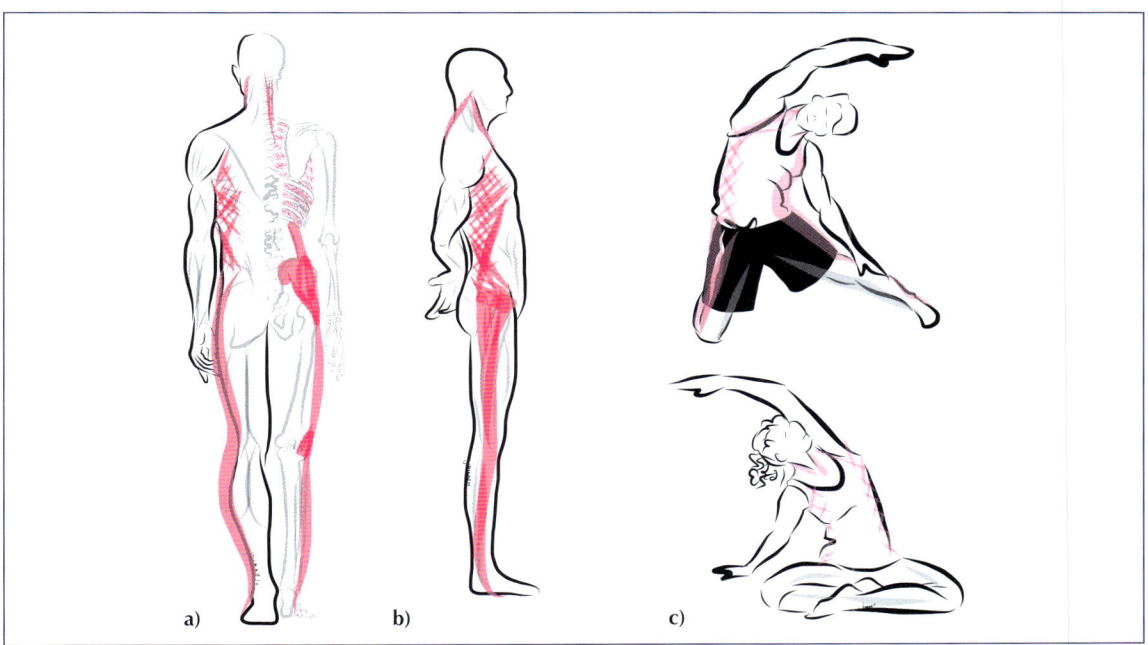

Figure 3.34. The lateral system: (a) posterior view; (b) lateral view; (c) in motion.
(Images: Joanne Avison, 2021).

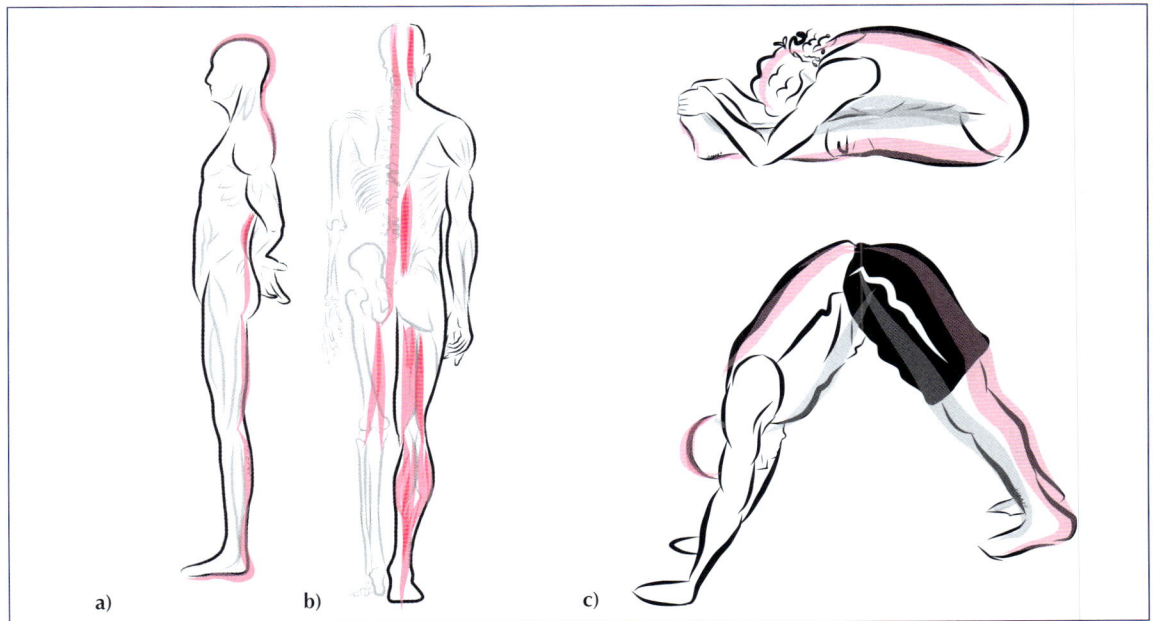

Figure 3.35. The posterior sagittal system: (a) lateral view; (b) posterior view; (c) in motion.
(Images: Joanne Avison, 2021).

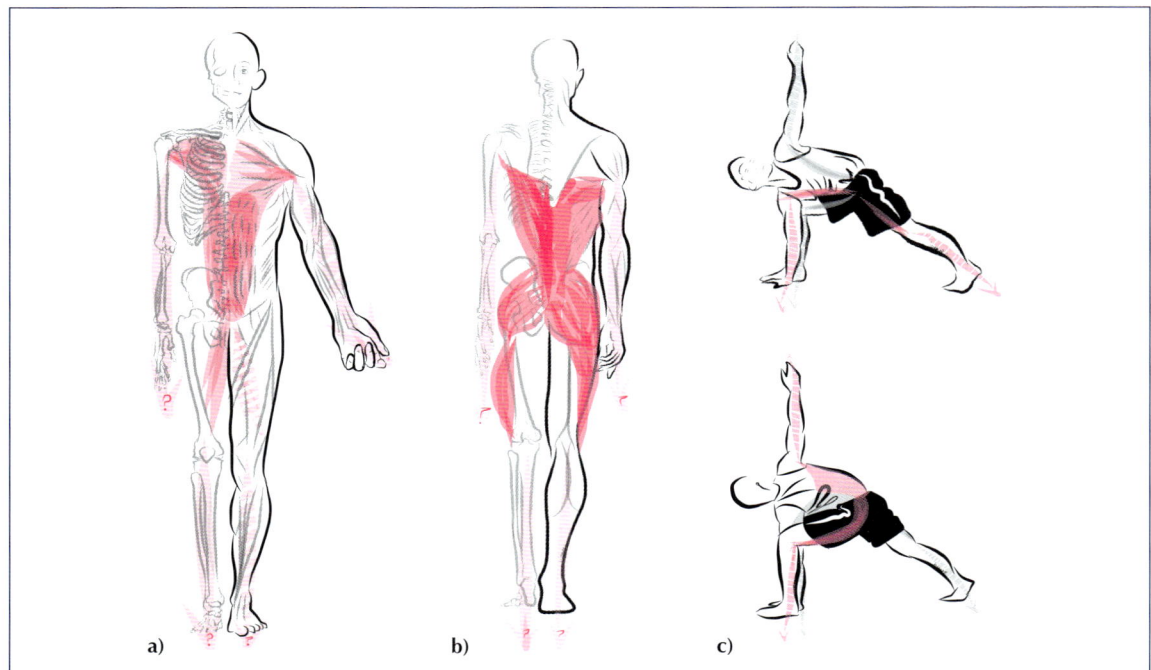

Figure 3.36. The posterior oblique links: (a) anterior view; (b) posterior view; (c) in motion. (Images: Joanne Avison, 2021).

sacrotuberous ligament, and biceps femoris (short head). This link can be continued to include the gastrocnemius and plantar fascia, offering movement and support to the joints of the periphery as well as to the spinal joints.

At the midsection, sublinks include the transversus abdominis and posterior fibers of the internal obliques. The pelvic floor muscles, including pyramidalis, multifidus, and lumbar portions of the longissimus and iliocostalis, as well as the diaphragm, are already described as the *core*. Of course, this joint support system is also present at the glenohumeral and lumbo-pelvic-hip (LPH) complex.

A deep posterior or sagittal linkage involves local, deep, segmentally related muscles, providing stiffness to a motion segment or joint (tonic type II).

A superficial oblique posterior linkage involves prime movers or more global muscles, which are, as the name implies, predominantly superficial. These muscles are primarily phasic or type I fibers with a high resistance to fatigue. The posterior oblique links (figure 3.36) include latissimus dorsi, contralateral gluteus maximus, and thoracolumbar fascia. This can be continued to include the iliotibial tract, tibialis anterior, and fibulares.

The Anterior Sagittal System

The anterior sagittal system (figure 3.37) includes the dorsal surface of the foot, tibial periosteum, rectus femoris (including articularis genu), AIIS (anterior inferior iliac spine), pubic tubercle, rectus abdominis,

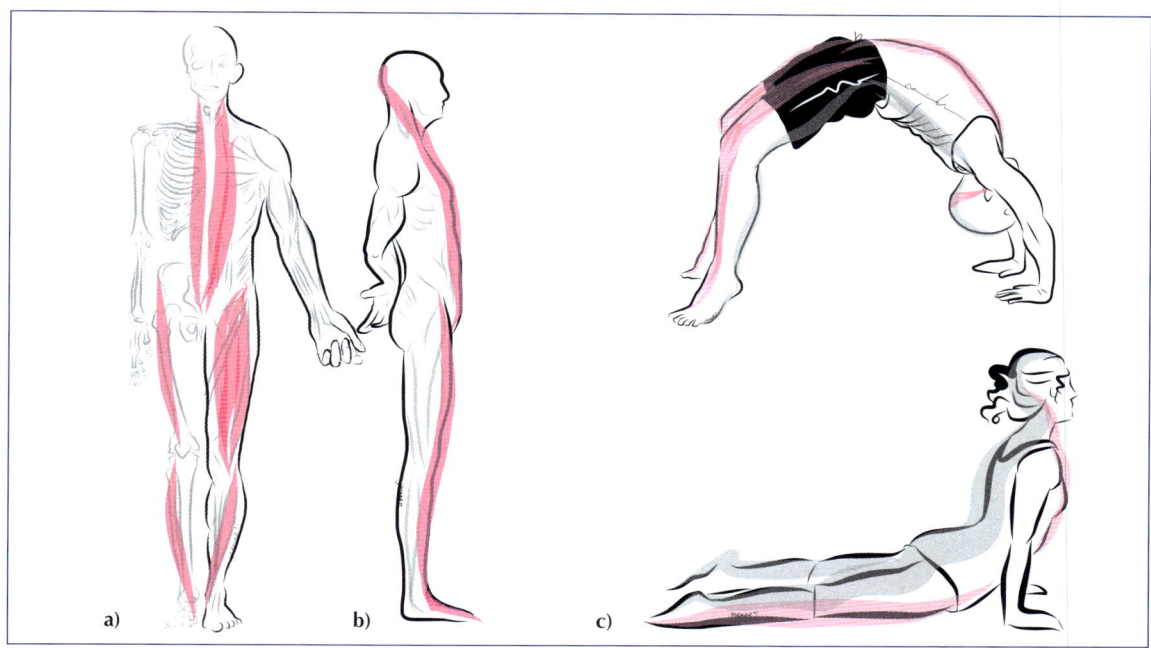

Figure 3.37. The anterior sagittal system: (a) anterior view; (b) lateral view; (c) in motion. (Images: Joanne Avison, 2021).

sternal periosteum, SCM, and periosteum of the mastoid process.

The Deep Anterior System

The deep anterior system (figure 3.38) includes the inner arch of the plantar surface (first cuneiform), tibialis posterior, medial tibial periosteum, adductors, linea aspera, ramus of the ischium and pubis, lesser trochanter, iliacus, anterior longitudinal ligament, psoas major, central tendon of diaphragm, mediastinum and pericardium, pleural fascia, prevertebral fascia, fascia scalenes, longus capitis, hyoid and associated fascia, mandible, occiput, and galea aponeurotica.

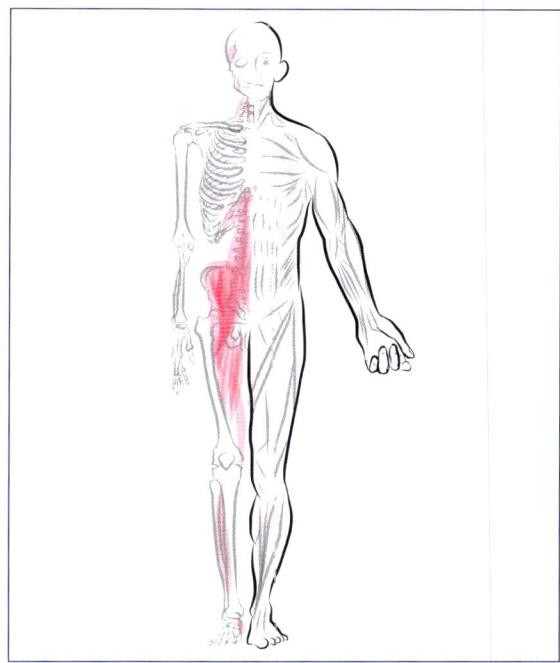

Figure 3.38. The deep anterior system. (Image: Joanne Avison, 2021).

A Little about Fascial Migration

There are typical migration patterns that you will see in most of your patients. Rounded shoulders are a good example. The posterior fascia migrates superiorly and laterally, with the anterior fascia migrating inferiorly and medially. One can visualize the closing down of the pectoral fascia (anterior) in such a situation (figure 3.39).

The elbow and forearm are excellent tools for picking the fascia off the shoulders and gathering up the tissue and slowly moving it medially toward the spine and inferiorly toward the sacrum. Hold the tissue in this position for several breath cycles. The abdominal fascia and lower back can be "hooked" or "scooped" up with the tips of the fingers. When injury occurs or in situations of repetitive stress, fascia becomes tacked down on the periosteum and thickens in the septal spaces between the muscles, where it acts as a partition.

The olecranon (tip of the elbow) is an ideal tool to encourage space within these partitions,

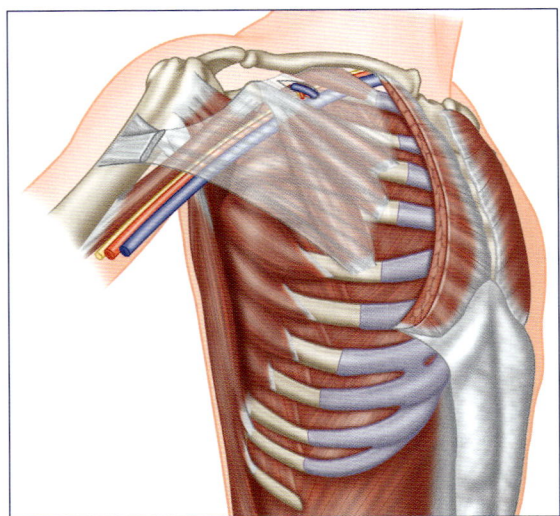

Figure 3.39. Pectoral fascia.

releasing the three layers of fascia: superficial, middle, and deep. As fascia clings to the periosteum, the therapist may feel sand-like particles beneath their fingertips. This tissue should be encouraged away from the bone while asking the patient to gently move the limb or body part involved. Fascial changes can take days, weeks, or even years from the moment of insult to the completion of migration. It is a type of contraction, but of course muscles have evolved to be the specialists in that department. Fascial contractions occur at a rate that is not always visible.

A Little about the Word *Dysfunction*

When fascia or muscle fibers change their resting status—that is, a muscle fiber shrinks or fascia migrates or thickens—we often refer to this as *dysfunction*. In reality, the muscle fiber and fascia are only doing what they have evolved to do. Try seeing it as a functional adaptation. The question to ask is, "Why is the muscle contracting?" or "Why has the fascia migrated?"

Fat, Skin, and Fascia

Fat is used for several functions, including shock absorption, insulation, energy provision (the capacity to do work), and hormonal production, to name but a few. The fat cells, or adipocyctes, that contain fatty glycerol are, interestingly, encapsulated by fascia. This fascia forms the superficial fascial layer.

I would like once again to highlight the importance of skin in human movement. The fascia is only one (very important) of the numerous interactive components of systems within systems within systems. From a simple example, it is easy to appreciate that movement at a point where there is a break or tear in the skin would not only be painful but also further damage the skin, as tensile and compressive forces act on the site of the tear causing a larger gap. Apart from the fascia, the skin is the largest organ system in the human body and must play a vital role in human movement, a role little understood but with great potential for research. Such research could help us better appreciate the integrative role that skin plays in providing stability to joints throughout the kinetic system and assisting in generating and dissipating forces necessary for controlled movements in conjunction with the retinacula cutis or skin ligaments, which provide anchorage of the skin to the deep fascia profunda.

Glossary of Arthrokinematic Terms

All acts of movement can be described with a mixture of the following arthrokinematic (*arthro-* = "joints"; *-kinematic* = "movement") terms.

Abduction To move a limb or body part away from the midline or to return from adduction; applies only to movement in the coronal plane

Adduction To move a limb or body part toward the midline; applies only to movement in the coronal plane

Circumduction Special combination of movement involving adduction, flexion, extension, and abduction; the resulting movement has a circular path

Depression Inferior movement or moving a body part down; the opposite of *elevation*

Elevation Superior movement or moving a body part upward; often applied to the shoulders—shrugging the shoulders is elevation

Extension Opposite of *flexion*, and there is an increase in the angle; applies only to movement in the sagittal or median plane

Flexion Where there is a reduction in the angle between bones or parts of the body; applies only to movement in the sagittal or median plane

Pronation Rotation of the hand so that the palm faces posteriorly; not medial rotation, as this must be performed when the arm is half flexed; *prone* means the hand is facing posteriorly

Protrusion Anterior movement of an object

Retrusion Opposite of protrusion

Rotation Movement of an entire limb clockwise (laterally) or anticlockwise (medially)

Supination Rotation of the hand so that the palm faces anteriorly; the hand is supine (facing anteriorly) in the anatomical position

Fascia Therapies and the Kinetic System

Fascia-focused therapy encourages a focus on the role of the CNS as it shapes and molds itself through movement experiences, providing the individual with the most efficient selection of neuromyofascial synergies so that they can perform integrated patterns of movement in the three planes of motion.

As explained, the kinetic system includes the muscle gasters, tendons, ligaments, the continuous fascia, and the joints involved (arthrokinematics), and works in a synergistic fashion providing eccentric contractions to decelerate, isometric contractions to stabilize, and concentric contractions to accelerate in the three planes of motion.

If one fascial tuning peg does not operate efficiently because of abuse, overuse, disuse, or neural inhibition, the result will involve an adaptational change in function and structure throughout the entire system. All tissues contribute to joint stiffness. For example, the joint capsule, comprising the associated ligaments, contributes 47 percent, the fascia 41 percent, the tendons 10 percent, and the skin the remaining 2 percent.

When a joint is not in correct alignment, tensional force is placed on the associated soft tissues, continuously changing the length-tension relationship of the muscles acting on that joint or joints. This in turn will alter muscle spindle activity, force couple relationships, RI, and synergistic dominance, and decrease neuromuscular efficiency throughout the entire body.

Fascia Tuning Pegs—Upper Limb

Awareness of the ubiquitous connectivity and mechanotransductive role of fascia provides the fascia-focused therapist with an appreciation of the expansive, decompressive, protective role that muscles and ligaments can play as site-specific fascia tuning pegs. Inhibited myofascial structures exacerbate inappropriate force exchange, resulting in greater compression of the fine neurovascular structures. Muscle fibers undoubtedly create forces for movement and produce heat; however, as muscle fibers are in continuity with fascia, inappropriate contraction or inhibition will have local and distant impacts on myofascial, neurofascial, and osseofascial structures.

The role of muscles—in additional to movement generation—can be clearly appreciated when examining the fascial continuity of a small muscle located at the posterior portion at the base of the head: rectus capitis posterior minor (RCPmi) (figure 3.40a). Interestingly, research has clearly demonstrated that fascia of the RCPmi is in continuity with the atlanto-occipital myodural bridge, a fascial structure in continuity with the dura mater of the spinal cord. This fascial continuity passes through the atlanto-occipital interspace and becomes integrated into the outer sleeve of the spinal cord.

The analogy of a fascia "tuning peg," similar to the tuning peg of a stringed instrument, is adopted to explain this new fascia-focused concept. An "out of tune" fascial system can lead to hypertonic or inhibited tissues, or, one could say, "dissonant notes." Hypertonic tissues increase the tensional forces operating within the local and global networks, leading to inappropriate densification of fascial structures, fibrosis, and neurovascular fascial adhesions. Inhibited tissues, unable to generate sufficient force to ensure appropriate fascial integrity, lead to excessive compression on neurovascular structures, similar to a wrong note striking a dissonant chord.

Supporting the model of site-specific fascia tuning pegs, it has been shown that RCPmi—its fascia and associated ligamentous elements (e.g., the to be named ligament, TBNL)—provides essential expansive tensioning to the dural sleeve (i.e., the thecal sac). Such fine-tuning creates a shape change in the dural sleeve conducive to reducing dural infolding and spinal cord impingement. In addition, it has been proposed that contraction of the suboccipital myofascial structures provides the main hydraulic source necessary for appropriate transportation of cerebrospinal fluid (figure 3.40b).

A comparable mechanism is proposed to be at play concerning site-specific fascia tuning pegs supporting normal neurovascular activity in the upper extremity. It is suggested that failure of these fascia tuning pegs to provide the necessary balance of tension and compression expresses dysfunction locally, or more globally in anatomical locations known as "places of perilous passage" ("the three Ps").

The brachial plexus (i.e., C5–C8 and T1) is a significant somatic nerve network formed by intercommunications among the primary ventral rami of the lower four cervical nerves and the first thoracic nerve. Comprising roots, trunks, divisions, cords, and terminal branches, the plexus is formed proximal to

distal. The lateral and medial cords of the brachial plexus merge to form the median nerve, traveling on the medial aspect of the arm, accompanied by the brachial artery and basilic vein (figure 3.41).

Based on fasciategrity-focused dissections, the bicipital aponeurosis and lacertus fibrosus (figures 3.42a and b) are hypothesized to play a site-specific fascia-tuning-peg role, offering decompression of the neurovascular structures that pass on the medial triangular interval at the antecubital fossa. In this hypothesis, teres major also provides expansive forces to the neurovascular structures proximally (including the radial nerve), in partnership with coracobrachialis (whose muscle gaster is proximal to the elbow joint), as its contractile expansive forces act to decompress the mid to upper humeral fascial compartments.

The axillary nerve arises from the posterior cord of the brachial plexus, formed by the C5 and C6 ventral rami, and divides into anterior and posterior divisions in the quadrangular space and extends to the inferior edge of subscapularis along the inferior aspect of the glenohumeral joint capsule. Posterior to the humerus, the axillary nerve courses around the surgical neck of the humerus, accompanied by the posterior circumflex artery, encased within the fascia profunda of deltoid. Omnidirectional forces produced by deltoid may act to expand fascia on the surgical neck leading to undue compression of the axillary nerve and associated vascular structures.

The muscles of the rotator cuff—commonly known as the SITS muscles—are supraspinatus, infraspinatus, teres minor,

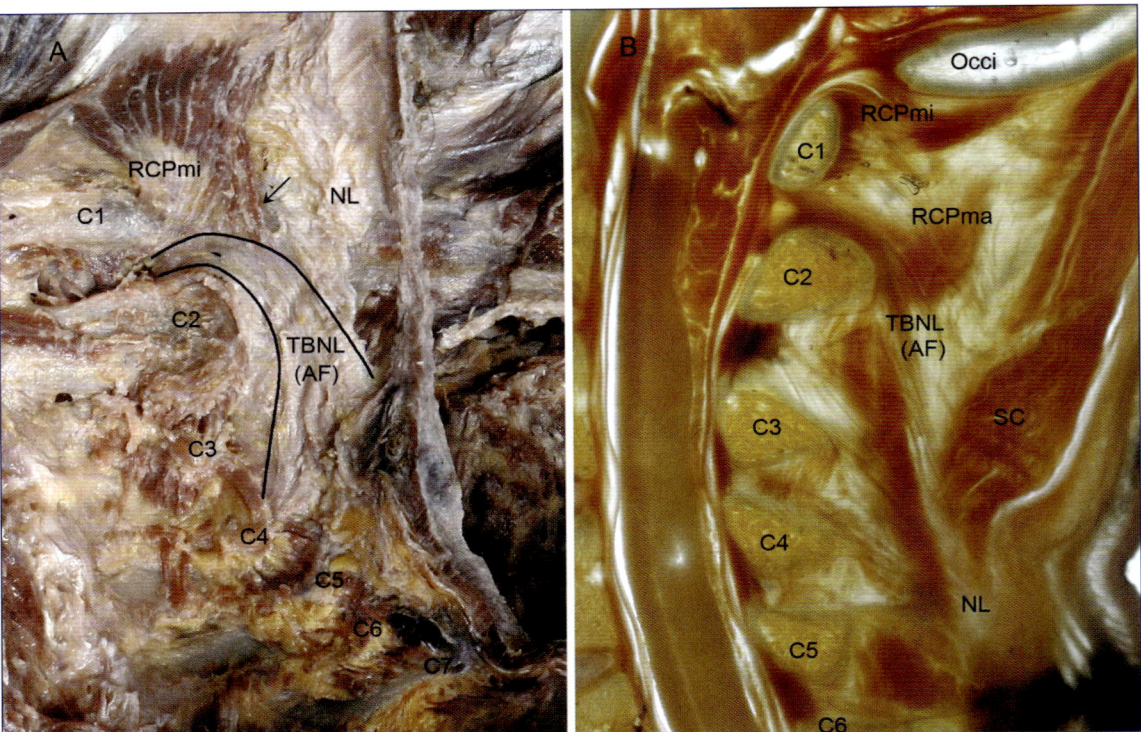

Figure 3.40. (a) Shows anatomical location, before plastination, of lateroposterior fascial and myofascial structures including the To Be Named Ligament (TBNL) located within the nuchal ligament (NL) and formed by arcuate fibers (AF) clearly in continuity with the anterosuperior atlanto-axial interspace attaching to the posterior aspect of the cervical dura mater (B).

(b) The plastinated specimen clearly demonstrates the fascial continuity of a small muscle located at the posterior portion at the base of the head, rectus capitis posterior minor (RCPmi), also in continuity with the atlanto-occipital myodural bridge, a fascial structure in continuity with the dura mater of the spinal cord. This fascial continuity passes through the atlanto-occipital interspace and becomes integrated into the outer sleeve of the spinal cord. The analogy of a fascia "tuning peg," similar to the tuning peg of a stringed instrument, is adopted to explain this new fascia-focused concept. An "out of tune" fascial system can lead to hypertonic or inhibited tissues, or, one could say, "dissonant notes." Hypertonic tissues increase the tensional forces operating within the local and global networks, leading to inappropriate densification of fascial structures, fibrosis, and neurovascular fascial adhesions. Inhibited tissues, unable to generate sufficient force to ensure appropriate fascial integrity, lead to excessive compression on neurovascular structures, similar to a wrong note striking a dissonant chord. B; Dura mater, Occi, C1, C7, first to seventh cervical vertebrae; Occi, occipital bone; RCPma, rectus capitis posterior major; SC, splenius capitis; NL, nuchal ligament.

and subscapularis. The fascia laminae of the SITS and associated axillary muscles, including latissimus dorsi and teres major, blend in an omnidirectional arrangement similar to the hub of a bicycle wheel. Dissection has identified multiple vectors with contributions from the fascicular arrangement of the SITS muscles, pectoralis minor, coracobrachialis, deltoid, trapezius, biceps brachii, triceps brachii, latissimus dorsi, teres major, and pectoralis major. It is proposed that these myofascial laminae coordinate forces as site-specific fascia

tuning pegs reducing compressive or tensional insult at places of perilous passage (i.e., the coracoid process). Fascial fine-tuning ensures the natural gliding, expansion, and decompression of the glenohumeral joint and axilla in three-dimensional fashion. To that end, it is proposed that fascial structures, including muscle fibers and ligaments, may operate as local or synergistically global fascia tuning pegs.

To underline and better appreciate this assertion, dissecting the brachial

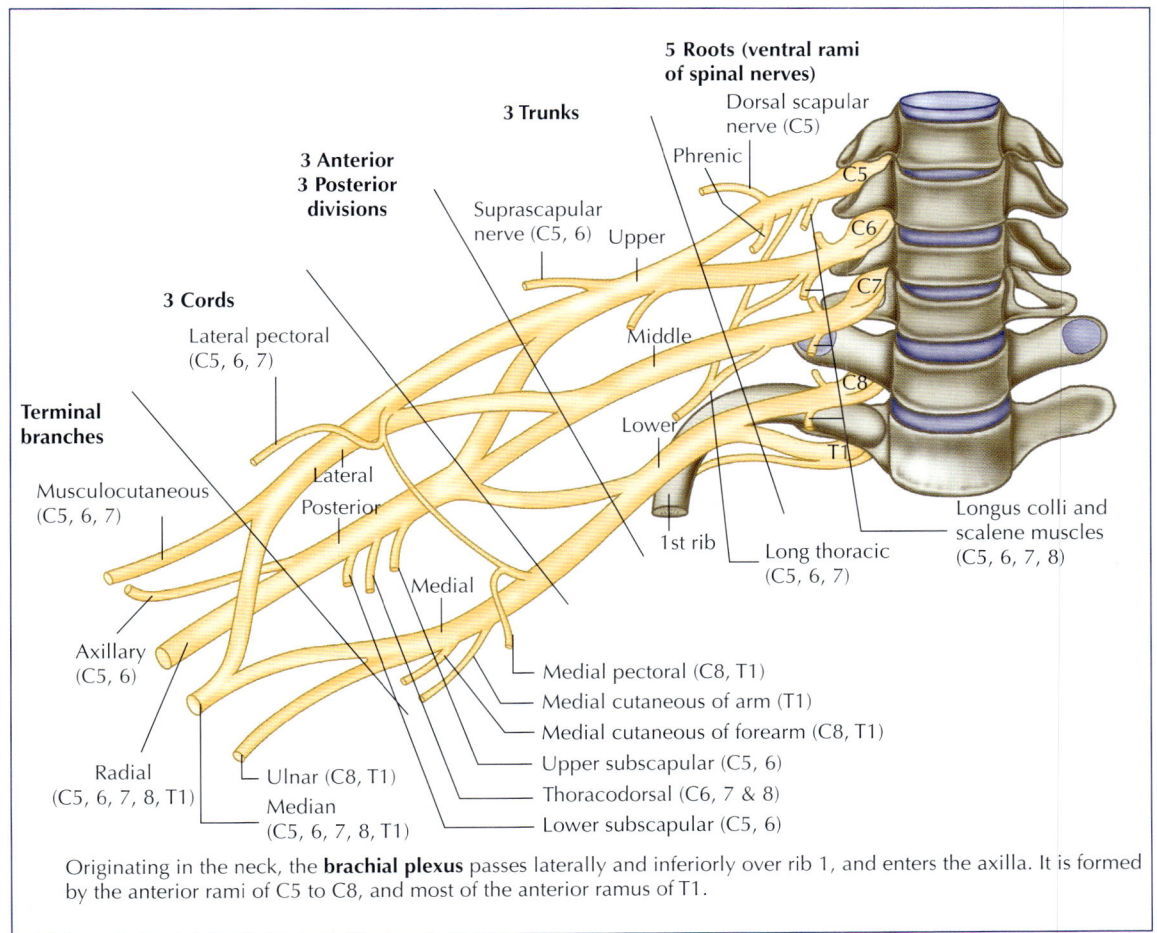

Originating in the neck, the **brachial plexus** passes laterally and inferiorly over rib 1, and enters the axilla. It is formed by the anterior rami of C5 to C8, and most of the anterior ramus of T1.

Figure 3.41. The brachial plexus.

plexus—including the path of the ulnar nerve—was completed in the dissection laboratory. The ulnar nerve arises from the medial cord of the brachial plexus at spinal levels C8 and T1. Traveling the length of the humerus on its medial border, the ulnar nerve enters an anatomical region slightly posterior and superficial to the medial intermuscular septum. This densified retrocondylar retinaculum tissue, called the *arcade of Struthers*, contains thickened fibrous dense fascial tissue found at variable distances proximal to the medial epicondyle.

Lacertus fibrosus and superficial and deep aponeurotic expansions are hypothesized to play a vital site-specific fascia-tuning-peg role in decompressing the deeper neurovascular structures (e.g., median nerve) passing on the cubital fossa and the distal portion of the arcade of Struthers and Osborne's ligament (see figure 3.42). Lacertus fibrosus spans in an omnidirectional fashion in continuity with the arcade of Struthers and Osborne's ligament, blending into the antebrachial fascia of the volar forearm. Supporting this expansive synergy are the intermuscular septa of pronator teres, flanked by the common flexor tendon and humeral head of the flexor carpi ulnaris. It is proposed that failure of the lacertus fibrosus to provide appropriate tension could lead to densification of the sublime bridge located deeper in the proximal forearm, representing a place of perilous passage specific to the ulnar nerve. Median nerve compression—also known as "eye of the hand" neuropathy—has also been implicated through sublime bridge compression.

The median nerve is of vital importance to overall wrist and hand function. Loss of nerve

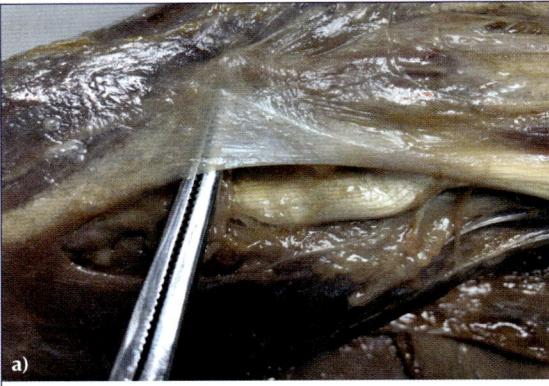

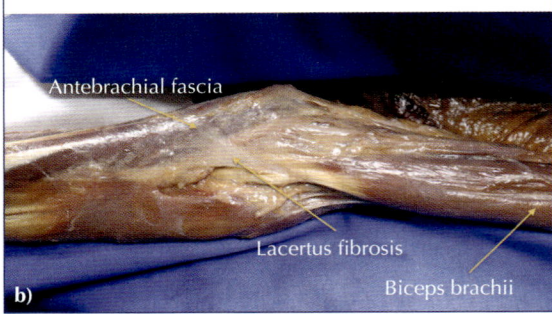

Figure 3.42a and b. Lacertus fibrosus and superficial and deep aponeurotic expansions are hypothesized to play a vital site-specific fascia-tuning-peg role in decompressing the deeper neurovascular structures (e.g., median nerve) that pass on the cubital fossa and the distal portion of the arcade of Struthers and Osborne's ligament.

function results in an inability to control thumb abduction, wrist flexion, and flexion of the digits, as well as sensory depreciation in digits one to three, and the radial half of digit four, and reduced palmar cutaneous sensation. A mononeuropathy entrapment of the median nerve results from excessive compression of the nerve within the carpal tunnel.

Dissection of palmaris longus highlights the crisscross interfascial relationship its tendon shares with the median nerve along its route.

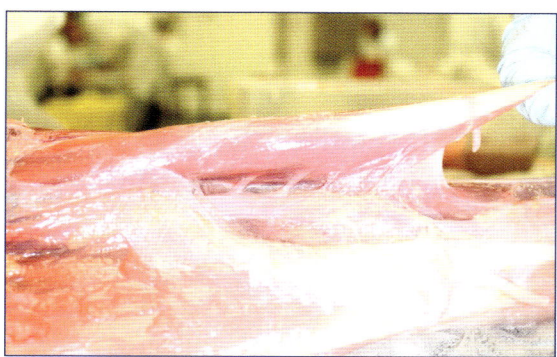

Figure 3.43. Placing traction on the distal tendon of palmaris longus highlighted the continuity of fascia and the transfer of forces by means of mechanotransduction via the epimysium.

In all cadavers dissected for the purpose of this investigation, the tendon of palmaris longus terminated in the palmar aponeurosis. The proximal tendon of this superficial fusiform, spindle-shaped flexor is associated with the medial epicondyle of the humerus, continuous with the antebrachial fascia of the forearm. The median nerve announces its arrival at the palm between the lateral and medial styloid processes.

Under cover of the palmar aponeurosis, the median nerve runs posterior to the tendon of palmaris longus, located outside the carpal tunnel. Lightly placing the fingertips above the palmar aponeurosis while gently providing traction to the gaster of palmaris longus resulted in a sensed lift, and expansion, relieving structures deep to the palmar aponeurosis overlying the carpus (figure 3.43). This observation supports the proposal of palmaris longus as a site-specific fascia tuning peg reducing decompressive forces on the carpal tunnel and, hence, the median nerve.

The ulnar nerve originates from brachial plexus ventral rami of C8 and T1, with

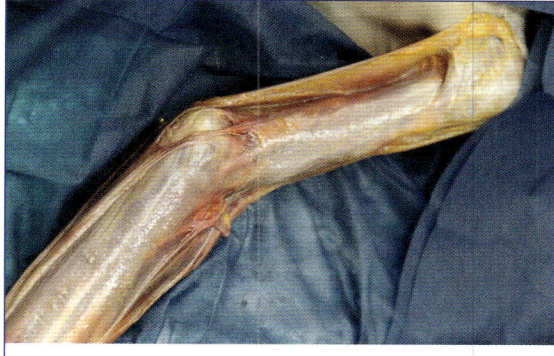

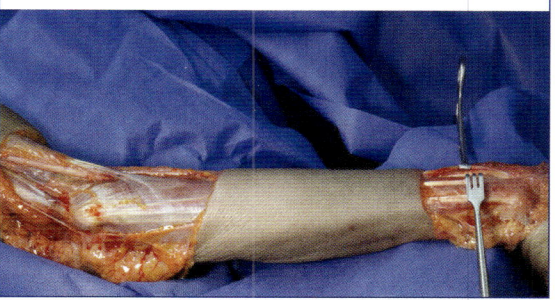

Figure 3.44. The ulnar nerve runs superficially in the medial arm. Traveling in close approximation to the medial tendon of triceps brachii passing through the cubital tunnel, a bony trough composed of the olecranon process and medial epicondyle. (Images: Andrzej Pilat from his personal collection.)

contributions occasionally from C7, and terminates in the distal phalanges of the fifth and half of the fourth digit, while innervating the forearm, wrist, and hand along its anatomical path. The ulnar nerve runs superficially in the medial arm (figure 3.44). Traveling in close approximation to the medial tendon of triceps brachii, the ulnar nerve passes medially to the cubital tunnel, a bony trough composed of the olecranon process and medial epicondyle. Places of perilous passage include the medial intermuscular septum as the ulnar nerve travels posteriorly to the cubital tunnel, the arcade of Struthers, and onward to Guyon's canal, prior to the hook of the hamate. On entering the forearm, the ulnar nerve traverses flexor carpi ulnaris, running superficially upon the oblique ulnar collateral ligament.

The humeral attachment of pronator teres, traveling within the cubital fossa, in conjunction with lacertus fibrosus is considered a site-specific fascia tuning peg providing a tensegral expansion at the medial supracondylar ridge of the humerus. Should this expansive fascial facilitation fail to occur, the ulnar, median, and interosseus nerves, with associated vasculature, may become irritated, resulting in pain, changes in sensation, and loss of ROM.

Changes due to hypertonicity or inhibition can lead to inappropriate tensional and compressional forces with subsequent morphological changes, possible densification of ligamentous structures, and dynamic ischemia. Fibers of the biceps brachii and brachialis contribute forces to the deep antebrachial fascia, diving to the depths of the floor of the cubital fossa (i.e., the elbow pit). The cubital fossa contains the brachial artery and median nerve, with the ulnar and radial nerves within the specific anatomical vicinity but not directly within the cubital fossa. Pulling on the humeral tendon of brachialis allowed observation of the mechanical effect, felt with the fingertips, downstream within the antebrachial fascia. It was observed that the distal attachment of brachialis associates with the tuberosity of the ulna, specifically the ventral surface of the coronoid process, by means of a splayed or pyramid-shaped aponeurosis. Distribution of forces through this thick, fan-shaped fascial structure is hypothesized to assist decompression at the internervous plane (between sartorius [femoral nerve] and tensor fasciae latae [superior gluteal nerve]).

As a major nerve of the upper limb, the musculocutaneous nerve is an extension of the lateral cord of the brachial plexus, containing fibers from the C5–C7 spinal nerve roots. The musculocutaneous nerve innervates biceps brachii and brachialis and supplies sensory branches to the integument over the lateral cubital and forearm regions via the lateral antebrachial cutaneous nerve. It is proposed that the specific location of the proximal portion of coracobrachialis supplies contractile forces resulting in fascia decompression of the neurovascular sheaths associated with the coracoid process.

The coracoid process, viewed as an osseofascial hub, provides the interface for mechanotransductive integration required for the facilitation of omnidirectional expansive forces. Such forces are proposed to act to protect the integrity of the neurovascular structures in the proximity of the axilla, in an omnidirectional fashion. It is further proposed that inhibition or spastic activity of the coracobrachialis would change the tensional-compressional relationship required for optimum neurophysiological function within the axilla.

Fascia Tuning Pegs—Lower Limb

Site-specific fascia tuning pegs—to return to the musical analogy—provide the appropriate frequency and note-specific tension and compression to ensure the combined forces operate in an omnidirectional manner, resulting in pain-free physiology, neurology, and motion. Numerous modest myofascial structures, including psoas minor, psoas tertius/accessorius, plantaris, and pyramidalis, are the source of debate concerning their precise function, with many considered to be vestigial fascial entities.

Fascia-focused dissection of the long posterior abdominal wall muscle psoas minor, carried out at the University of Dundee, revealed its relationship to the iliopectineal eminence and pelvic fascia located superior to the acetabulum—ideally placed to coordinate the decompression of local and more global neurovascular and lymphatic vessels. The lumbar plexus is prisoner to the fascia of the psoas major anteriorly and quadratus lumborum posteriorly, as the L1 to L4 roots of the ventral rami emerge posterior to the psoas muscle before penetrating its muscle belly (figure 3.45). Nerves emerge medially and laterally to the psoas major as follows:

Laterally   iliohypogastric, ilioinguinal, genitofemoral, lateral femoral cutaneous nerve

Medially   obturator, lumbosacral trunk

Fascia-focused dissection of the lumbar plexus confirmed it as a bilateral interweaving of six peripheral nerve branches exiting at the T12 to L5 spinal cord levels, located in front of the corresponding transverse process. The intervertebral foraminal entrance zone represents the earliest peripheral location or place of perilous passage where lumbar nerves can be insulted and/or compressed. Nerve insults to the sciatic, pudendal, genitofemoral, obturator, femoral, or lateral femoral cutaneous nerves can occur at

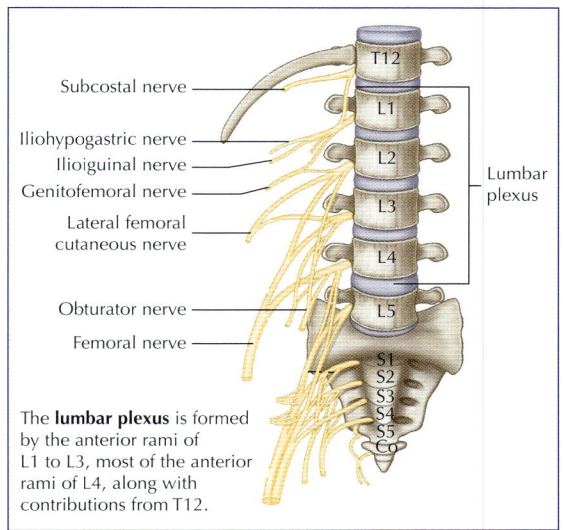

Figure 3.45. The lumbar plexus.

numerous locations along their course before and after they exit the pelvis, owing to a lack of appropriate tissue gliding.

One branch—the nerve to the obturator—exits through the obturator foramen, a possible site of perilous passage. One should consider double or multiple crush compressions culminating in a complex and possibly confusing picture during clinical assessment. Intervertebral disc pathology should be ruled out as the primary or a contributing cause of the patient's complaint, as well as checking site-specific fascia tuning pegs such as psoas minor fascia dysfunction leading to compression of neurovascular structures, such as the genitofemoral nerve.

The psoas major fascia is in direct continuity with the endopelvic fascia, including the iliolumbar ligament and the fascia overlying iliacus. Fascia integrity, provided by mechanotransductive forces

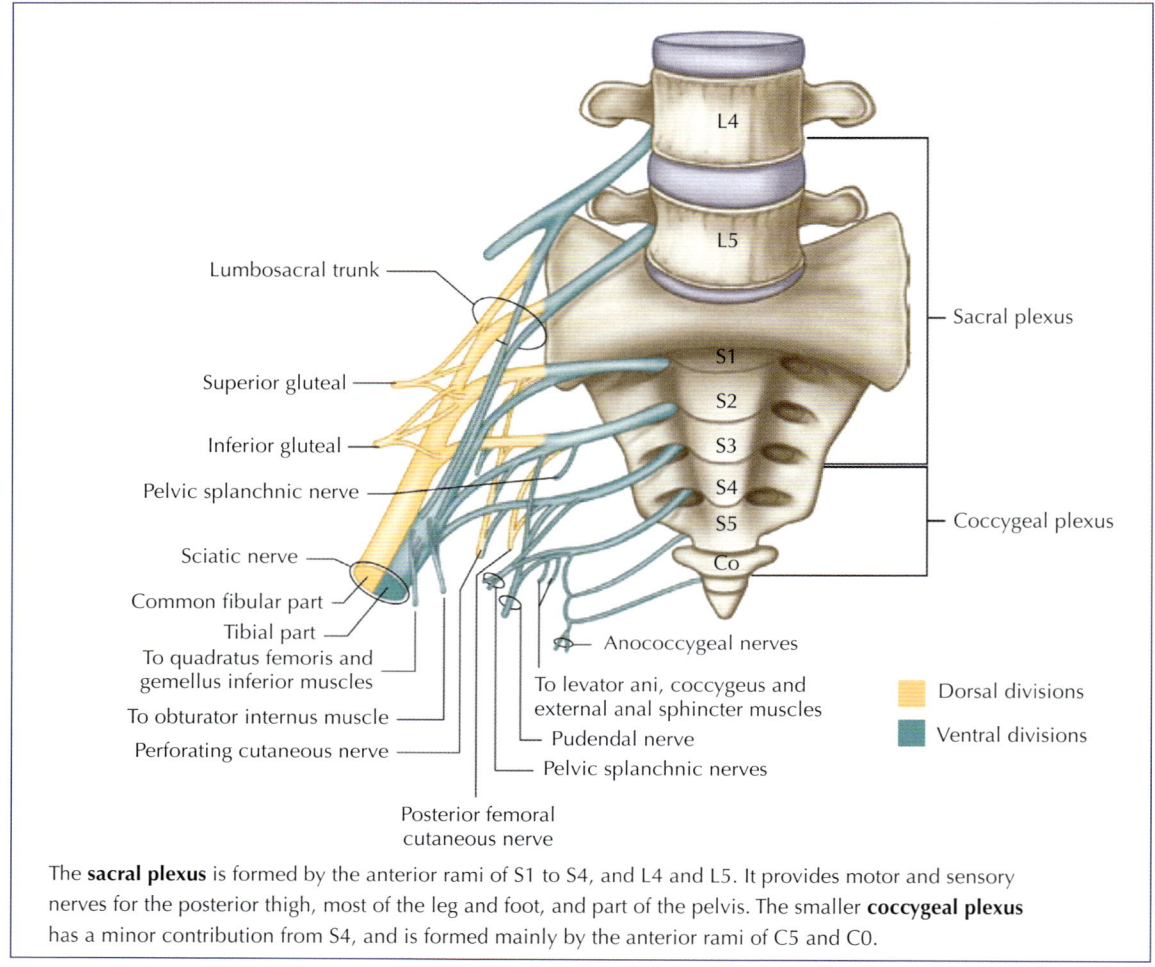

The **sacral plexus** is formed by the anterior rami of S1 to S4, and L4 and L5. It provides motor and sensory nerves for the posterior thigh, most of the leg and foot, and part of the pelvis. The smaller **coccygeal plexus** has a minor contribution from S4, and is formed mainly by the anterior rami of C5 and C0.

Figure 3.46. The sacral plexus.

from quadratus femoris and psoas major, are hypothesized to reduce excessive compressional forces on the subcostal nerve, iliohypogastric nerve, ilioinguinal nerve, lateral femoral nerve of the thigh, and femoral nerve.

The lumbosacral plexus (L4–S3) and its various branches, including a unique converging of lumbar and sacral nerves via the furcal nerve, typically arises at the level 4 nerve root and innervates the lower

limb (figure 3.46). The primary nerves for our consideration regarding lower-limb places of perilous passage are the sciatic and femoral nerves.

During fascia-focused dissection, the lumbosacral trunk was traced inferiorly upon the sacral ala contouring the osseofascial pelvic brim and joining the first sacral nerve. The first sacral nerve was seen to be invested in the parietal fascia overlaying piriformis. Innervation of the posterior thigh, portions

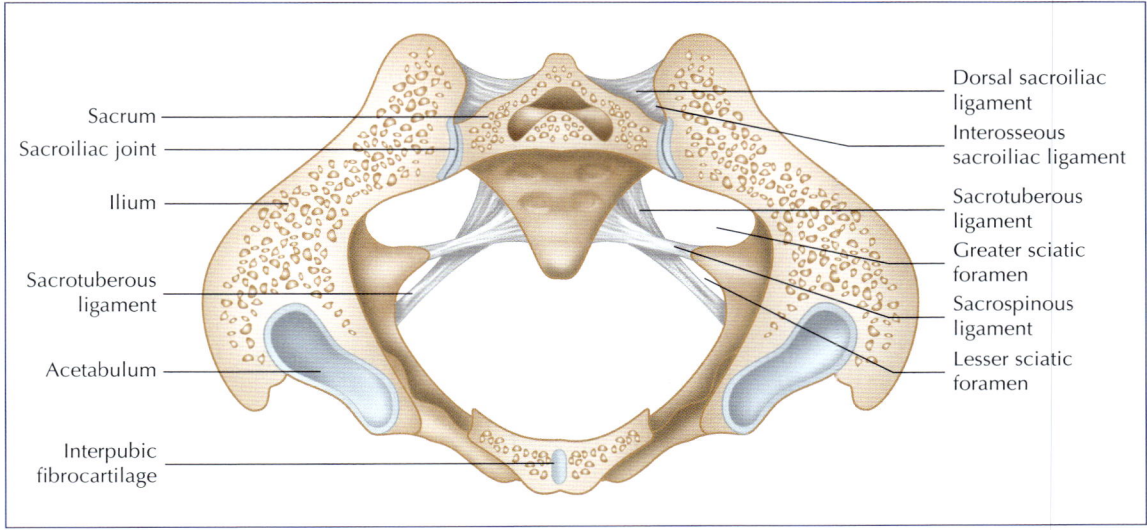

Sacrum

Sacroiliac joint

Ilium

Sacrotuberous ligament

Acetabulum

Interpubic fibrocartilage

Dorsal sacroiliac ligament

Interosseous sacroiliac ligament

Sacrotuberous ligament

Greater sciatic foramen

Sacrospinous ligament

Lesser sciatic foramen

Figure 3.47. Transverse section of the pelvis.

of the pelvis, the majority of the anatomical leg, and the entire foot comes from the sciatic, tibial, and fibular nerves, which are all major branches of the sacral plexus.

The large sciatic nerve can be palpated by the experienced therapist as it exits through the greater sciatic foramen of the pelvis and dives beneath the muscle piriformis (figure 3.47). It is clinically important to appreciate the location of the greater sciatic notch: this is a significant passage point where the fascia-focused therapist can garner therapeutic benefit owing to the large number of neurovascular structures that can be compressed or adhered at this junction.

These structures include the superior and the inferior gluteal vessels and associated nerves, the sciatic nerve, posterior femoral cutaneous nerve, the internal pudendal nerve and associated blood vessels, the nerve to obturator internus, and, importantly, the nerve to the unique fascia tuning peg that is quadratus

femoris (L4, L5, S1). The sciatic nerve dives deep on exiting the sciatic notch. The therapist can once again safely palpate and manipulate the sciatic nerve when it reaches the level of the gluteal crease, after which it once again dives deep to the hamstrings.

Like the "one muscle" concept, you could say there is only one nerve in the body. However, in anatomical terms, the named sciatic nerve officially terminates shortly before arriving at the apex of the popliteal fossa, at which point it bifurcates into the tibial and common fibular nerves. The sciatic nerve can be effectively mobilized by engaging the fascia profunda of the hamstring muscles with a "pin and move" technique such as soft tissue release (STR), although this may leave the patient with a feeling of low-level soreness for a period of hours after the session (figure 3.48).

The lumbar plexus is formed by the anterior rami of the L1–4 spinal nerves (see figure 3.46). The femoral nerve is one of the

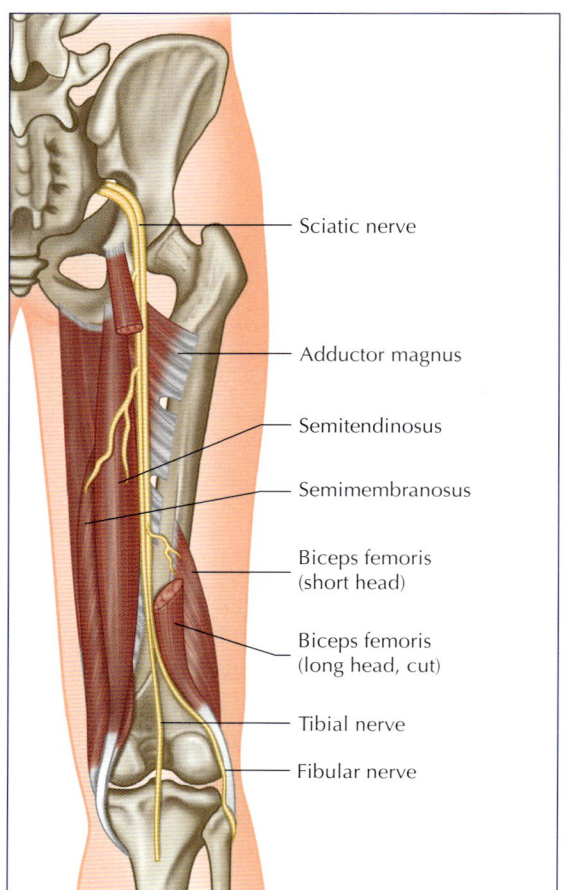

Figure 3.48. The sciatic nerve, posterior view.

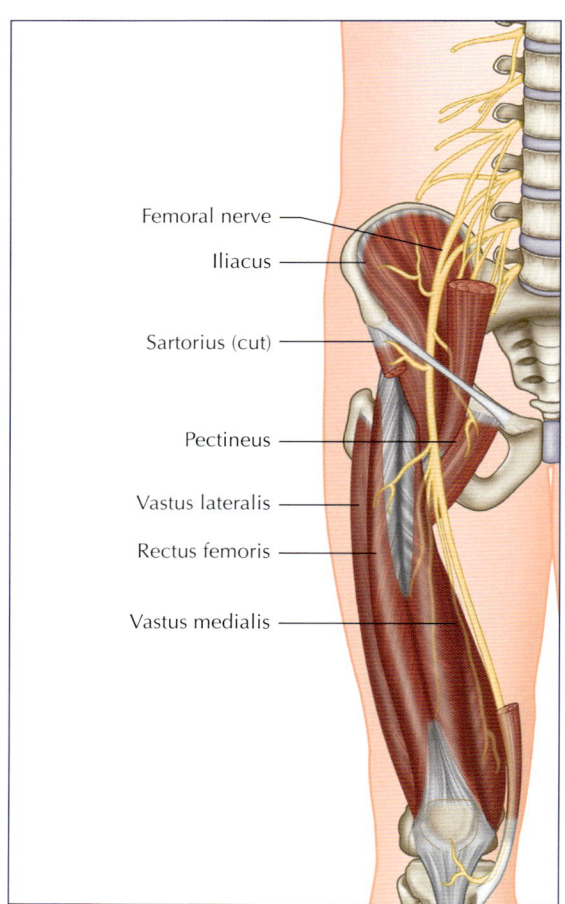

Figure 3.49. The femoral nerve, anterior view.

major nerves that originates from the lumbar plexus, and it provides innervation to the anterior compartment of the thigh, emerging from the posterior aspect of psoas major at the level of the L2–4 vertebrae, before descending along the medial border of the muscle (figure 3.49). It then passes through the pelvic brim and enters the thigh via the femoral canal—a passage formed by the femoral ring and the cribriform fascia.

The cribriform fascia is a dense connective tissue that lines the femoral canal of the thigh and covers the femoral vessels and the femoral

nerve as they pass through it. It is formed by fusion of the iliac fascia, the transversalis fascia, and the psoas fascia. The cribriform fascia is perforated by the great and small saphenous veins, as well as by other structures such as cutaneous nerves, lymphatic vessels, and blood vessels, resulting in it being a slightly weaker anatomical location.

An important consideration in the surrounding location is the density of the fibrous bands of fascial tissue, retinacula cutis or skin ligaments, serving to anchor the skin to the underlying deeper fascia. Adhesions in this area restrict blood and nerve supply and have an adverse effect on movement of the skin, while having an impact upstream and downstream in the kinetic system.

In fascia-focused dissections carried out at the University of Dundee, three arrangements of retinacula cutis were clearly observed in the thigh. A medially located retinaculum attaches to the deep fascia of the adductor muscles, including a portion of sartorius. A site-specific lateral retinaculum attaches to the iliotibial tract, and a third intermediate retinaculum is found located in the anterior thigh attaching to the epimysium of the so-called quadriceps. These vital fascial structures prevent the skin from moving excessively during motion and irradiating friction and shear forces that would lead to damage and injury. Insults to the retinacula cutis and superficial fascia include

morphological changes in the extracellular matrix resulting from hyperglycemia, repetitive trauma, adhesions, skin pathologies, postural misalignment, and scars due to surgery or other trauma.

As the femoral nerve passes through the cribriform fascia, it is closely related to the femoral artery and vein, which lie medial and lateral to it respectively. The nerve then divides into its terminal branches, which innervate the muscles of the anterior thigh, as well as the skin over the anterior and medial aspects of the thigh and the knee. Due to the unique anatomy of this region and high quantity of superficial skin ligaments prone to adhesions, therapists should pay close attention to the impact of the ascending and descending fascia on more distant sites.

PART II

PRACTICE

Myofascial Trigger Points—Assessment and Treatment

MTrP Formation—a New Hypothesis

In this text, I refer to MTrPs exclusively as hyperirritable localized spots (sarcomeres) found in taut bands within muscles (figure 4.1). These spots are painful to touch and can provide referred pain, or a change in sensation distally or proximally, which is often the patient's primary complaint (numbness, itching, burning, pain, or coldness).

Latent or active MTrPs can mimic everything from headaches to toothaches. Autonomic responses to MTrPs include excessive sweating

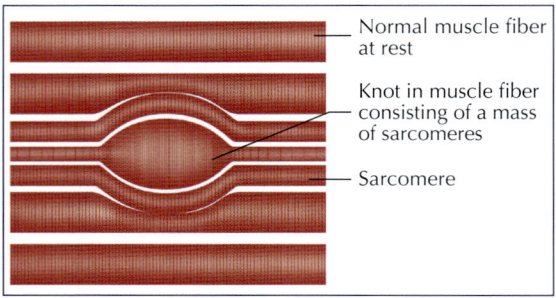

Figure 4.1. A trigger point complex showing shortened sarcomeres without nerve stimulus, and the associated taut band (also called a contracture).

and salivation, goose pimples (pilomotor reflex response), or redness on the skin at the site of the MTrP. For example, MTrPs located in the paraspinal muscles can lead to hair loss in the associated dermatome. Currently, MTrPs are considered to be a result of end plate dysfunction.

For example, rectus abdominis contains several bellies (four or more on both sides) and can potentially contain MTrPs in each belly. All MTrPs have the potential to refer pain. When an MTrP is created within the pain referral zone of another muscle, it is called a *satellite MTrP*. Active MTrPs will refer a pain that the patient will recognize, and latent MTrPs will refer pain but it will not be a recognized pain, although it may contribute 15, 20, or 30+ percent of the patient's primary pain. Reducing pain by only 5 percent will be much appreciated by all patients.

Research and clinical experience have improved our knowledge of why and how MTrPs form and their mechanisms of referral (Simons, Travell, and Simons 1999, 2017).

The following theoretical platform concerning the mechanisms of MTrP formation and referral is based on sound physiology.

A dysfunctional end plate activity occurs, commonly associated with a strain caused by unaccustomed physical activity or other soft tissue insult. Stored calcium is released at the site, and the neurotransmitter acetylcholine (ACh) is released through calcium-charged gates at the synapse, leading to an abundant and constant presence of this neurotransmitter. Ischemia results and creates an oxygen/nutrient deficit accompanied by a local energy crisis. Energy (ATP) is needed to remove the excess calcium. ATP availability is decreased by the ensuing tissue tightness (figure 4.2). This in turn restricts local blood supply.

The persistent high calcium levels maintain the release of ACh, resulting in a vicious cycle (figure 4.3).

ACh transmission causes the actin and myosin elements of myofibrils to slide into a shortened position, resulting in the

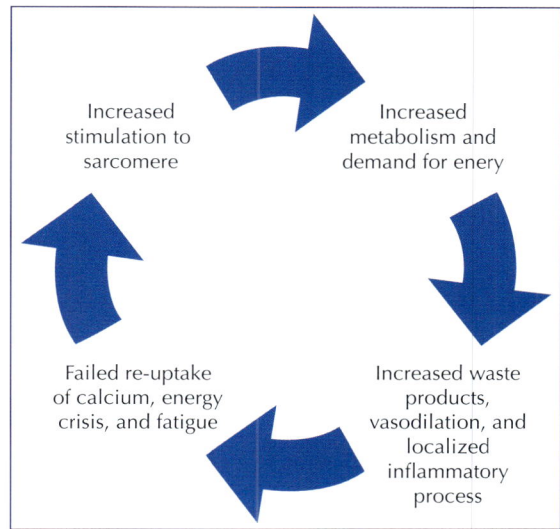

Figure 4.3. Vicious cycle of MTrP physiology.

formation of contractures (involuntary, without action potential). Removal of the excessive calcium requires more energy than sustaining the contracture, so the contracture remains. The contracture is sustained by the chemistry at the innervation site, not by action potentials. These should be differentiated from contractions (voluntary with action potentials) and spasms (involuntary with action potentials). The actin/myosin filaments slide into a fully shortened position (a weakened state) in the immediate area around the motor end plate (positioned at the center of the fiber). As the sarcomeres shorten, a *contracture nodule* forms, which is a palpable characteristic of an MTrP. The remainder of the sarcomeres, to either side of this nodule within the fiber, are lengthened, thereby creating a palpable taut band, another common MTrP characteristic. Other characteristics are spot tenderness of a nodule in the taut band, and the patient's recognition of pain or sensation when applying pressure on the tender nodule.

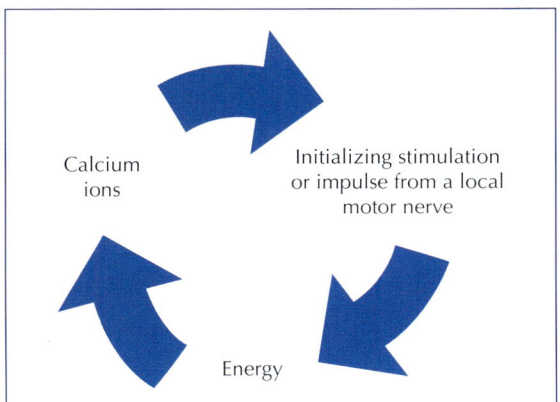

Figure 4.2. Flow chart showing how a nerve impulse causes a muscle contraction.

Additionally, there may be:

- visual or tactile evidence of local twitch response (LTR); imaging of this may be induced by needle penetration of the tender nodule
- pain or altered sensation in the target zone associated with the MTrP when provoked
- Electromyography (EMG) demonstration of spontaneous electrical activity (SEA) in the nidus (nucleus) of the MTrP
- a painful limit to full stretch and reduced range of motion
- weakness in the muscle housing the MTrP on testing
- altered cutaneous humidity (dry or moist), temperature (cool or hot), or texture (rough)
- a "jump sign" or exclamation by the patient owing to extreme tenderness of the palpated tissues, including central and attachment MTrPs

In this new edition, I will describe an expanded hypothesis concerning the pathophysiology of MTrPs, which I call "rigor trigger." *Rigor trigger* describes the MTrP expressed within the sarcomere due to high levels of calcium ions. As a clinical anatomist, I am experienced in working with cadavers generously donated to science, and with the rigor contractions—or stiffening—that occur in muscle fibers shortly after death. I propose that in living muscles, at the level of the sarcomere, a MTrP is in effect a rigor contracture. What this means is that the shrinking or contracting of the sarcomeres is purely electromagnetic. Therefore, the contracture requires neither neural input nor ATP.

This could partially account for the success of needles in the treatment of MTrPs,

as the introduction of a metal needle in close proximity to a cluster of MTrPs results in an immediate twitch response and electromagnetic phase change of the sarcomeres. Such dysfunction or functional adaptation in the living muscle results in a shortening of several sarcomeres (approximately a hundred per MTrP), creating a palpable nodule in the muscle.

Muscles can develop not just one but multiple MTrPs. MTrPs create both a nodule and an associated taut band on either side. As an MTrP can occur anywhere within a muscle fiber, "X" is no longer used nor useful in identifying the location. Knowledge is needed regarding the arrangement of the fibers and number of muscle bellies in any given muscle, alongside excellent palpation skills. *Contracture* describes when a sarcomere (or several sarcomeres) shortens without the input of a nerve stimulus or the need for ATP.

Types of Myofascial Trigger Points

Central MTrPs

The previous description of a centrally located nodule describes a *central MTrP*, which usually forms in the center of a fiber's belly and is most likely associated with motor end plate activity. The central MTrP is therefore defined as a palpable nodule at the center of a taut band of fibers, which, when properly provoked, will refer pain, tingling, numbness, itching, or a variety of other sensations. The site of the referred sensations is referred to as a *target zone*. The target zone is usually located distally to the MTrP, although it can also be more central or, more rarely, within the local tissue where the MTrP is housed.

Attachment MTrPs form where fibers merge into tendons or at periosteal insertions. Although attachment MTrPs are not directly the result of end plate dysfunction (like the central MTrPs), they are presumed to be indirectly caused by the central MTrPs since they develop at the attachment sites (periosteal, myotendinous junction) of the shortened, contractured bands associated with a central MTrP. Active MTrPs form at attachment sites where muscular tension provokes inflammation, fibrosis, and eventually deposition of calcium.

As noted, central MTrPs are located in the center of muscle fibers, while attachment MTrPs form at the myotendinous junction or the periosteal attachment. This classification of MTrPs will greatly influence the therapeutic application. During dissection, I regularly find isolated muscle fibers that have migrated over the tendon. This is what I suggest is the underlying basis for attachment MTrPs. I call these isolated fibers *muscle islands.*

Satellite MTrPs

MTrPs can also develop within the pain referral zone of active or parent MTrPs. When such MTrPs develop, we refer to them as either *satellite* or *baby MTrPs.*

It is important when treating MTrPs to treat all the muscles that refer pain within the target zone but limit the number of muscles in any treatment to between three and five. If treatment is not having the desired result, immediate referral to the patient's general practitioner is advised.

MTrPs in the smallest of muscles can cause extreme, debilitating pain. A 2007 study by

Hsieh and colleagues found that dry needling evoked inactivation of a primary (key) MTrP situated in its zone of pain referral. This supports the concept that activity in a primary MTrP leads to the development of activity in satellite MTrPs, and the suggested spinal cord mechanism responsible for this phenomenon.

Types of MTrP

Active	Produces a pain recognized by the patient as their primary complaint and is active when the patient is at rest
Latent	Produces pain when palpated; this pain may not be recognized as the primary pain
Primary	Forms in response to trauma or insult
Key	Responsible for activating satellite MTrPs
Satellite	Activated by key MTrP in its kinetic area of referral
Central	Located near the center of the gaster or muscle fibers
Attachment	Located in the tendon of a muscle

Factors Affecting Myofascial Trigger Points

Work Environment Considerations

Repetitive strains can result from manual working activity. Appropriate posture and correct arthrokinematics (or biomechanics) are essential for avoiding undue muscle

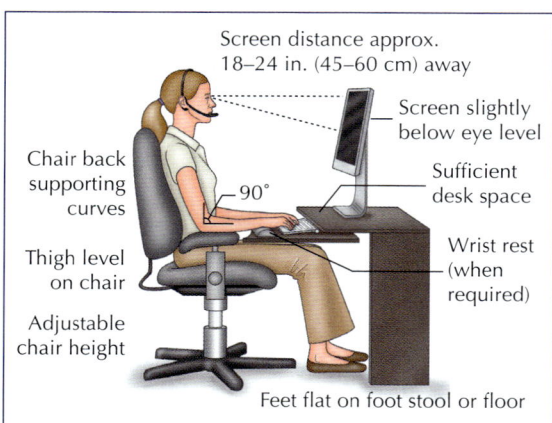

Figure 4.4. Ideal sitting posture for reducing stress while working.

stiffness and resulting compensations, which can quickly lead to the formation of MTrPs. Just sitting causes harmful forces and compressions, without the added stress that working at a computer station can place on the neck, forearms, wrists, and lower back. The height of the work desk and the position of the computer relative to eye level and degree of neck flexion or extension are pivotal (figure 4.4).

Dietary Influences

Adequate quantities of minerals and vitamins are essential for healthy muscles and tissues. Many patients presenting with chronic pain are found to be deficient in a number of vitamins and minerals.

Vitamins B1, B6, and B12, along with vitamin C and folic acid, are important in the war on pain. Calcium, magnesium, iron, and potassium are critically important also. All too often people are confused as to why they are deficient in these important minerals and vitamins, as they will report that they eat well and have normal dietary habits when compared with other family members. The problem may not be their diet but rather their personal health choices, such as smoking or drinking alcoholic or caffeinated drinks. Smoking, for example, annihilates vitamin C, while oral contraceptives affect vitamin B6 levels. Antacid medication can leave people with symptoms of chronic fatigue, where even signing their signature becomes an effort.

Patients with vitamin and/or mineral deficiencies may report symptoms such as feeling unusually cold, bouts of diarrhea, restless leg syndrome, headaches, disturbed sleep, and MTrP pain. Other symptoms include feeling fatigued, muscle cramping, and depression. Metabolic disorders should not be ruled out, particularly thyroid problems and hypoglycemia, and referral is recommended.

Contraindications to Myofascial Trigger Point Therapy

- Avoid open wounds or broken skin.
- Should a patient state that they have a malignancy, their medical practitioner must give written permission before any treatment can be given.
- Do not use MTrP therapy on a patient with an aneurysm.
- Never press, massage, or stretch a hematoma.
- Due to the risk of blood clot formation, medical practitioner approval must be provided in writing if arteriosclerosis is present. Information regarding all medications should be provided.
- If the patient has osteoporosis, this is particularly serious if using dry needle techniques owing to the risk of

fenestrations (small holes that occur in bones such as the scapula, through which the needle could contact the lungs if care is not taken).

Visceral pain has a temporal evolution, and in its early stages can be insidious and difficult to identify. Due to the low density of sensory innervation of viscera and the extensive divergence of visceral input within the CNS, what is called "true visceral pain" is a vague, diffuse, and poorly defined sensation, regardless of the specific internal organ of origin. It is usually perceived in the midline at the level of the lower sternum or upper abdomen. Whether the origin is the heart, esophagus, stomach, duodenum, gallbladder, or pancreas, visceral pain in the early phase is perceived in this same general area.

Additional stimuli such as local compression applied to this area fail to worsen the pain. True visceral pain can easily be overlooked. This is due in part to the fact that the patient cannot clearly describe the pain. It is often described as a vague sense of discomfort, malaise, or oppression. It is typically associated with marked autonomic phenomena, such as pallor, profuse sweating, nausea, vomiting, changes in blood pressure and heart rate, gastrointestinal disturbances (e.g., diarrhea), and changes in body temperature. Strong emotional reactions are commonly present, including anxiety, anguish, and sometimes even a sense of impending death.

Sometimes, visceral pathology may manifest principally through vegetative and emotional reactions, with minimal pain and discomfort. A typical example is painless myocardial infarction, which may produce a sense of gastric fullness, heaviness, pressure, squeezing,

or choking. As a general rule, in these early stages the intensity of visceral pain bears no relationship to the extent of the internal injury. Visceral pain should always be suspected when your patient presents with vague midline sensations of malaise. This is particularly important when the patient is elderly.

As visceral pain continues to progress (minutes to hours) it may refer to the dermatomes whose innervations enter the spinal cord at the same level as the visceral organ involved. This can be misinterpreted by the brain as joint, muscular, or nerve pain, manifesting itself as sharp, localized, deep somatic pain. For example, liver pathology can lead to referred pain in the right upper shoulder (figure 4.5). Peripheral nerve pathology such as irritation of the C7–C8 spinal nerves may present as pain in the fourth and fifth fingers (ulnar nerve).

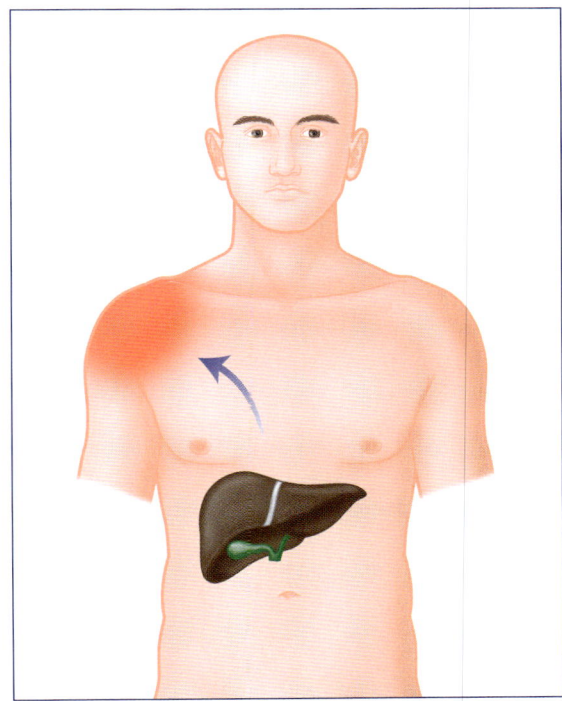

Figure 4.5. Site of pain referral from the liver.

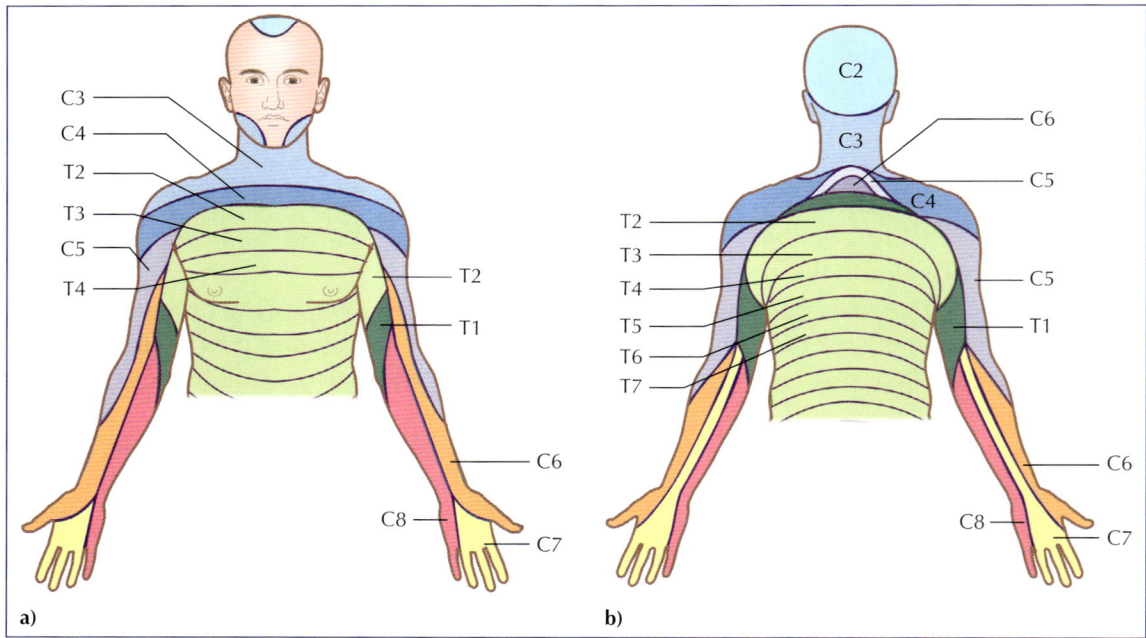

Figure 4.6. Dermatomes of the upper body.

This type of pain can be accompanied by hyperalgesia (increased sensitivity, pain on light stimulation) or hypoalgesia (decreased sensitivity, numbness) (figure 4.6).

Detailed questioning of patient is required to clarify their compliance and level of discomfort. During this assessment stage, you must determine the characteristics of the pain, the pathways of pain radiation or referral, its form and dependency from active, active resisted, or passive movements. Feedback from the patient concerning neurological signs, skin sensitivity, pain and referral, and other symptoms including heat, cold, tingling, itching, and mood swings is vital information that will ensure you refer the patient to the appropriate medical practitioner.

Once your patient returns to you, they must supply a letter from their medical practitioner stating that fascia-focused therapy is appropriate in this specific case, and that pathology is not suspected or has been ruled out. Fascia-focused therapists, unless medically qualified, cannot diagnose pathologies, although for many patients, their therapist may be the first practitioner they visit. As time can be such a crucial factor in pathology, referral on suspicion of any pathology, without delay, is always in the patient's best interests.

General Rules for the Treatment of MTrPs

- Treat the most severe MTrPs.
- Treat MTrPs that are more medial and superior before those that are distal (inferior) and more lateral.
- Treat those areas that have a cluster of MTrPs as a priority.

- When a muscle has several MTrPs, initially treat the ones located in the center of the gaster (muscle belly) or muscle fibers.
- Only treat between three to five muscles in any one treatment, especially in the earliest stages of treatment intervention.

Shoulder Anatomy, Arthrokinematics, and MTrP Considerations

Shoulder Biomechanics (Arthrokinematics)

The glenohumeral articulation is exceptional because of its unique degree of mobility throughout its ROM, having three degrees of freedom (figure 4.7):

- Flexion–extension
- Abduction–adduction
- Medial–lateral rotation

Stability is maintained in the shoulder joint by the glenohumeral ligamental complex (figure 4.8), the compressive forces of the rotator cuff, the glenoid labrum, negative intra-articular pressure, and normal scapular kinematics as part of the scapulohumeral rhythm (figure 4.9). The scapula moves in coordination with the moving humerus, so that the center of rotation of the joint remains within a safe zone.

MTrPs can affect correct glenohumeral positioning. Coordinated muscle activity will reduce maximum concavity compression. Scapular retraction allows for full cocking, ensuring an efficient and explosive forward acceleration of the arm (figure 4.10). Scapular protraction allows for maintenance of proper glenohumeral positioning and facilitates deceleration in follow-through.

The coupled motion of the arm and scapula provides dynamic stability for the glenohumeral joint in the various positions encountered in activity. It is easy to see how MTrPs can interfere with this force couple action. Latent MTrPs have been shown to

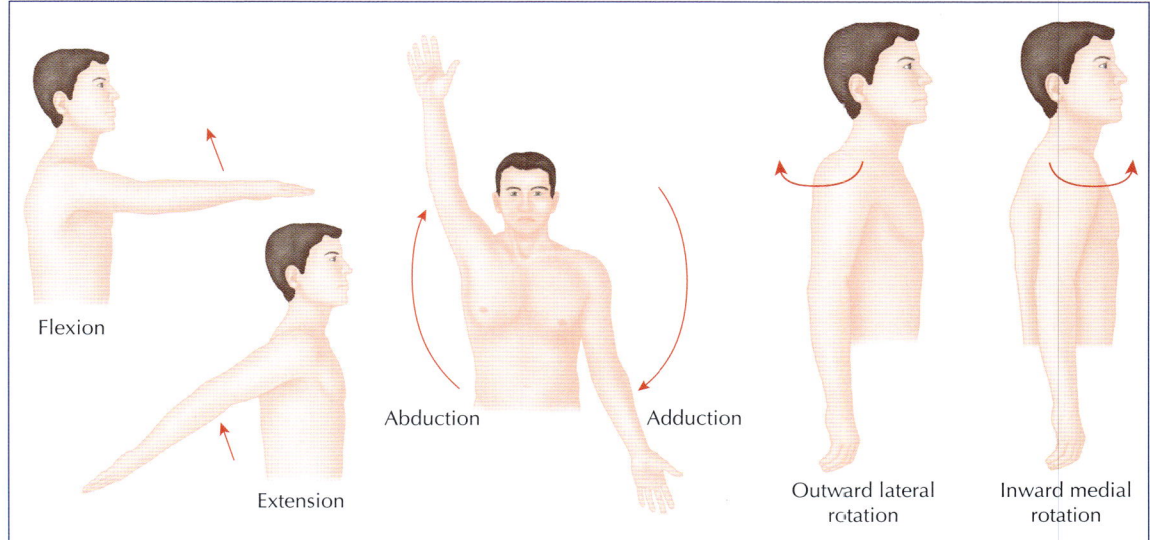

Flexion

Extension

Abduction

Adduction

Outward lateral rotation

Inward medial rotation

Figure 4.7. Movements of the shoulder.

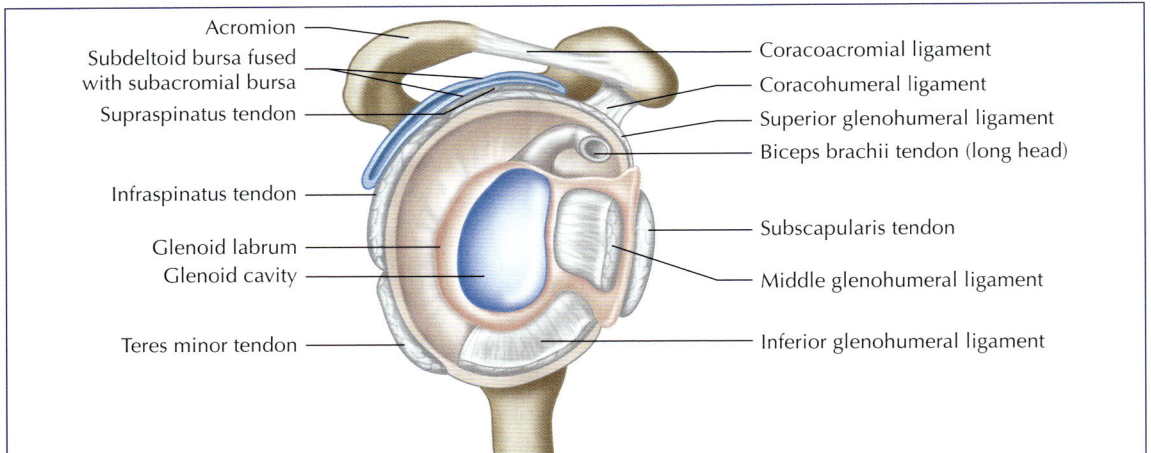

Figure 4.8. Ligaments of the glenohumeral joint.

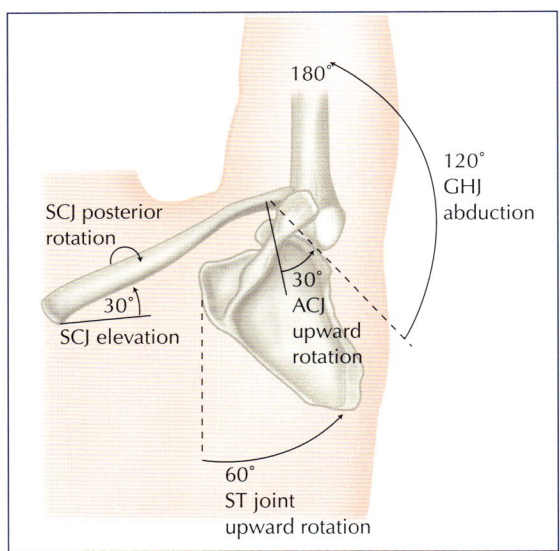

Figure 4.9. Scapulohumeral rhythm.

interfere with this finely tuned mechanism, resulting in muscles firing out of their normal and appropriate neurological sequence.

Acromial elevation, necessary to prevent rotator cuff impingement, may be disrupted by fatigue of the serratus anterior, lower trapezius, and the rotator cuff muscles owing to MTrP formation or loss of fascial integrity (e.g., the spiral system, see p. 132). The scapula

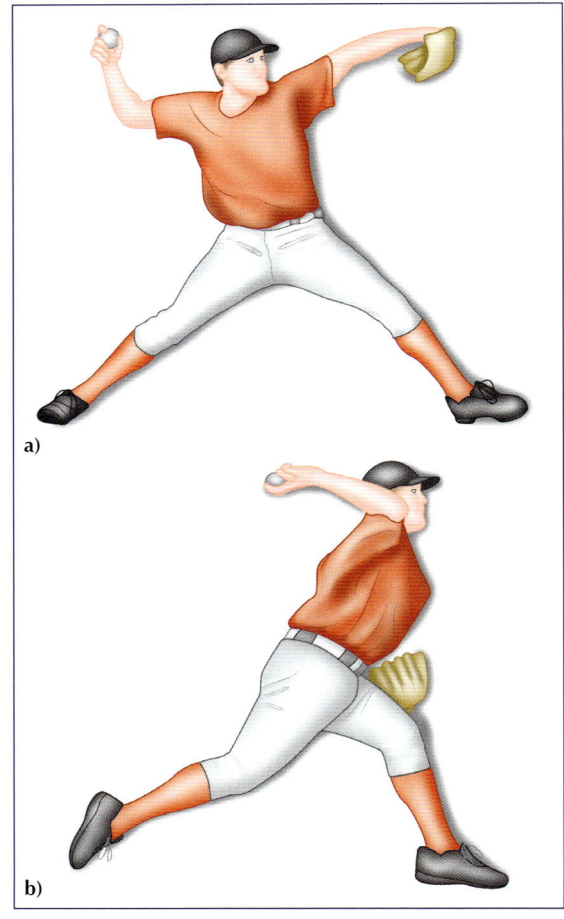

Figure 4.10. The cocking phase of throwing: (a) early phase; (b) late phase.

therefore forms an important link in the kinetic mechanism in which large forces are generated in the proximal segments (legs, hips, and trunk) and transferred through the scapula into the shoulder and ultimately to the arm and hand (upper sleeve) for execution of some movement. Maintaining a stable scapular platform, in conjunction with core neuromuscular efficiency, allows for the most appropriate shoulder function.

Evaluation of the Shoulder

The glenohumeral (GH), scapulothoracic, suprahumeral, acromioclavicular, sternoclavicular, and costovertebral articulations are the key joints (both true and false) affecting the shoulder (figure 4.11).

Structures that are anterior and medial to the glenohumeral joint include the biceps brachii and musculotendinous units including the pectoralis major, pectoralis minor, and subclavius. They also include the bony coracoid process.

Intra-articular structures include the supraspinatus and infraspinatus, the labrum, capsule, bursa, and ligaments. Posterior structures include the scapula and the rotator cuff (SITS) and scapular stabilizing muscles, which include the triceps brachii, rhomboids, serratus anterior, trapezius, and levator scapulae.

Depending on the patient's presentation, the assessment can be expanded to examine the cervical and upper thoracic spine, the brachial plexus and its branches, the sternoclavicular

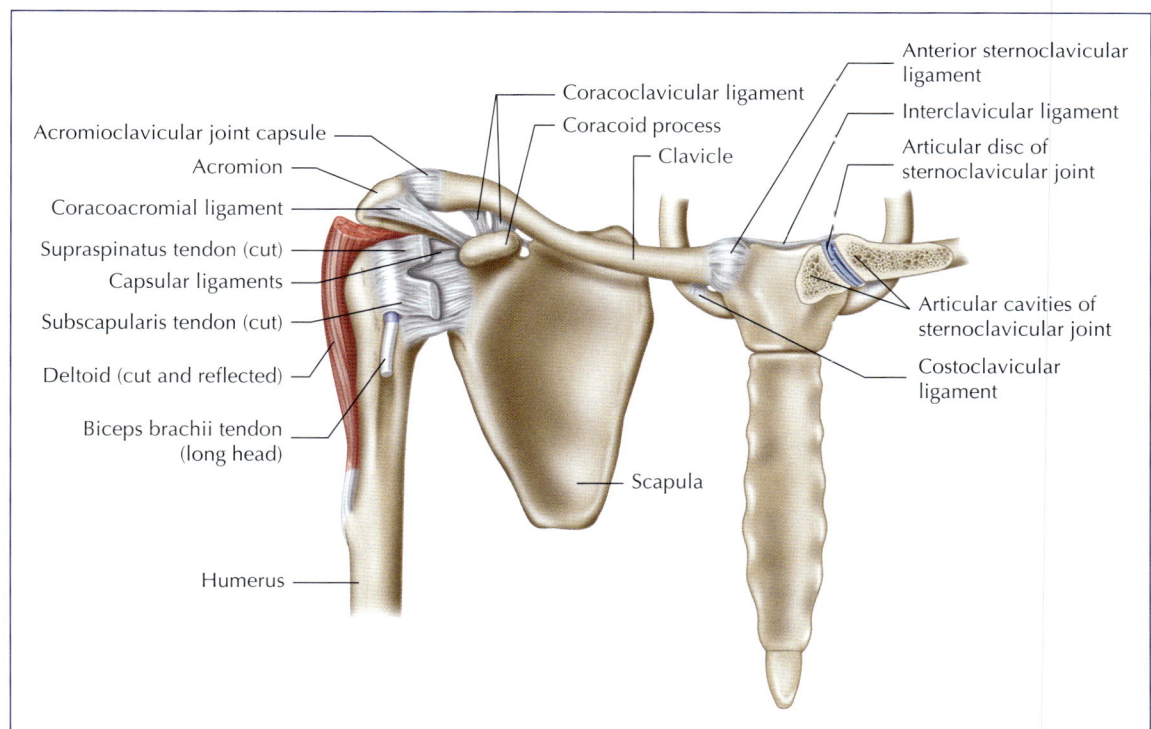

Figure 4.11. The anatomical landmarks of key shoulder articulations.

joint, and muscles such as the paraspinals and scalenes.

It is essential to utilize neuromuscular thumb or finger techniques to assess skin, muscle tone, and autonomic changes (i.e., sweating, texture, spot soreness, fibrosis, dryness) as well as monitoring and comparing pulses such as the brachial and radial. MTrPs housed in these muscles can squeeze both blood vessels and nerves, leading to loss of sensation or hypersensation, including burning, tingling, or itching. MTrPs can lead to a retardation of blood supply and cause cramping or swelling. Such body parts often feel cold. In the long term, reduced blood supply can lead to serious pathological conditions.

If the SITS muscles are not performing their role in drawing the head of the humerus into the glenoid during an action—like abduction of the humerus—it is possible to envisage a slipping posterior–inferior or anterior–inferior of the humeral head. This will result in a subluxation, or in the more serious case a dislocation of the glenohumeral joint (figure 4.12). This change in joint positioning and arthrokinematics is the basis for the formation of functional MTrPs.

Functional MTrPs will evolve to provide tension or stiffness within the joint facility, and likely in the most inhibited musculotendinous structures. The body produces this stiffness or tension as a short-term protective facility. Unfortunately, MTrPs can persist and become the source of unrelenting pain and reduced ROM.

In frozen shoulder conditions, it is regularly noted that the pectoralis major is spastic,

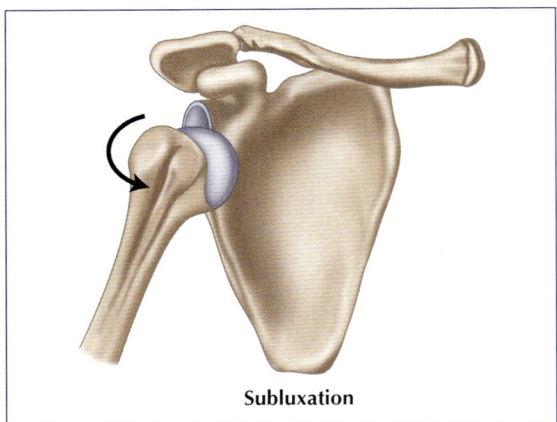

Subluxation

Figure 4.12. Subluxation of the glenohumeral joint.

drawing the humerus into the side of the body and internally rotating the humerus in the GH joint. This has the effect of closing down the blood supply to the GH region and provides the foundations for a sequence of events that compounds the frozen shoulder syndrome (figure 4.13). Upper trapezius will be short and over-contractured, and the scapula will not demonstrate normal scapulohumeral rhythm.

A thorough history is important and should include the mechanism of injury, location of pain, identity of MTrPs, position of the arm when pain occurs, relieving and aggravating factors, activity modifications, prior injuries to the shoulder and kinetic structures, treatment update, sport or functional demands, and a general medical history. If there is a risk of dislocation, fracture, or serious pathology present, no special tests are required and the patient should be referred without delay.

As stated earlier, the proximal structures of the kinetic system (legs, hips, and trunk) and the scapula are very much connected

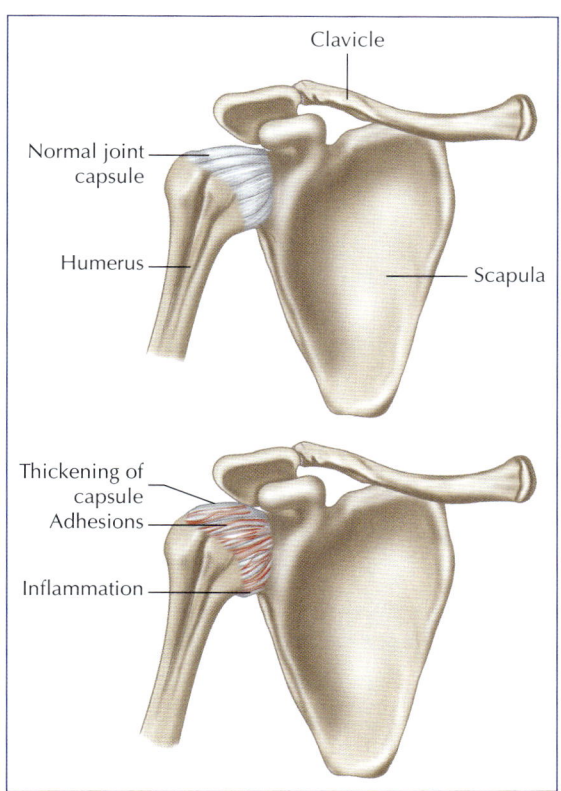

Figure 4.13. Frozen shoulder (adhesive capsulitis).

with shoulder function and should also be evaluated. Leg/trunk strength can be screened with one-legged stability tests. Such tests could include the one-legged stance, the one-legged squat, and the simple lunge test.

Factors to look out for are the Trendelenburg sign (dropping of the contralateral hip), knee valgus, pelvic rotation, increased lumbar lordosis, and forward lean. In general, these signs suggest weakness of the core lumbo-pelvic-hip muscles, which are the muscles of the abdomen and diaphragm, back, pelvis, and superior portion of the lower limb.

Thoracic and cervical posture should be assessed for thoracic scoliosis, or excessive kyphosis or cervical lordosis. Look for tenderness and MTrPs by palpating on the spinous processes, paraspinals, levator scapulae, vertebral scapular border, rotator cuff muscles, serratus anterior, coracoid process, pectoralis minor, and biceps brachii tendon.

Supraspinatus strength can be assessed by resisted abduction in the scapular plane. Infraspinatus strength can be tested by resisted external rotation with the elbow at 90 degrees and the arm by the side. Both these muscles should be tested with the scapula retracted, to eliminate the appearance of muscular weakness that can result from a protracted position, which does not allow the scapula to provide a stable base for muscle action.

Subscapularis strength can be tested by internally rotating the shoulder and pressing the hand into the gaster, by internally rotating the shoulder and lifting the hand off the back against resistance, and by doing an uppercut maneuver against resistance.

The shoulder should be examined in flexion, abduction, and internal/external rotation at 0 degrees and 90 degrees. This test should be repeated with the therapist offering compression from both sides to the sacroiliac joint (assisted force closure).

If the patient's pain reduces by at least 70 percent with increased ROM when the test is repeated, the therapist can assume that the patient has reduced core stability. A medical exercise program to address this neuromuscular inefficiency should be put in place. Particular attention should be paid to determine the presence of glenohumeral internal rotation deficit (GIRD), which is associated with labral and rotator cuff injury.

An assessment of GIRD can be done by comparing side-to-side differences in internal rotation, measured using a goniometer, with the scapula stabilized and the shoulder abducted to 90 degrees and then internally rotated to the point of tightness.

Abnormalities of winging, translation, and rotation are best assessed at rest and during shoulder abduction or flexion. Muscle weakness causing scapular dyskinesis—deviation in the normal resting or active position of the scapula during shoulder movement—is often seen as a hitch or jump, seen more in the descending phase of arm movement. This may be due to latent MTrPs in associated muscles and can often be a red flag for lack of sacroiliac force closure and reduced core stability. Dyskinesis is often present in more than one plane, and it is more important to identify the presence or absence of dyskinetic patterns. A whole-body kinetic system perspective is required.

Based on the position, the dyskinetic pattern can be categorized into one of three visual positions, which can help to identify involved kinetics (figure 4.14):

Type 1　(lower trapezius weakness), with the inferomedial border prominent

Type 2　(serratus anterior weakness), with the medial border prominent

Type 3　(upper trapezius weakness), with the superomedial border prominent

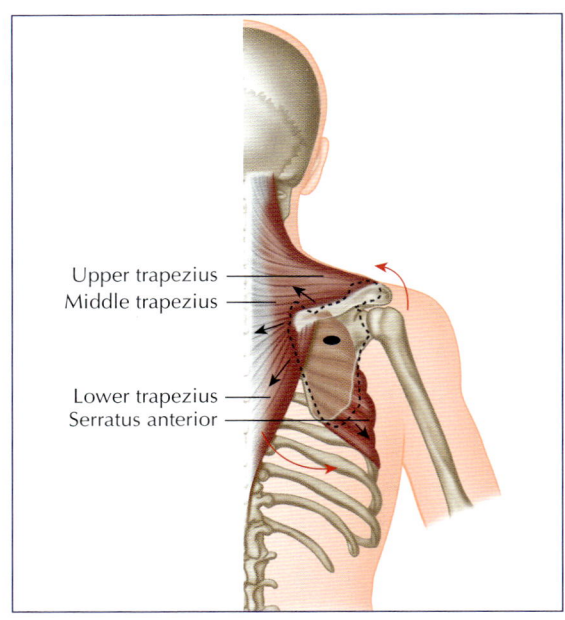

Figure 4.14. Trapezius–serratus anterior relationship.

Arm abduction that elicits painful crepitus over the superomedial or inferomedial borders is suggestive of scapulothoracic bursitis, although MTrPs must be ruled out as the true source of the symptoms. A treatment plan involving vigorous cryotherapy is recommended, which should be applied for 6 to 10 minutes several times a day, especially in the morning and last thing at night.

The scapular assistance test evaluates local scapular and acromial involvement in subacromial impingement (figure 4.15). To perform this maneuver in patients with signs of impingement, the superior border is stabilized and then the inferomedial border is assisted to facilitate upward rotation, posterior tilt, and external rotation of the scapula during elevation of the arm. This procedure simulates the force couple activity of the serratus anterior and lower trapezius. Elimination or

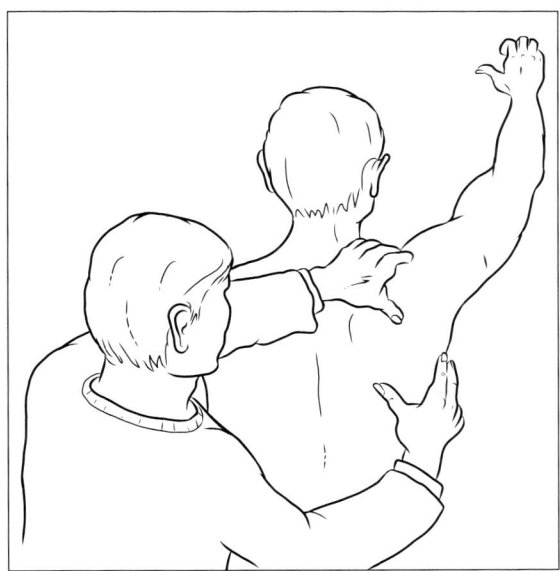

Figure 4.15. Scapular assistance test.

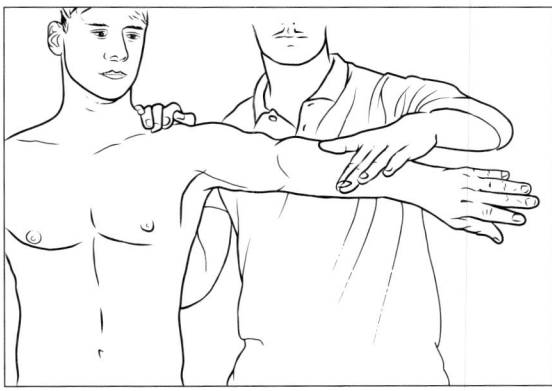

Figure 4.16. Scapular retraction test.

reduction of impingement symptoms indicates that these muscles should be a focus of local rehabilitation.

The scapular retraction test involves stabilizing the scapula in a retracted position on the thorax (figure 4.16). This position provides a stable base of origin for the rotator cuff muscles and will often facilitate an improvement in supraspinatus strength.

It may also decrease pain related to internal impingement from to scapular and glenoid involvement, as the glenoid has been removed from the excessively protracted position that causes impingement. These findings indicate that subsequent rehabilitation should focus on endurance strength of the rhomboids and trapezius.

Quantitative measurement of scapular stabilizer strength can be achieved by means of a lateral scapular slide test (figure 4.17). This test compares the position of the scapula on the injured and noninjured sides in relation to a fixed point in three different positions: arm

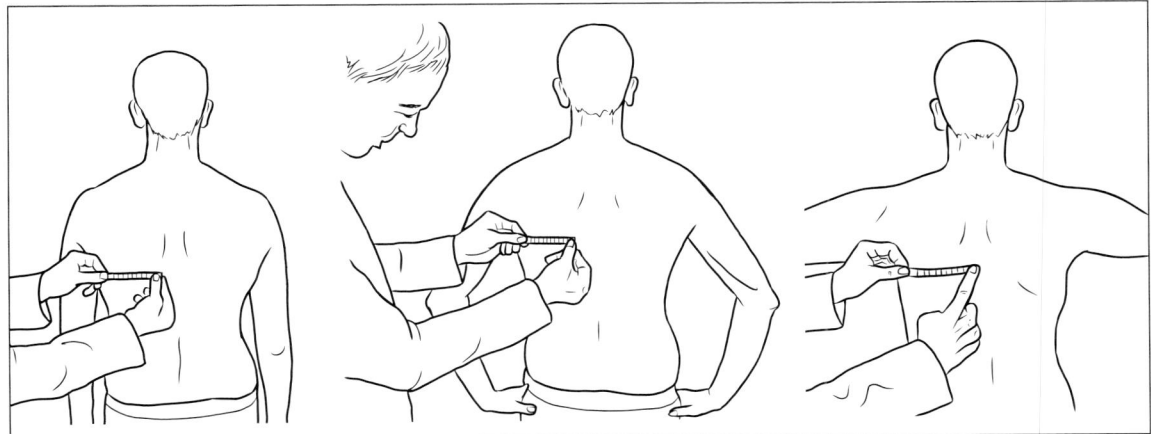

Figure 4.17. Lateral scapular slide test.

at the side, hands on the hips with the fingers anterior and thumb posterior with about 10 degrees of shoulder extension, and arms at 90 degrees of elevation with maximal internal rotation of the glenohumeral joints.

In each position, the distance between the inferior angle of the scapula and a fixed bony point on the spine is marked on each side. A side-to-side difference of ¾ inch (1.5 cm) or more in any of these positions can be considered abnormal.

Glenoid labrum integrity can be clinically tested by palpating for tenderness along the anterior and posterior joint lines while moving the joint through its ROM, and by the following maneuvers.

The anterior slide test is undertaken with the patient's hand on their hip, fingers anterior, thumb posterior, and the shoulder in about 10 degrees of extension (figure 4.18). The examiner applies an upward force to the elbow while the patient resists this motion.

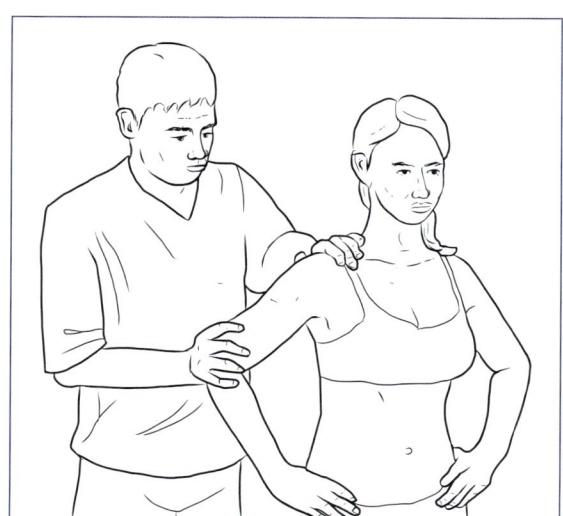

Figure 4.18. Anterior slide test.

Test 1

With the patient's shoulder flexed to 90 degrees and internally rotated, the examiner applies a downward force to the elbow while the patient resists this motion.

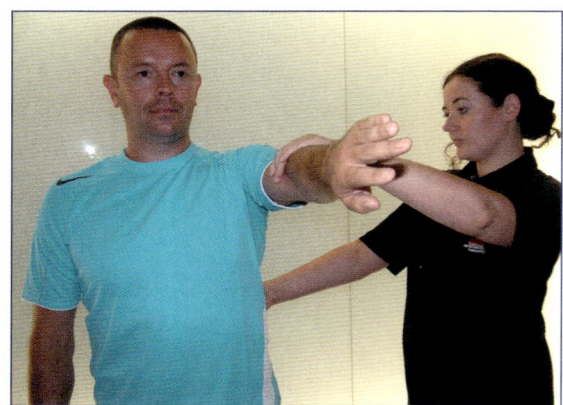

Figure 4.19. Test 1.

Test 2

With the patient's elbow flexed, shoulder abducted to 90 degrees, and externally rotated, the patient resists the examiner's attempt to extend the elbow.

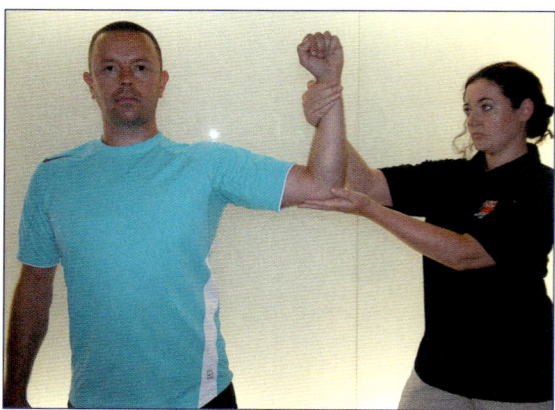

Figure 4.20. Test 2.

Shear Test

With the patient's shoulder placed into a 90-degree angle of abduction, then passively externally rotated and pulled down, the examiner palpates the posterior joint line.

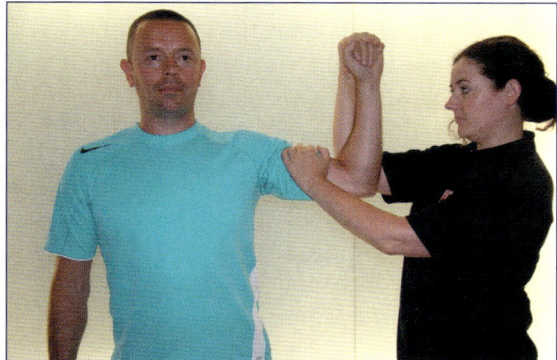

Figure 4.21. Shear test.

The tests described are considered positive if there is a reproduction of pain. Glenohumeral instability should be assessed by including an anterior and posterior drawer or compression test. Inferior instability is assessed using a sulcus test.

For all these tests, the scapula is stabilized and the two sides compared. Then the arm is held and translated anteriorly for anterior instability and posteriorly for posterior instability. For the sulcus test, the arm is distracted inferiorly to create a sulcus (groove or furrow) between the acromion and the humerus. A test is considered positive if the translation generates pain and/or there is increased laxity in comparison with the other shoulder.

Medical Exercise, Balance, and Proprioception

Medical exercise has been advocated to restore motor control to the upper and lower extremity. In the clinic, the term *balance* is often used without clear definition. Details such as static and dynamic conditions, equilibrium, and biomechanical stress and strain must be considered. Efferent or motor response to sensory information results in activities affecting muscle tone, motor execution programs, cognitive somatic perceptions, and reflex joint stabilization.

Proprioceptors or mechanoreceptors are located in and surround each joint, and are composed of Ruffini cells, Golgi tendon organs (GTOs), muscle spindles, and free nerve endings (figure 4.22). Each of these sense organs plays a different role in the type of information it sends to the CNS. They are found in the joint capsule, the muscle gaster, tendon, and retinaculum, as well as in the various ligaments supporting a joint. The ankle has the most mechanoreceptors, followed by the hip and knee.

Sherrington first described the term *proprioception* in the early 1900s, and it has been defined in many ways. Current thinking divides it into two categories. The first is the ability to know where a joint is in space and time, as well as how to reposition a joint to a previously experienced position either actively or passively. The second is called *kinesthetic awareness*, which is the ability to detect motion at a joint.

These are two very important hallmarks of skilled movement. Proprioceptive information is transmitted to the spinal cord via afferent, or sensory, pathways. The information travels at 70 to 100 m/sec. This is much faster than pain signals, which travel at only 1 to 3 m/sec. This information contains details such as static and dynamic conditions, equilibrium, and biomechanical stress and strain. Efferent, or motor, response to sensory information results in activities affecting muscle tone, motor execution programs, cognitive somatic perceptions, and reflex joint stabilization. Typically, ligament loading and rupture can occur in the 70 to 90 m/sec range, while reflex arc reactions occur in the 40 to 80 m/sec range. Cortical response can take up to 120–150 m/sec to be elicited after ligament loading, therefore it is important that any neuromuscular response delay is eliminated with medical exercise to reduce the risk of injury.

The relationship between proprioception and balance is important. The body uses three systems to keep itself upright against gravity. The vestibular system centered in the inner ear is the foundation of the balance mechanism, is enhanced by visual input, and is further assisted by information from the mechanoreceptors. However, injury can damage the mechanoreceptors, which will cause a diminished ability to know where the joint is in space and time and an inability to detect motion. This directly affects skilled movements and indirectly affects balance.

Detecting this loss is important to the medical exercise rehabilitation process, which for lower or upper extremity injuries should center on proprioception, endurance, ROM, strength, flexibility, power, and agility.

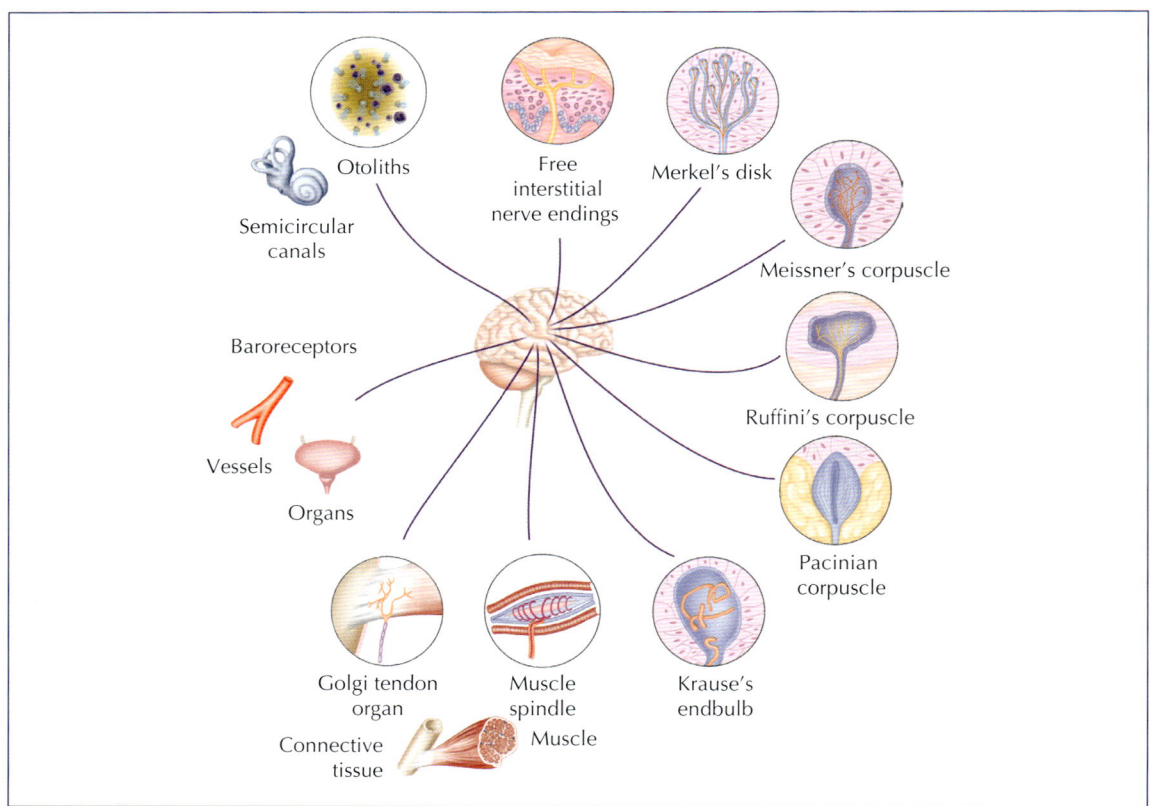

Figure 4.22. Anatomy of the muscle spindle, GTOs, Ruffini cells, and free nerve endings.

The fascia-focused therapist should keep in mind that, as professor of anatomy and embryology Jaap van der Wal noted, mechanoreceptors have no idea about muscles or ligaments. Proprioceptors react to the change in the shape of the fascia and the resulting change in tension and compression, including velocity in change within the connective tissue architecture. Proprioception is a specialized variation of sensory modality, described as body awareness. It is a sense that people rely on daily yet are frequently unaware of. More easily demonstrated than explained, proprioception is the unconscious awareness of where the various regions of the body are in relation to one another at any given time.

Proprioception and balance are separate entities, yet intricately related, and I recommend training both combined as an integral part of medical exercise to restore motor control. Proprioception is the forerunner of appropriate balance and function. Balance can be described as the process by which we control the body's center of mass with respect to the base of support, whether static or moving. This can include the ability to maintain a position, the ability to move voluntarily, and the ability to react to a perturbation.

The three components of balance that are important in the maintenance of an upright posture, include:

Static balance	An individual's ability to maintain a stable position against gravity at rest by maintaining the center of mass within the available base of support
Dynamic balance	Involves automatic postural responses to the disruption of the position of the center of mass
Reactive postural responses (RPR)	Activated to recapture stability when an unexpected force displaces the center of mass

RPR can be demonstrated by anyone closing their eyes and moving their leg around in a circle (i.e., circumduction). Assuming proper proprioceptive function, at no time will the person lose awareness of their leg, even though it is not being detected by any of their other senses.

To fully comprehend proprioception and proprioceptive training, you must appreciate that as you perform physical actions, the overall muscular activity, joint ROM, and posture are all products of sensory nerve activities received, coded, and acted on by the CNS (figure 4.23). The CNS receives the information needed to control movements from three subsystems within the body:

- Somatosensory system
- Vestibular system
- Visual system

The somatosensory system contains nerves located in the skin, bones, musculotendinous junctions, and joints, and can detect touch, pressure, pain, and joint motion and position. In joints, the somatosensory system possesses both quick-adapting (QA) and slow-adapting (SA) mechanoreceptors, nerve endings that detect physical actions. Should a joint be stimulated continuously by pressure or

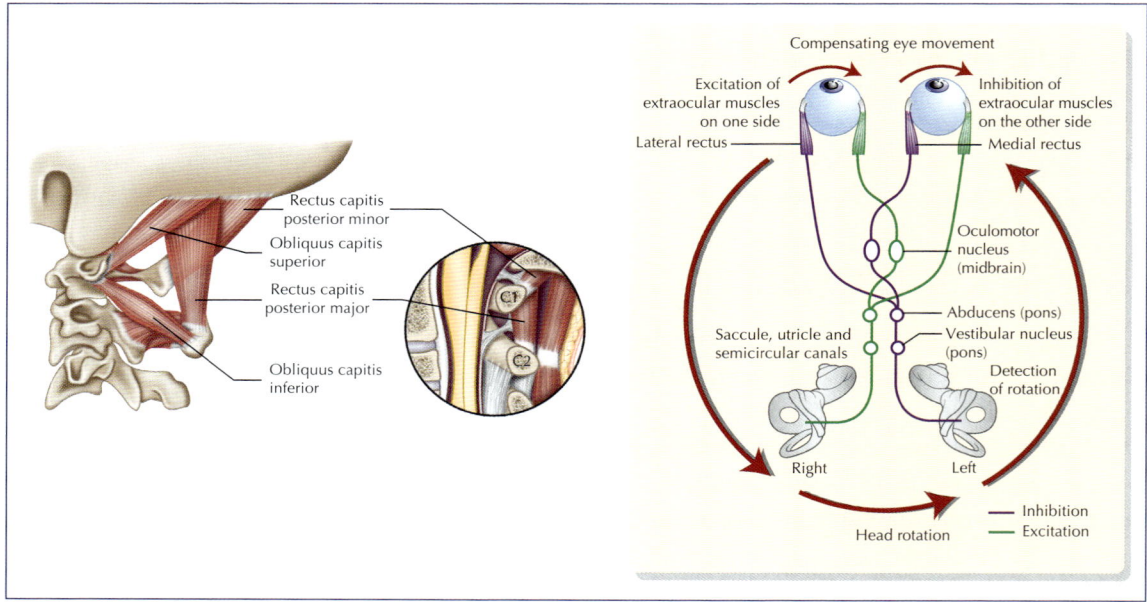

Figure 4.23. Vestibular system and vestibulo-ocular reflex.

motion, the QA mechanoreceptors decrease their signaling to the CNS, while the SA mechanoreceptors keep the CNS fired up.

Mechanoreceptor experts believe that the sensation of joint motion is mediated primarily by QA mechanoreceptors, with SA mechanoreceptors playing more of a role in telling the CNS about joint position and sensation. For example, in the human knee joint, mechanoreceptors have been identified that respond specifically to joint acceleration and deceleration.

Human muscles contain mechanoreceptors that report to the CNS concerning muscle length and tension—spindles and GTOs—and that work with the joint QA and SA mechanoreceptors to give the brain and spinal cord comprehensive information about what is happening elsewhere in the body. Proprioception is referred to as the collection

of sensations regarding joint movement (kinesthesia) and joint position at any given time in space.

As mentioned above, injury to tissues or joints can cause a diminished ability to know where the joint is in time and space and an inability to detect motion, which directly affects skilled movements and indirectly affects balance. Special tests are required to detect this loss so that a graduated program of physical activities can be provided as part of the medical exercise rehabilitation process.

Three levels of the CNS are activated with this medical exercise rehabilitative balance-based training.

The spinal reflex is the simplest (figure 4.24). It is used in reactive situations triggered by external stimuli. The response regulates muscle responses that are highly stereotyped.

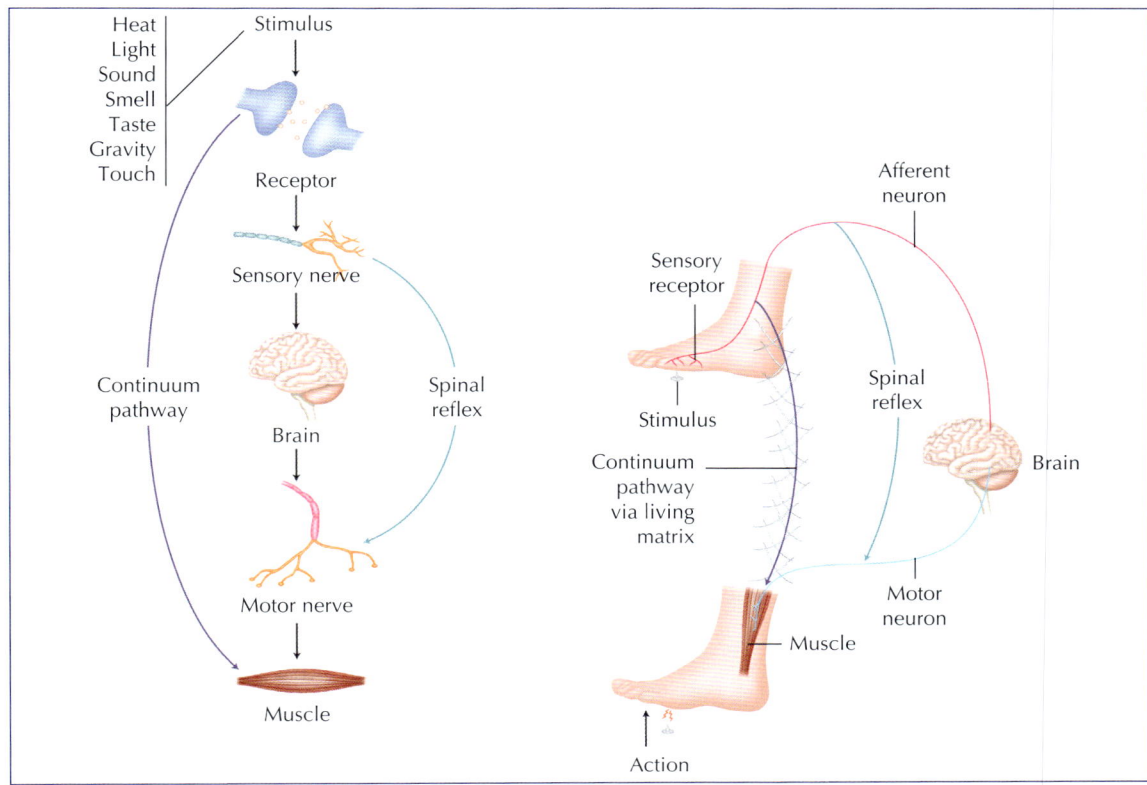

Figure 4.24. The spinal reflex.

These activities are characterized by sudden alterations in joint position that require reflex muscle stabilization. In medical exercise, we recommend the use of rhythmic stabilization activities, as they stimulate the spinal reflex arc.

Perturbation activities are also an excellent way to develop this facility. They can be done while the patient is balancing on either one or both legs or while standing on an unstable surface. The brain-stem level is also triggered by external stimuli. The response is automatic and is not as stereotypical, therefore can be impacted by medical exercise balance training.

Response time is within the 90–100 m/sec range and composed of coordinated movement patterns. Medical exercise balance training activities with and without visual input will enhance motor function at the brain-stem level. Neuromuscular balance activities at this level should be progressed from bilateral stance to unilateral stance, from eyes open to eyes closed, and from a stable base to an unstable base. The cerebral cortex is the highest level of control, where mechanoreceptor information interacts with and influences cognitive awareness and movement, and motor commands are initiated for voluntary movements. These activities take place in the 120–150+ m/sec range.

Training at the level of the cerebral cortex stimulates the conversion of conscious programming to unconscious programming—taking the conscious mind out of the activity. Examples of training at this level would include throwing a small ball to the patient while they are trying to balance on an unstable surface.

Motor coordination is the product of a complex set of cognitive and physical processes, often taken for granted. Smooth, targeted, and accurate movements, gross and fine, necessitate the harmonious functioning of sensory input, central processing of this information in the brain, and coordination with the higher executive cerebral functions (e.g., volition, motivation, motor planning of an activity), and finally, carrying out of a certain motor pattern. These elements must work in a coordinated and rapid way to enable the execution of complex movements with the different parts of the body. Adequate realization of a motion or sequence of movements requires the convergence of numerous pathways and a central system in charge of integrating the information. The motor cortex, cerebellum, and vestibular system (providing input about directionality, gravity, motion) are all part of this central mechanism.

Proprioceptive information (sensation of where the body is in space and the positions of the various limbs and parts of the body), visual input (seeing where the body is in space and where it should go), and an adequate degree of alertness (i.e., the reticular formation being activated to an optimal degree) are ingredients that provide information to the CNS. If one of these systems is not functioning adequately, the resulting planned movement may not be satisfactory or smooth, and the risk of injury and formation of MTrPs increases.

Medical exercise is used to offer a progressive program of functional physical activity that is critical for restoring the synergy and synchronicity of muscle firing patterns required for dynamic stability and fine motor control. The main objective of medical exercise is to return patients to their preinjury activity level as quickly and as safely as possible. Fascia-focused therapists achieve this by enhancing the dynamic muscular stabilization of the joint while increasing the cognitive appreciation of the relevant joint in regard to both position and motion. This is achieved following appropriate intervention with fascia-focused applications such as MTrP deactivation.

Medical exercises are designed to restore joint functional stability and enhance motor control skills. Program design must include a graduated manipulation of the environment to facilitate an appropriate response and make use of balance and proprioception. Control is provided over the joints that dominate the plane in which the activity is taking place.

Medical exercise programs designed to comprehensively address proprioceptive aspects of the joint may protect against injury. Specific proprioceptive training can help to fine-tune the afferent-efferent arcs. Such activities should include repetitive, consciously mediated movement sequences performed slowly and deliberately as well as sudden, externally applied perturbations of joint position to initiate reflex, subconscious muscle contraction. It is not possible to single out specific mechanoreceptors to train, but certain activities can enhance mechanoreceptor activation and therefore influence the CNS pathway.

Reestablishing neuromuscular control is a critical component of medical exercise in the rehabilitation of pathological joints. The objectives of the medical exercise activities are to integrate peripheral sensations relative to joint loads and process these signals into coordinated motor responses. This muscle activity serves to protect joint structures from excessive strain and helps prevent recurrent injury. Neuromuscular control activities as part of medical exercise are intended to complement rehabilitation protocols.

Elements crucial for reestablishing neuromuscular control and functional stability include joint proprioception and kinesthesia, dynamic stability, preparatory and reactive muscle characteristics, and conscious and unconscious functional motor patterns. Dynamic joint stabilization exercises additionally encourage preparatory agonist/antagonist coactivation, whilst efficient coactivation restores the force couples necessary to balance joint forces and increases joint congruency, thus reducing the loads imparted onto static structures.

Focus on stimulating the reflex pathways from articular, muscular, and tendinous receptors. Although preprogrammed muscle stiffness can enhance reflex latency, the objective is to induce joint perturbations that are not anticipated and will stimulate reflex stabilization. The last element requires preprogrammed adaptations to functionally specify motor patterns and joint loads.

Restoring dynamic stability, an important component of functional movement, requires challenging the proprioceptive and balance systems. In injury, pain free should not be mistaken for cured. If the proprioceptive deficit is not addressed, complete rehabilitation will not have been accomplished. Correction of a damaged static restraint (e.g., surgical correction of mechanically disrupted tissue) may not maximize the C-tactile afferent neuromuscular input needed to enhance dynamic joint stability. Mechanically stable joints are not necessarily functionally stable, especially in less constrained systems such as the shoulder. Dynamic stability allows for the control of abnormal joint translation during functional activities. Neuromuscular balance training through medical exercise is essential to enable patients with upper extremity orthopedic injury to return to physical activity.

These activities incorporate all the available resources for stimulating peripheral afferent nerves, muscle coactivation, reflex control, and motor programming, and emphasis should be placed on sports or life-specific techniques. With repetition and controlled intensity, muscle activity (preparatory and reactive) gradually progresses from conscious to unconscious motor control. The lower extremities function in a closed manner during daily life activities and sporting activities. In the upper extremities, exercise application of graded, multidirectional manual resistance can provide proprioceptive feedback in a closed fashion.

Open-manual resistance exercises with rhythmic stabilization (rapid change in direction of applied pressure) are also considered proprioceptively rich. In either case, resistance can be modified, depending on pain, as the patient progresses. Prescribing appropriate and effective exercise requires knowledge of the process known as the "stages of learning." Understanding the stages of learning is crucial for patients to perform exercises efficiently and appropriately as it provides insights into the cognitive and motor processes involved in acquiring a new skill. The stages of learning, typically categorized as the cognitive, associative, and autonomous stages, help fascia-focused professionals to tailor their approach to meet the patient's evolving needs.

Stages of Learning

The first stage of learning is the *cognitive stage*, which is the initial training stage and requires a high level of cognitive awareness regarding the patient. This is the time when the patient is improving their perception of the skill, understanding the task, and getting to know what it feels like. Clear instructions and demonstrations are essential.

For example, cognitive awareness is necessary to isolate the cocontraction of the transversus abdominis and multifidus without substitution of the global muscles (e.g., rectus abdominis, obliques, and thoracic portion of erector spinae). The objective of the first stage is to train the specific isometric cocontraction of transversus abdominis with lumbar multifidus at low levels of maximal voluntary contraction, including appropriate breathing, in weight bearing within a neutral lordosis. The therapist needs to provide instructions, visual cues, mental imagery, and optimal body positions or postures, and use various facilitation/feedback techniques to encourage the ideal response.

The second phase of motor learning is the *associative stage*, where the focus is on refining specific movement patterns that have been identified as faulty and/or pain provocative. The objective is to identify a small number of these movement patterns during examination, so that during rehabilitation they can be broken down into component movements and performed for a nonspecific number of repetitions. The patient is taken through these component movements whilst isolating the cocontraction of the local muscle system. Patients will begin to detect errors independently and work towards improving their technique. Guidance from the fascia-focused therapist remains valuable, however, emphasizing subtle adjustments and honing specific aspects of the exercise.

Initially, exercises are performed whilst maintaining the spine in a neutral lordotic posture, and the patient subsequently progresses to normal spinal movement. At all times, segmental control and pain control must be ensured. Some of the movement patterns identified during examination may include sit to stand, walking, lifting, bending, twisting, extending, and so on. The patient is prescribed independent exercises that focus on the movement components, which are performed daily, with pain control emphasized. Physical activities are progressed as speed and complexity of the movement pattern are increased. In time, these movements should be performed in an efficient neuromuscular manner. The patient should also perform exercises like walking while maintaining correct postural alignment, low-level transversus abdominis and multifidus cocontraction, and appropriate breathing.

A key issue in pain control is focusing on muscle control (performing the cocontraction) during movement patterns throughout the day that a patient would typically anticipate resulting in lower back pain and instability. This is fundamental to ensure that the cocontraction during these movement patterns becomes automatic and subconscious. This stage can last from two to four months. Rehabilitation time depends on motivation and compliance of the patient, along with intensity of practice, and depends upon the degree and nature of the pathology.

The third and final stage is the *autonomous stage*, where the patient requires a low degree of attention to perform the motor task correctly. This stage involves specific exercise intervention, whereby subjects can dynamically stabilize their spines appropriately in an automatic manner during the functional demands of daily living. Multiple studies show that changes to automatic patterns of muscle recruitment can be achieved. The key is a decrease in recurrence of symptoms and better functional outcome.

How to progress:

1. Independent activation of transversus abdominis and multifidus
2. Independent coactivation of transversus abdominis and multifidus
3. Improve precision
4. Coordination of breathing (paradoxical breathing is a common problem and needs correction)
5. Function—simple to more difficult static tasks
6. Function—easy to difficult dynamic tasks
7. Local and global coactivation
8. Specific progressive functional retraining

Integrating Local and Global Muscle Units

Local muscles are those involved in providing support for joints in the form of stabilization (figure 4.25). Such muscles are located throughout the body and are less involved with specific movement. Local muscles provide the stability and increased stiffness required to ensure safe and effective joint movement.

Global muscles are ultimately responsible for creating movement (figure 4.25). Such muscles are larger in size and attach the pelvis to the costal bones, providing a link between the lower limbs and upper quarter. A muscle creates force when it contracts. This force in turn creates stiffness. Force creates joint torque, supporting postures and creating movement.

There are times when the force will enhance joint stability, while at other times it will compromise stability. It all depends on the magnitude of the force and its degree relative to all other muscle forces acting at the joint. In contrast, the role of muscle stiffness is always to provide stability. A stiff muscle supports against perturbations in all planes. Stiffness at one joint supports the development of explosive power at another. Stiffness is also improved by positional techniques of the body segment linkage, where one segment can be stiffened against another. When all muscles that act on a joint stiffen together, a superior stiffness occurs. The total stiffness provided at the joint by all the muscles contracting together will provide more stiffness than any one muscle could on its own.

As an example, let us look at the abdominal wall in creating core stability.

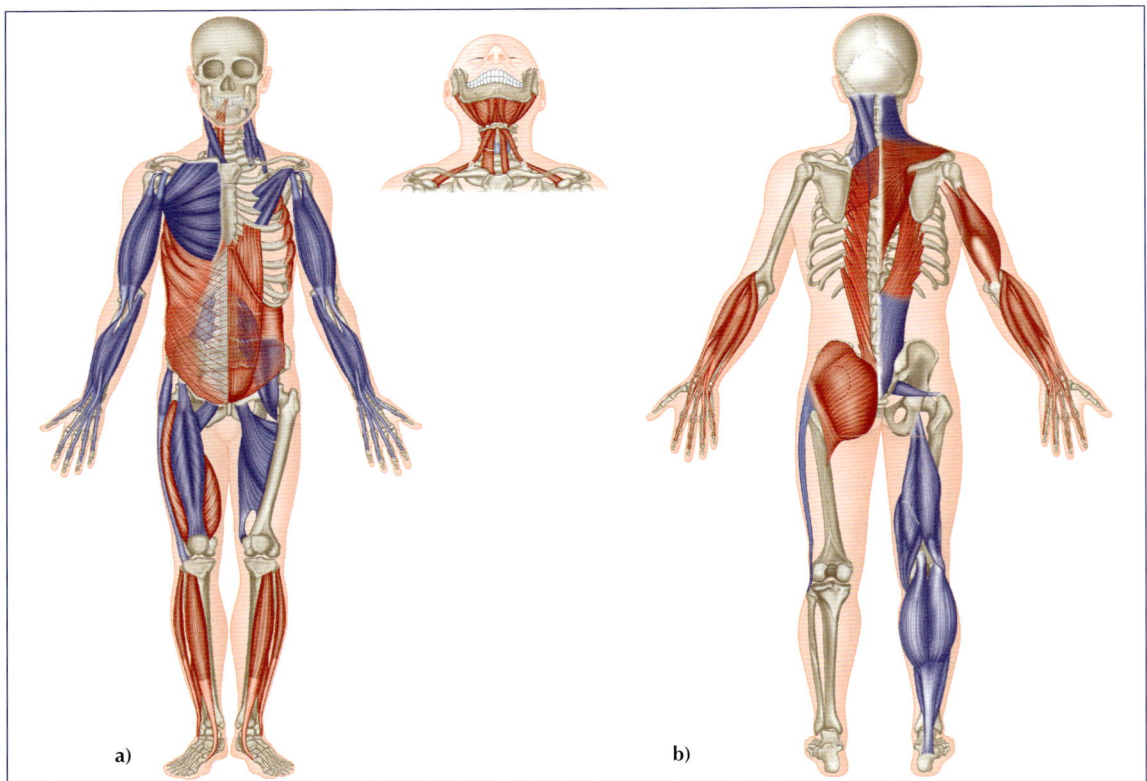

Figure 4.25. Local (blue) and global (red) muscles.

Rectus abdominis, the obliques, and transversus abdominis work together as a unit to create this superior stiffness, which is greater than the sum of each individual muscle. In the neck this superior stiffness is provided by the infra- and suprahyoids and the sternocleidomastoid (SCM) during activities such as sit-ups. If the tongue is not placed in its physiological resting position behind the front teeth in the roof of the mouth, the hyoid muscles cannot contract to create the level of stiffness required to offer cervical joint support.

The SCM will contract even more to make up the stiffness deficit, resulting in shortened SCM, forward head posture, rounded shoulders, and full-body kinetic implications.

In higher intensity activities that demand greater core stability, all muscles must be activated. High performance in athletics requires rapid muscle activation and force development, together with equally rapid reduction of muscle force. Superior stiffness needs to occur only briefly in such cases, but if it needs to be brief, the motor control system must be highly tuned to ensure optimal superior stiffness.

Form and Force Closure

Form closure addresses how the topography of the contacting surfaces of a joint and its ligaments contribute to stability and reduce

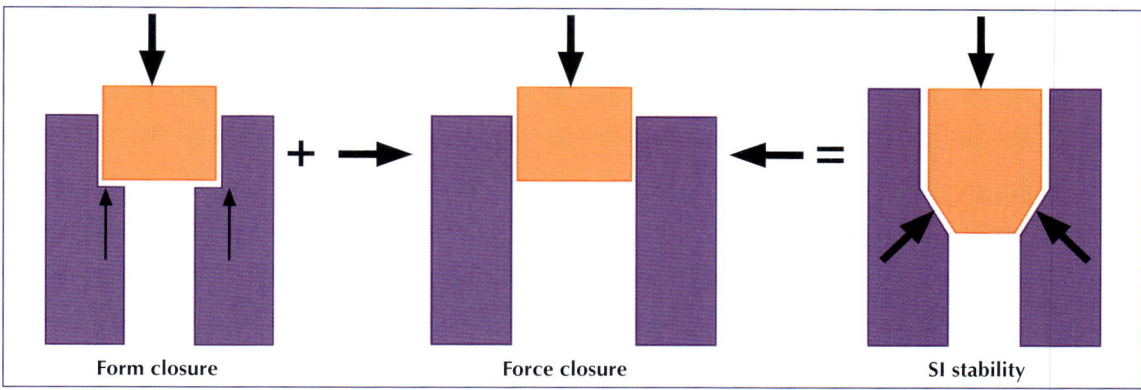

Figure 4.26. Form and force closure.

or prevent shearing and excessive translation between the two joint surfaces when under load (figure 4.26).

Force closure addresses the forces necessary to control translation between two joint surfaces when under load (figure 4.26). For example, at the SI joint, the force required for controlling shear is compression. The stabilizing muscles of the lower back and pelvis in conjunction with the fascia through the sacrotuberous ligament provide this compression. They include the transversus abdominis, multifidus, pelvic floor, and biceps femoris of the lower limb.

Machine-Based Exercise

Medical exercise includes machine-based exercise; however, if an individual does not integrate whole-body kinetic system functional exercises into their program, the risk of muscle dominance, neuromuscular inefficiency, adaptive postural changes, and injury may increase. Machine-based exercise can promote neuromuscular inhibition, resulting in the nervous system shutting down prime movers.

To avoid this, a focus on stabilizing the core with functional or life-specific physical activity through the LPH complex is included.

Machine-based exercises are usually unidirectional, while all functional movements are triplanar—that is, movement occurs in all three planes. Triplanar movement requires acceleration, deceleration, and dynamic stabilization. However, many machine-based exercises have no functional relationship to how humans move or live. For example, you would never reach for an item in the way you move your arms while performing an abdominal crunch. Couple that with the fact that your trunk and hips are flexed while generating substantial forces, and one can visualize and appreciate how this repetitive action could promote poor motor patterns and poor posture—for example, rounded shoulders.

Muscle Synergies

This, however, does not mean that machine-based exercises are necessarily bad. The CNS recruits muscles in groups or synergies, allowing movements to be organized in such a way as to reduce unwanted movements. The result is a smooth economical action. Over time and through a sequence of learning synergies, movement becomes more anatomical and fluent. Understanding muscular synergies will enable you to appreciate functional anatomy and related biomechanics. The human body is ultimately designed to provide movement through an integrated and connected system. Physical activities such as exercise and training should reflect this.

Muscle synergies, or "links," organize movement in a coordinated manner to minimize the amount of unwanted movement at a joint or joints. Once a motor pattern has been learned, the CNS will fine-tune and automate this alliance, ensuring its fluency with time and practice; an example of the law of facilitation. For example, a child eating an ice cream cone gets more ice cream on their face than in their mouth. Of course, as they mature and grow, so too does their nervous system. With practice and experience, they learn to accurately place the ice cream in their mouth. This requires timing, coordination, reaction time, balance, and a collective "integration" of neural activity. Ice cream ending up on the face is not the required result, and the child learns from augmented feedback known as "knowledge of results" or "knowledge of performance." These relate specifically to the outcome of a performance and the quality of the overall movement sequence or plan. Of course, relearning how to perform an action in a manner that does not stress the muscular, myofascial, articular, or neural system will require reeducation.

Once a person has established a neuromuscular synergy specific to a task, they will always perform that task utilizing the same muscles in the same sequence. Over time this may pr-dispose that individual to postural adaptations, inappropriate neural activity, muscular inhibition, joint stress, and ultimately injury. In other words, if a person learns to perform something incorrectly, they will always perform it incorrectly. Once the movement or posture is learned, the neurological engram is established, and muscles will be recruited in a specific sequence, the same sequence every time that person performs that task. Learning to do it correctly will feel odd and uncomfortable.

Atrophy

Atrophy of muscles is the progressive loss of muscle mass (or wasting), caused by a reduction in the size or number of muscle cells.

Hypertrophy

Hypertrophy involves an increase in both the size and diameter of muscle fibers. This occurs when the components of muscle fibers, including structures such as mitochondria, increase their size and number/quantity in the sarcomere.

General and Local Adaptation Syndromes

Changes at a local level will in turn affect the larger global picture. Changes are occurring all the time, moment to moment in the human body. Some changes lead to positive adaptations, whilst others create problems, termed "bad gas" (bad general adaptations). The cumulative effect of a small number of local minor areas of stress can result in more global adaptations because of the demands being made on a constant basis.

Inflammation

Inflammation is the body's reaction to tissue injury (figure 4.27). Although it is often seen as something to be avoided, it plays a vital role in the repair of and recovery from injury. Inflammation is a protective facility that provides the first step in repair of damage from burns, cuts, tears, and chemical irritation, as well as invasion by bacteria or viruses.

A potential problem exists in that the rate or level of inflammation is in direct proportion to the extent of trauma the tissue undergoes.

When tissue damage occurs, a series of reactions takes place, including the release of histamine and other inflammatory chemicals such as kinins. This results in vasodilation at the injury site and an increase in permeability of the walls of the capillaries. This increase in blood flow results in a temperature increase and redness. Excess swelling results from changes in the capillary walls that allow blood plasma to escape into the interstitial fluid. This in turn increases the pressure within the affected tissue, irritating special pain receptors (nociceptors) and resulting in pain.

Pain and swelling will obviously limit ROM, which reduces the risk of further damage. The tissue fills with plasma, and an increase in phagocytes and other white blood cells is seen in the damaged tissue. Phagocytes engulf any damaged cellular debris, cleaning the area and removing any foreign invaders that could cause infection. Specialized clotting

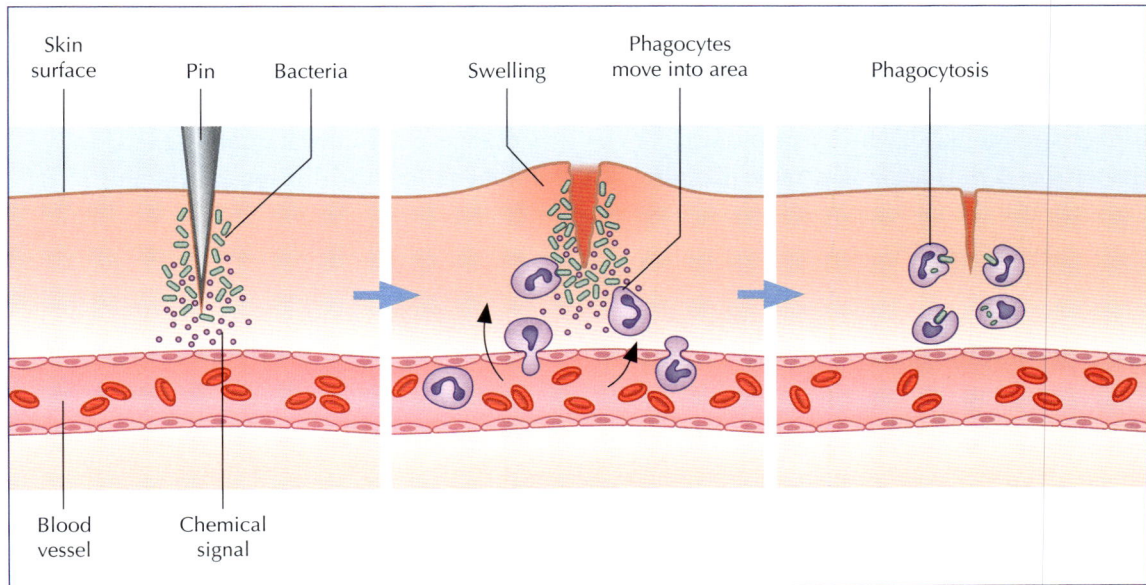

Figure 4.27. The inflammatory process. Courtesy of Emily Evans.

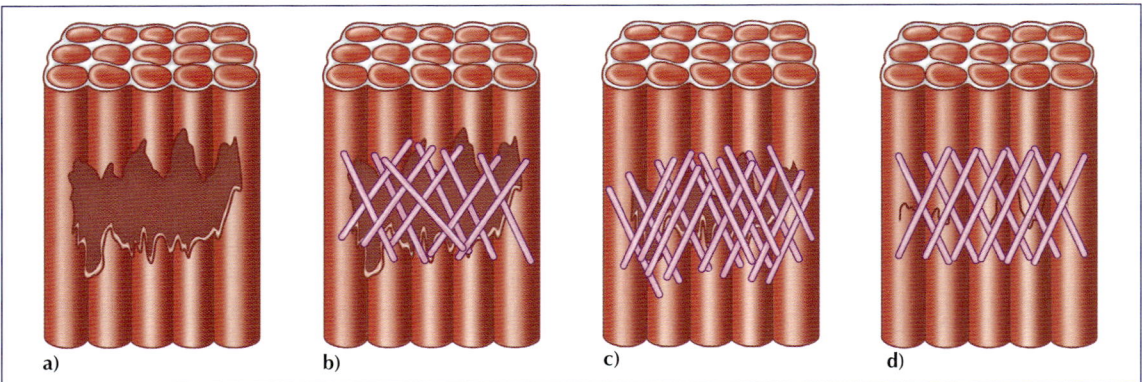

Figure 4.28. Scar tissue: a) tear in the tissue, b) scar tissue lays down in random fashion, c) too much time and lack of movement cause tension to build around area of repair, d) scar tissue better aligned to the natural tension in the tissue.

agents stick together to reduce blood loss and seal any leaks, allowing the tissue to begin regenerating.

As is often the case, the body lays down additional collagen fibers as a specific adaptation to the original tissue damage (figure 4.28). This is a protective mechanism to reduce the risk of injury reoccurring at the same site. However, although the initial collagen is organized along the axis of the muscle fiber arrangement, additional collagen is often unorganized, which leads to scar tissue. This is the reason why movement in the earliest stages of injury recovery, to ensure correct collagen orientation, is so vital. Many people rest the injury for far too long and, in the case of upper limb injuries, may avoid involving the limb in daily activities. This is detrimental and not only prolongs recovery but can lead to increases in scar tissue and loss of ROM.

The sequence of events following tissue injury usually includes muscular splinting or spasm. While the initial inflammation is an integral stage in correct healing, it does need to be controlled. The resulting protective spasm (with possible formation of MTrPs) is the real culprit and needs to be addressed and returned to homeostasis before any additional exertion or physical activities are encouraged. The introduction of exercise without addressing this spasm will only offer temporary relief. Once the physical activities stop, the patient usually finds that their problem returns. The missing link is to treat the spastic tissue first and then reeducate the muscles through graded functional physical challenges.

Patient Assessment and Treatment Protocols

t helpful to keep in mind certain physiological considerations when providing fascia-focused therapy.

Ten Physiological Considerations of Fascia-Focused Therapy

Regardless of our chosen field, whether it's osteopathy, structural integration, medical studies, neuromuscular therapy, physiotherapy, fascia therapy, chiropractic, or massage, our goal is to reshape our perception of muscles and movement. The shift required is from a focus on singular muscles and isolated contractions to acknowledging the involvement of multiple muscles (myofascial synergistic units) in a whole-body kinetic system. In essence, movement isn't a solitary note but a harmonious combination of finely tuned body-wide notes, culminating not just in a singular melody of motion but in a symphony of movement. But specific fascial structures can experience inhibition or hypertonicity, leading to inappropriate neuromuscular patterns, a perspective known as "fascia tuning pegs" (see chapter 3).

As you read through the anatomy and neurophysiology sections, I would like you to consider the sequence and use of neuromuscular, fascia-informed techniques and phased introduction of medical exercise, based on the following models, A and B.

Model A: The Ten Considerations

Considering the following factors when treating a patient can give you a comprehensive and holistic approach to healthcare. Each of these factors plays a role in the overall well-being of the individual. Understanding them can contribute to a more effective and targeted treatment plan. Here is a breakdown of each consideration:

1. Monosynaptic Reflex Arc

Understanding the monosynaptic reflex arc (see figure 3.12) helps in assessing and addressing the body's rapid, involuntary responses to stimuli. This can be crucial in neurologic assessments and rehabilitation.

2. Ischemia

Ischemia refers to inadequate blood supply for current physiological demands. Restoration of appropriate blood supply is essential for healthy, pain-free fascia.

3. Myofascial Trigger Points (MTrPs)

Identifying and addressing myofascial trigger points is crucial in managing myofascial pain. These specific points can mimic neurological and discogenic pain, as well as being a source of headaches and elbow and foot pain. It is essential when treating unresolved chronic pain to give due consideration to the possibility of MTrPs being the true source or a significant contributing factor.

4. Fascial Considerations

Fascia changes morphology and can migrate based on changes in tension and compression.

5. Nerve Insult

Nerve insults, such as compression, stretching, or tethering, can result in various neurological symptoms. Addressing nerve health is crucial in the treatment and management of insults like neuropathies or radiculopathies. Keep in mind the three Ps—places of perilous passage—locations of high risk for nerve compression and adhesions.

6. Posture

Poor posture can contribute to various myofascial issues, affecting the spine, joints, and muscles. The most common posture of the twenty-first century is forward head posture. As a very general statement, postural influences can be a bottom-up or head-down issue, requiring expert intervention from the therapist, who needs to translate the information gained during assessment.

7. Alignment

Proper alignment is crucial for optimal function and movement. Tissues out of alignment fail to receive or dissipate forces in a nutritious or healthy manner.

8. Nutrition/Hydration

Nutrition and hydration are fundamental for overall health. Considering the patient's nutritional habits and fluid intake is essential for promoting healing, tissue repair, and overall well-being.

9. Stress (Strain)

Both physical and psychological stress can impact the body. A little stress is good for all of us; however, too much results in strain on the fascial net; nervous, endocrine, and immune systems; and mental health.

10. The Individual

Recognizing the uniqueness of each patient, including their medical history, lifestyle, and other preferences, is essential for tailoring treatments to their specific needs. A personalized approach contributes to better patient outcomes.

Model B: The Temporal Sequence of Tissue Insults

Injury or insult with resulting protective spasm leads to:

1. reciprocal inhibition,
2. synergistic dominance (altered force couple relationships),
3. arthrokinetic dysfunction (altered joint motion),
4. neuromuscular inefficiency,
5. myofascial fatigue,
6. cumulative injury cycle.

Changes in posture coupled with repetitive movements can be the basis for dysfunction in the myofascial and musculoskeletal systems and the formation of MTrPs. The fascia-focused approach is to achieve optimum neuromuscular efficiency by restoring length-tension relationships, force couple relationships, and correct arthrokinetics. When postural alignment is not correct, the body will not effectively cope or deal with the forces generated through its tissues. Rather than being effectively dissipated, these forces will now provide ongoing traumas throughout the myofascial and osseofascial systems, not only resulting in faulty movement patterns but also causing excessive breakdown or overproduction of tissues. The result is pain and changes in sensation (e.g., numbness, itching, tingling, or burning).

This text teaches that certain myofascial tissues become hypertonic when stressed, resulting in an inhibition of others. In turn, this creates muscular imbalances, which must first be identified and treated before the patient is encouraged to challenge the muscles through physical activity. To appreciate the wonderful techniques of fascia-focused therapy, and other modalities, will require an expert understanding of anatomy, and so this is where we will start.

Patient Assessment

Before prescribing medical exercise, such as in a rehabilitative program, or performing any type of fascia-focused therapy, conduct a complete and comprehensive patient assessment, including a kinetic postural assessment and a detailed patient health history.

The cornerstone of any assessment must be to include a postural component. Of course, motivational interviewing is essential to get to know your client or patient. There is little point in asking a patient to participate in water-based physical activities if they do not like being in water. It is vital to listen to your patient. Discover what they wish to achieve, their likes and dislikes, and their current daily tasks. This will allow both of you to identify an appropriate, effective, yet safe rehabilitative medical exercise program that fits their lifestyle. Realistic goals can be identified within an appropriate time frame.

A framework is required, involving testing muscles for shortness, relative weakness, ROM, neuromuscular reflexes, and postural (a)symmetry. Such deficiencies may be the cause of, or a contributor to, pain and change in respiratory function. Nutritional and psychosocial influences should also be considered.

Muscles that shorten owing to stress include gastrocnemius, soleus, the adductors, psoas major, tensor fasciae latae, rectus femoris, piriformis, quadratus lumborum, erector spinae, pectoralis major/minor, teres major, upper trapezius, levator scapulae, and SCM.

Muscles that tend to be inhibited include tibialis anterior/posterior, serratus anterior, vastus medialis oblique, middle/lower trapezius, articularis genu, the rhomboids, transversus abdominis, teres minor, internal oblique, infraspinatus, multifidus, posterior deltoid, and the deep cervical muscles.

Ask your patient to shade in areas of pain referral or changes in sensation on the silhouette (figure 5.1). This will provide a visual aid in determining which muscles

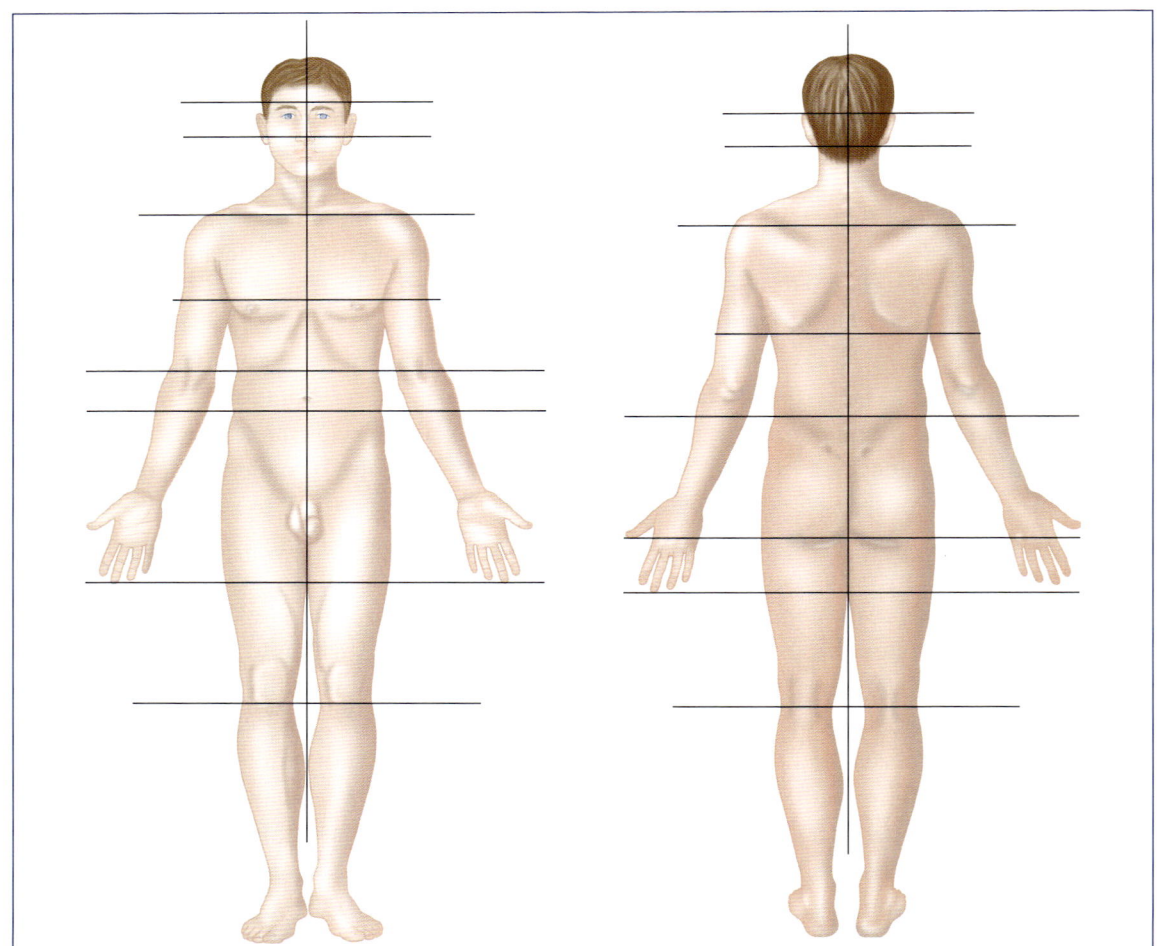

Figure 5.1. Body outlines on which the patient should shade areas of pain referral or changes in sensation.

may be housing MTrPs responsible for, or adding to, the patient's condition.

Training Principles

Physical activities can provide health and/or skill-related components of fitness. Our primary focus in rehabilitation is to provide the correct mix to offer improved joint health and neuromuscular efficiency. Consideration must be given to the principles of progressive overload, specificity, reversibility, variation, and individual difference.

Progressive Overload

An appropriate physical activity is provided to produce optimal physical, physiological, and performance adaptations. A program of medical exercise will provide the effective and safe level of physical effort to ensure appropriate progressive adaptations. The components include the volume (number of repetitions and sets), intensity, contraction velocity, muscle action, recovery period, training frequency, plane of motion, exercise selection, and order of performance.

Specificity

Adaptations that occur owing to physical activity are specific to the kinematic and kinetic demands placed on the person. The outcomes of the chosen activities will be specifically related to the motor unit synchronization, rate coding, motor unit involvement, and rate of force production (neuromuscular specificity).

Choosing movements that mimic, or are related to, the patient's daily activities ensures improved movement patterns that are relevant to their lives. This is known as *specific adaptation to imposed demands*, or SAID.

Reversibility

This principle has two variations on the theme. The first refers to the loss of gained improvements and neuromuscular efficiency should the patient cease their involvement in physical activity. The second refers to reversing the status of damaged, weak, or dysfunctional tissues to homeostasis/allostasis. Once successful rehabilitation has occurred, the focus of physical activity can be to maintain neuromuscular efficiency and provide the basis for a reduced risk of injury in the future.

Variation

Changes are required concerning the type of stimulus provided. Changes involving speed of movement (acceleration and deceleration) and stabilization within all planes of motion should be provided. Medical exercise should provide the patient with the multiplanar, multidimensional training necessary to ensure a progressive and systematic scale of physical activities.

Individual Difference

Designing a medical exercise program requires consideration of the patient's needs and realistic goals. Consideration, therefore, must be given to their age, medical and health status (and history, including injuries), and gender. Consider the following points for progressing a program of physical activity:

- Set up the program with simple, familiar movements and progress to more complex ones involving all three planes of motion.
- Begin with simple static challenges and progress to more dynamic movements.
- Move slowly at first, then add speed.
- Provide tactile, visual, and verbal support to ensure effective and appropriate force couples.
- Low forces are appropriate for beginners, rising to high forces.
- Start with one arm movement, and then progress to both arms.
- Begin with two leg movements and progress to one leg.
- Initiate with stable surface movements, moving on to unstable surfaces.
- Once your client/patient loses form, the exercise is finished. Remember that it is not about repetitions. It is quality not quantity.
- Ensure your patients avoid breath holding.
- Avoid static stretching and encourage dynamic range of movement (DROM).
- Hands must be properly washed with soap and lukewarm water and be clean before every session.

General Standards and Guidelines

Step 1

A health history questionnaire with signed consent is required. The therapist should discuss the treatment with the client/patient and provide a reasonable description of what they should expect from and during the session. If a client has a history of blood pressure, coronary heart disease, or any other life-threatening chronic illness, they must get clearance, in writing, from their doctor.

The therapist or medical exercise specialist must be aware of any medications the client is taking, because of the impact certain medications can have on the patient's physiology and metabolism. The patient's doctor should be consulted for any special guidelines or contraindications. Learning about your patient's health history provides you with vital information to help you make the best-informed decisions regarding treatment strategies and appropriate physical activities and tasks.

For example, low back pain can cause decreased neural control of stabilizing muscles to the lumbo-pelvic-hip (LPH) complex, resulting in reduced stabilization of the vertebral column. Injuries to the lower limb, in particular the ankle, may decrease neural control of gluteus maximus and medius, while shoulder injury is related to neuromuscular retardation of the SITS muscles. Any letters or documents pertaining to your client/patient should be affixed to their file. It is imperative to tell patients that the treatment can lead to a feeling of soreness sometime afterward (usually the next day). This must also be provided in written form and signed by the patient.

A Few Words on Client Records

Your clients' records are strictly private and confidential, and they are, in effect, the clients' property. You can share their information with other professionals only once your client has given you written permission to do so. All records must be secured under lock and key and must be retained for no less than seven years (please check with a professional authority in your geographical location for guidelines specific to licensing). All patients and clients must give written consent to participate in fascia-focused therapy and state they have had all their questions and concerns adequately addressed. It is worth repeating that therapists must inform the patient/client both verbally and in writing that treatment using NMTq can result in tissues feeling sore during or sometime after the treatment. The therapist must have the client sign a consent form to that effect.

Step 2

Interview your patient regarding their reason for treatment. It is essential to get a clear picture of what the patient requires and to ascertain if those expectations are both within your scope of practice and realistic. At this stage the patient should shade in any areas of pain or heightened sensation on the silhouette provided. A red felt-tip pen should be used for this purpose. This information can provide a visual impression of the patient's experienced pain patterns or change in sensation. These may also provide a link to MTrP referral patterns.

Step 3

Postural assessment and kinematic system evaluation begins the moment you meet your patient. Careful observation of your patient's movements, and static posture, can provide valuable insights. You should observe the manner in which your patient walks. For example, do the arms swing evenly with a matched pace and rhythm, or is one arm held short, or perhaps closer to the body? When standing still, do the arms hang down by the side with the hands semi-supinated and the little finger in line with the seam of their trousers? Observe the space between the line of the elbow and rib cage. Is more light seen through one side than the other?

Anatomical landmarks can be used to assess symmetry. Very small differences exist in all of us, but significant differences can help identify short, spastic, or hypertonic tissues and assist in recognizing inhibited muscles.

To help your patient avoid feeling self-conscious, the use of distractions can be helpful. Ask your patient to march on the spot for sixty seconds, and then repeat this with their eyes closed. On stopping, some patients have a tendency to pull their body up and suck their tummy in. Turning your patient around while their eyes are closed can result in a slight disorientation and often allows a more realistic image of their true posture to be witnessed. Global and local compensations may be identified standing 10 to 15 feet (3–4.5 m) away from the patient.

Postural Considerations

Examples might include head tilt, forward head, rotated head, shoulder level difference, pro/retracted shoulder girdle, standing on one leg in preference to the other, locked knees, accentuated or flat spinal curves, scoliosis, level of the ends of fingers with arms hanging by the side, kneecap positioning, flat feet, or feet turned out/in.

Anterior Midsagittal Plane

Includes the nasal septum, sternum, belly button (umbilicus), and symphysis pubis.

Anterior Transverse Horizontal Plane

Includes the crown of the head, eyes, ears, acromion, anterior superior iliac spine (ASIS), crest of the ilium, crease of the elbows, tips of fingers, patellae, head of fibula, and medial malleolus.

Coronal Plane

Includes the auditory meatus, head of humerus, greater trochanter, head of fibula, lateral malleolus, and ASIS relative to posterior superior iliac spine (PSIS).

Posterior Midsagittal Plane

Includes the occipital protuberance, spinal processes, sacral tubercles, and coccyx.

Posterior Transverse Horizontal Plane

Includes the acromioclavicular (AC) joints, inferior angles of scapulae, crest of ilium, PSIS, gluteal fold, creases of knee, and straight calcaneal tendon.

Two calibrated scales can be used side by side, with the patient standing on the scales with one foot on each scale. Weight bearing should be bilaterally close to even, although a small differential is normal (optimal posture is being sought). Significant differences to look out for include:

- Is the head erect or leaning/turning to one side?
- Are both eyes level?
- Are both ears level (mastoid process)?
- Is the distance between the ear lobe and the acromion symmetrical bilaterally?
- Is the nose straight?
- Does the midline of the mandible track in a smooth and straight (vertical) line when opening and closing?
- Are the AC joints level?
- Is there any obvious internal/external rotation regarding the position of the arms?
- Is there a slight bend in the elbows?
- Are the fingertips level?
- Are the hands slightly pronated with the dorsal surfaces facing 45 degrees anteriorly?
- Are the fingers relaxed and slightly curved?
- Is the space between the arm and torso bilaterally symmetrical?
- Is the general appearance of the torso balanced?
- Is the rib cage bilaterally symmetrical?

- Is the distance between the inferior angle of the ribs and the iliac crest even on both sides?
- Is the ASIS level on both sides?
- Are the greater trochanters level with each other?
- Do the patellar bones look even, level, and symmetrical?
- Are the anterior fibular heads level?
- Are the malleoli even?
- Do the feet look turned in/out?
- Are the arches normal/high/fallen?

Step 4

Implementation of a treatment plan based on stages 1, 2, and 3, including supportive medical exercise for rehabilitative purposes.

Massage

Massage is a useful adjunct to fascia-focused therapy, as a preparatory intervention to warm up tissues, to disassociate stuck, convoluted, or adhered tissues, to increase blood supply, to lower sympathetic tone, or to influence fascia. It can be used in the intermediate stage to complement fascia interventions or to finish a treatment.

Massage can be dangerous if used in the wrong or inappropriate situation, such as with cancer conditions, stroke, or osteoporosis to name a few. In the case of cancer, due to new research, I recommend that cancer patients should not receive massage. Some massage techniques, such as friction, are used to break down fibrotic or scarred tissues and can cause local inflammation. This approach requires

much skill and knowledge and should not inflict undue pain on the patient. The notion of sticking an elbow deep into a patient's muscle and frictioning the tissues is enough to make anyone cringe. This is a dangerous and uninformed way to treat tissues. It will in most cases lead to inappropriate tissue damage, irritation, bruising, and increased stress for the patient.

Fascia-focused therapists should, when appropriate, make use of T-bars to apply ischemic pressure and/or mild friction, rather than developing repetitive strain injury to their own thumbs and fingers. T-bars are relatively inexpensive and can be purchased on the internet.

Massage includes variations on the following techniques.

Effleurage

These are generally warming techniques with a broad surface such as the palm of the hands. Techniques can be fast, slow, long, or short, depending on the desired physiological effect. Faster and shorter are stimulating, while slower and longer are more relaxing. Other variations include faltering, compressive, or combined. Friction is created between the therapist's hands and the patient's skin. The less oil or cream that is used, the greater the frictioning effect.

Petrissage

These include a multitude of variations, such as gently lifting muscles up and away from the bones, rolling, and squeezing muscles. Petrissage generally involves kneading and compression motions to enhance deeper circulation. These techniques help to stimulate circulation and assist clearing out of energy by-products from muscle and nerve tissue.

Tapotement

This consists of briskly applied percussive movements, using the hands alternately to strike or tap the muscles, to provide an invigorating effect. There are numerous variations on this stroke, including using the edge of the hand, the tips of the fingers, or a closed fist. Tapotement attempts to release tension and cramping from muscles in spasm.

Neuromuscular Laws

The fascia-focused therapist provides a physical therapy operating under a system of neurological laws. These laws illustrate both acute and chronic pain patterns and demonstrate how pain is dispersed throughout the body. The nervous system is designed to produce normal muscle tonus at thirty stimuli per second. If the nervous system is suddenly innervating the damaged tissues, because of trauma, at perhaps seventy-five stimuli per second, it must respond in a more creative, allostatic way to distribute the pain.

The Law of Unilaterality

If a mild irritation is applied to one or more sensory nerves, the movement will take place

usually on one side only, which is side that is irritated.

As an illustration, if a person were involved in a myofascial insult injuring their left hip and they did not receive treatment, the hip area would be painful within a relatively short period of time.

If they continue without treatment and take a painkiller and perhaps a hot shower to ease the pain, not only would the initial injury site still be in pain the following day, but so equally would be the and opposite side. This illustrates the second law, the law of symmetry.

The Law of Symmetry

If the stimulation is sufficiently increased, the motor reaction is manifested not only to the irritated side but also in similar muscles on the opposite side of the body.

From a practical perspective, if a fascia therapist can treat the unaffected side, it is possible that the injured, painful area can be addressed to some degree without initial direct application of fascia therapy to that side.

Without correct treatment of this injury, the pain would now have intensified at the original injury site, with a lesser pain present on the contralateral hip. This describes the third law, the law of intensity.

The Law of Intensity

Reflex movements are usually more intense on the side of irritation; at times the movements of the opposite side equal them in intensity, but they are usually less pronounced.

The fourth law is the law of radiation.

The Law of Radiation

If the excitation continues to increase it is propagated upward, and reactions take place through centrifugal nerves coming from the cord segments higher up.

This means that the pain will radiate upward from the site of the original injury toward the brain and then, failing alleviation, will radiate outward, creating a general contraction of all the muscles in the body.

If left untreated, the patient would at some future time find it difficult to move without pain or be unable to move without intense headache, accompanied by a general contraction of all the myofascial tissues from head to toe (e.g., fibromyalgia). The nervous and myofascial systems would now be adversely affected, including all other systems in the body, such as the respiratory, cardiovascular, lymphatic, digestive, and endocrine systems. This illustrates the fifth law, the law of generalization.

The Law of Generalization

If the irritation becomes very intense, it is propagated in the medulla oblongata, which becomes the focus from which the stimuli radiate to all parts of the cord, causing a general contraction of all the muscles of the body.

Acute injury (i.e., compression), chronic injury (i.e., repetitive micro trauma), muscle imbalances, joint dysfunctions, and poor posture provide the foundation for negative changes in pose and compromise the integrity of neurofascial tissues. The neurogenic reflex mechanism is initiated by tissue trauma, as is the cumulative injury cycle. Such changes result in morphological disturbances at the micro level, leading to chemical irritation from intraneural edema, tissue hypoxia, microvascular starvation, and the formation of MTrPs.

Other laws include:

The Law of Facilitation

When a neuron takes its course through a specific group of neurons to the exclusion of others it will tend to repeat the same course on future occasions, and each time it travels this pathway the resistance decreases. Facilitation occurs when a pool of neurons (premotor neurons, motor neurons, or in spinal regions preganglionic sympathetic neurons) are in a state of partial or subthreshold excitation. This results in a lesser degree of afferent stimulation being required to trigger the discharge of impulses.

Arndt-Schultz's Law

Weak stimuli excite physiologic activity, moderately strong ones favor it, and strong ones retard it. Very strong ones arrest it.

Davis's Law

Ligaments or any soft tissue when placed under even a moderate degree of tension will elongate by the addition of new material, if that tension is unremitting. Conversely, when ligaments or other soft tissues remain uninterruptedly in a loose or lax state, they will gradually shorten, as the effete (by-product) material is removed, until they come to maintain the same relationship to the bony structures with which they are united as they did before their stretching.

Head's Law

A painful stimulus applied to a body part of low sensitivity (such as an organ), when in close central connection (i.e., the same segmental supply) with an area of higher sensitivity (such as a part of the soma), will cause pain to be felt at the point of higher intensity rather than where the stimulus was applied.

Hilton's Law

A nerve trunk that supplies a joint also supplies the muscles of the joint and the skin over the insertions of those muscles. Each nerve root also serves blood vessels, organs, and glands. Therefore, excitation along a nerve pathway to any of these tissues can spill over to facilitate the other tissues also served by that nerve, creating dysfunction or pain in those secondary tissues as well. For example, excitation to a diseased gallbladder could excite the muscles overlying the area, which are innervated by the same nerve that serves that organ.

Hooke's Law

The stress used to stretch or compress a body is proportional to the strain, as long as the elastic limits of the body have not been exceeded.

Sherrington's Law

Every posterior spinal nerve root supplies a specific region of the skin (a dermatome), which is invaded above and below by fibers from the adjacent spinal segments (figure 5.2).

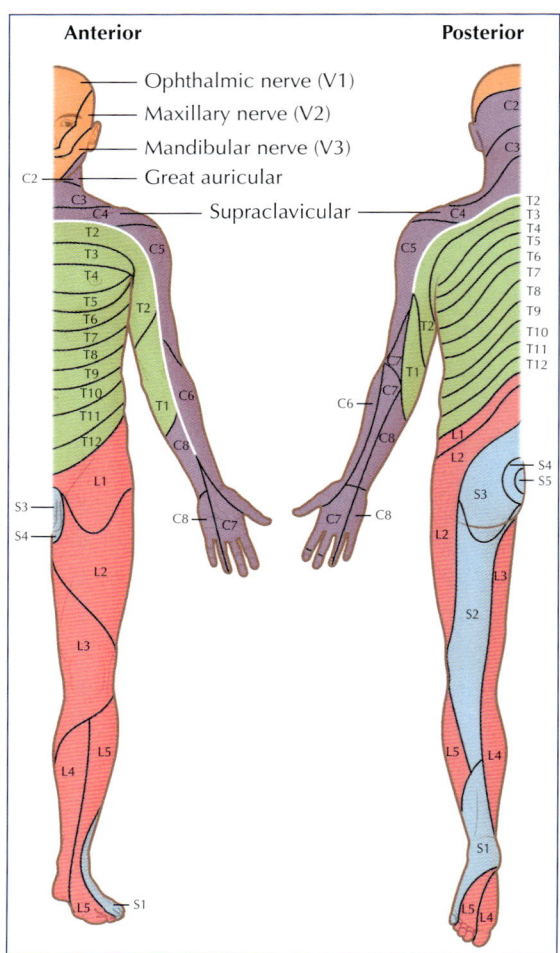

Figure 5.2. Anterior and posterior dermatomes.

Wolff's Law

Every change in the form and function of a bone, or in its function alone, is followed by certain definite changes in its internal architecture and secondary alterations in its external conformation; these changes usually represent responses to alterations in weight-bearing stresses.

Use of Oils, Creams, Sprays, and Lotions

Before attempting any of the techniques outlined below, to avoid the risk of anaphylactic episodes, the fascia-focused therapist must ensure that their patient has no known adverse reaction to topical applications. In any circumstance, a small sample of the oil or cream to be used (if needed) can be applied to the surface of the skin before a larger amount is applied.

A common mistake made by therapists concerns the application of heat creams. One can imagine that, depending on the circumstances—for example, a pre-event massage—a therapist might want to apply a heat-producing topical cream to several individuals. Some athletes look for such applications before a competition. The problem lies in the fact that one application to one individual is fine, but if the therapist is applying the cream to several people, the therapist too is absorbing the cream into their body with each application. Steps need to be taken to avoid this, such as wearing latex-free gloves.

Always consult an athlete's doctor, trainer, or coach regarding the use of any creams, sprays, or oils. Some oils, creams, or sprays, used unwittingly by therapists, have been discovered to contain banned substances. It is often best if the athlete provides you with a cream or oil of their own choice.

Neuromuscular Techniques

The term *neuromuscular techniques* (NMTq) should be understood to refer to the assessment and treatment of local myofascial dysfunction, mainly involving MTrPs, fascia dysfunction, tender points, areas of congestion, scar tissue, fibrosis, edema, hypersensitivity, and numbness utilizing finger and/or thumb techniques.

NMTq start in the assessment mode (in the chronic stage) but can, at any stage, move to a treatment mode as the therapist sees fit. NMTq are used to identify altered states in the tissues beneath the thumb or fingers of the therapist. Digital pressure (ischemic pressure) and strokes are used to locate, identify, and treat focal points. Engaging the tissues by meeting and matching the return tension, the therapist combs the tissues, observing any differences in tissue texture, sensitivity, contour, temperature, moisture, and pain points, whilst encouraging feedback from the patient. In particular, a VAS (visual analog scale) should be established (0–10) for the level of pain or discomfort or change in sensation experienced by the patient (figure 5.3). The fascia-focused therapist should work at a level that causes mild discomfort (5–8) and avoid major pain (9–10 plus).

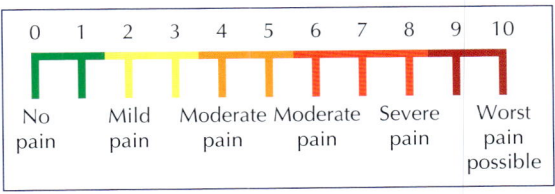

Figure 5.3. The VAS for pain measurement.

It is important to avoid rushing when using NMTq. The tissues will begin to melt beneath the therapist's fingers, allowing deeper tissues to be palpated and investigated. NMTq is excellent for identifying MTrPs, as they are located in the muscle fibers. When using the thumb technique, the fingers act as a fulcrum or axis around which the thumb moves (figure 5.4a).

Search the tissues over a 4-inch surface area at a time (approximately 1.5 seconds every 4 inches), then move the fingers to the next position in whatever direction the therapist wishes to direct the thumb. Forces running through the thumb should run down the long axis of the arm (figure 5.4b). These forces are generated in the lower limbs and translated through the core to the arm.

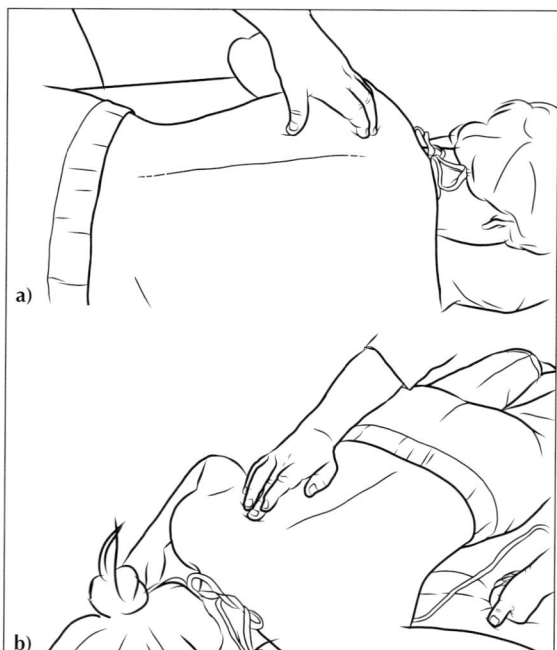

Figure 5.4. (a) Thumb drag technique: the digital/ thumb method utilizes four aspects of the thumb with various degrees of pressure to assess or treat areas of induration, tenderness, or myofascial trigger points. (b) Single drag technique: the middle finger is used to apply gentle uniform traction to the skin over a 4-inch (10 cm) area for 4 seconds, and this is repeated a number of times.

Muscle Energy Techniques

Muscle energy techniques (MET) are gentle resistive applications where the patient is requested to provide a gentle contraction of specific myofascial synergists, from a precisely controlled position in a specific direction, against a mild (25–30 percent) counterforce for a specific period of time (usually 10 seconds).

Types of contractions (figure 5.5) include:

Isometric Contraction

The distance between the origin and insertion remains the same. No movement occurs; the muscle fibers shorten but only initially.

Isotonic Concentric Contraction

The length of the muscle shortens. The patient gently overcomes the resistance offered by the therapist.

Isotonic Eccentric Contraction

This is also called an *isolytic contraction*— whereby the length of the myofascial tissue increases. The patient allows the therapist to overcome their resistance through a specific ROM. This variation is the most intense

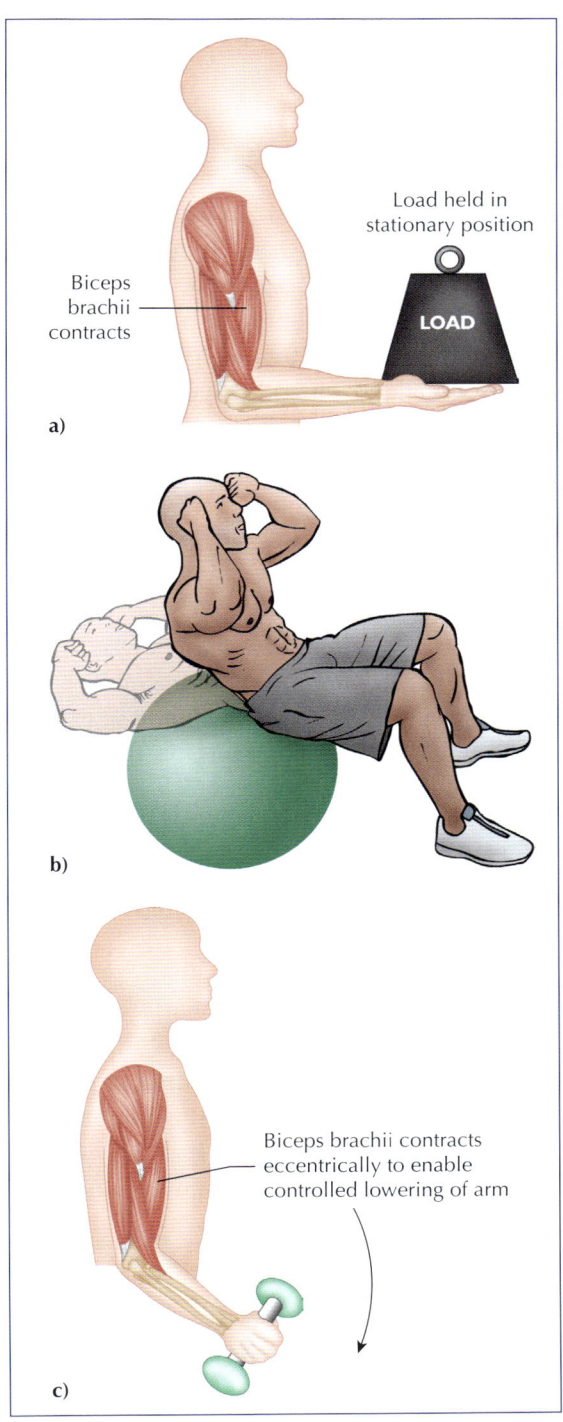

and can lead to slight structural damage (if performed correctly) as adhesions are broken down. As already stated, some soreness may be expected after treatment.

MET require the patient to have the capacity to offer a gentle force against a specific resistance of low intensity provided by the therapist (figure 5.6). Having established the first barrier (the first sign of resistance to movement), within a specific ROM in a specific plane, a number of variations can be used, depending on whether the situation is acute or chronic. In an acute situation, a low-intensity contraction is requested from the position where the first sense of restriction is perceived (targeting type 1 fibers).

In the chronic stage this barrier should be avoided, and the therapist should back off a small amount to provide the patient with a contractile advantage. MET techniques are

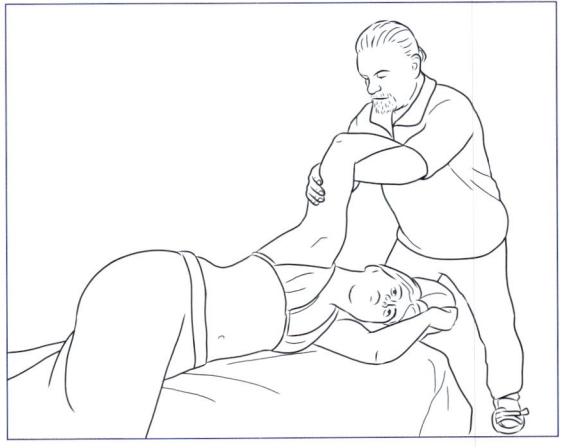

Figure 5.6. With the patient in a side-lying position, the therapist stands at the head of the plinth and supports the patient's upper limb using the opposite upper limb. The therapist takes the humerus through abduction and adduction at the glenohumeral joint, assessing for the first area of bind.

Figure 5.5. Contraction examples: (a) isometric contraction; (b) isotonic concentric contraction; (c) isotonic eccentric contraction.

slightly different when a joint is the target. When treating a joint (or in the acute stage) no increase in length is employed following a mild contraction.

Most muscle energy procedures use post-isometric relaxation (PIR). After an isometric contraction, there is a refractory period during which passive lengthening of the target muscle may be achieved without strong resistance from the target muscle owing to lowered muscle spindle activity (figure 5.7).

Another popular variation on the theme is reciprocal inhibition (RI). This takes advantage of the fact that when a target myofascial synergy's antagonists are contracted, the target myofascial synergies are inhibited and therefore reduce contractile forces (figure 5.7). One example of this is a contraction of the quadriceps muscles to inhibit the hamstring muscles.

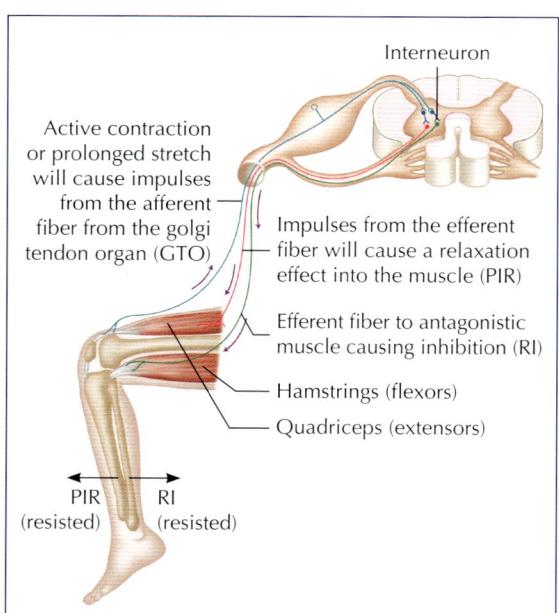

Active contraction or prolonged stretch will cause impulses from the afferent fiber from the golgi tendon organ (GTO)

Interneuron

Impulses from the efferent fiber will cause a relaxation effect into the muscle (PIR)

Efferent fiber to antagonistic muscle causing inhibition (RI)

Hamstrings (flexors)

Quadriceps (extensors)

PIR (resisted)   RI (resisted)

Figure 5.7. Post-isometric relaxation and reciprocal inhibition.

Indications for MET

- To mobilize restricted joints
- To return normal length to shortened muscles and fascia
- To return neuromuscular efficiency to an asymmetrically weak, or inhibited, muscle or to decrease hypertonicity
- To improve circulation, respiration, and neuromuscular relationships
- To provide therapeutic input to rectify a more distal pain in the kinetic system

Contraindications for MET

MET are not advised if pathology is suspected; for example, if there is a fracture or other serious bone health pathology. The neuromuscular therapist should refer for accurate diagnosis to be established. Once a diagnosis has been confirmed, the correct level or intensity of application can be tailored to suit the specific situation—for example, arthritis, osteoporosis, and so on.

Following a mild contraction, it is advisable to allow a rest period of about five seconds so that the patient's muscles can reduce in tone and to allow for the dissipation of any contractile residue before lengthening. In acute settings the physical therapist should avoid stretching or lengthening the muscle after the contraction phase.

Pulsed MET

This method requires a series of rapid, yet gentle, pulsating contractions against a resistance provided by the therapist.

A contraction rate of one every second is usually sufficient. The therapist can work at one specific angle to the joint or move slowly through a range by gently overcoming the patient and slowly moving the limb or body part through a new ROM. It may be useful to provide some support to the limb to ensure the patient does not overexert. Some body parts are better suited than others for this technique. Patients can be instructed to perform this technique at home if appropriate. Stretching of the tissues following the contractile effort is optional. Patients should be encouraged to avoid holding their breath. Correct positioning of the targeted limb will ensure a mechanical advantage and will allow the patient to provide a contraction without additional stress to the tissue or related joint(s).

Upper-Crossed Syndrome: A New View

In upper-crossed (and, indeed, the same will apply in lower-crossed) syndrome, both the short and lengthened myofascial synergies will be weaker than their potential (figure 5.8). In other books, the muscle relationship in upper-crossed syndrome is described as one muscle being tight and short, while opposing muscles are weak.

It is important to realize that both will be weak. One muscle will be short, spastic, or contracted and weak—for example, pectoralis major and minor, upper trapezius, levator scapulae, and SCM—while the opposing muscle will be inhibited, lengthened, tight, and weak: lower and middle trapezius, deep neck flexors, serratus anterior, and rhomboids.

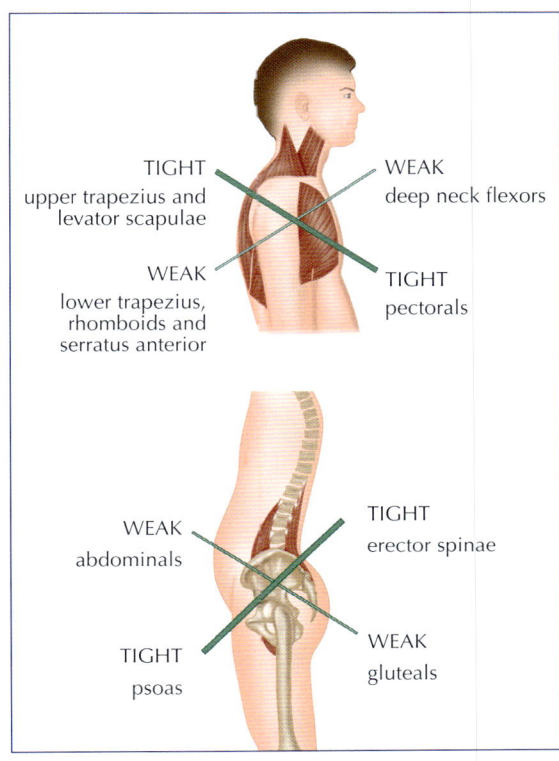

Figure 5.8. Upper- and lower-crossed syndrome.

The following occurs in kinetic-system terms when the upper-crossed pattern is noted: Occiput with C1 (atlas) and C2 (axis) hyperextend, with the head translating anteriorly. The lower cervical vertebrae down to the fourth thoracic vertebra are now stressed. Rotation and abduction of the scapula occurs as the upper trapezius and levator scapulae become shortened and hypertonic (contracted, contractured, or spastic). As a result, the scapula loses stability, which places excess demands on the humerus, now involving the levator scapulae, upper trapezius, and supraspinatus to maintain functional efficiency. This will predispose the person to increased risk of rotator cuff injury, shoulder instability, biceps tendinitis, thoracic outlet/inlet syndrome, and headaches.

Further Kinetic-System Implications

With the neck in hyperextension and the scapula rotated and abducted, this rounds out the shoulders and closes down the anterior chest wall, reducing the possibility of a full functional breath, and compresses the viscera and abdominal contents. Erector spinae will be inhibited, and the deep cervical muscles—including the anterior and middle scalenes—will be shortened. Short scalenes will have an effect of pulling up the first and second ribs, while SCM pulls the clavicle. This pulling up will be opposed by a pulling down by the psoas muscles, causing an internal rotation to the femur, and the resulting change in the lower kinetic system in the lower limb affecting the position of the feet.

In fascia-focused therapy, we will identify the short muscles first using special tests and then offer interventions that will have a muscle-spindle deactivation and GTO response (includes slow, deep ischemic work, MET, and PR). The inhibited muscle requires stimulation of the muscle spindles. This work may include placing the target muscle under lengthening and then stimulating or firing up the muscle spindles with up-tempo techniques such as hacking or cupping.

Positional Release and Strain/ Counterstrain (SCS)

Movement is life, and sleeping is an activity involving movement. If you were to see a time-lapsed recording of a person sleeping, you would see that sleep is far from being inactive or static. On the contrary, we shift and move into and out of various positions.

Many of us start our sleep in some version of the fetal position. During the night, we move many times, rotating, turning, twisting, bending, and so on. (In my opinion this is mother nature's version of PR). This could be seen as a "resetting" of the neuromuscular programming, or parameters, after an active day.

Ruffini receptors are located in the joint capsules and report aspects of joint position and velocity, as well as direction of movements (see figure 4.22). This information is dealt with by higher brain function within the cerebral cortex and therefore has no direct influence at the local segmental level. The GTOs and muscle spindles previously mentioned deal with tension and moment-to-moment changes in length and velocity (respectively) of muscles. GTOs and muscle spindles are connected directly to the spinal cord by gamma and alpha neurons, providing influence specifically at the local spinal level. The muscle spindle is of primary concern in PR and SCS.

Neuromuscular feedback systems, including the muscle spindles, GTOs, and Ruffini receptors, are at the core of many somatic spasm and pain disorders. Ruffini receptors are located within the joint capsule, and are responsive to position, velocity, and direction of motion. Sudden changes in the rate of change in length of muscle lead to larger than normal neural discharges, with tissue tearing, resulting in an immediate contractile response ending in a spastic muscle. The parameters of homeostasis specific to the resting length of the muscle will now be changed. Any attempt to lengthen the already short muscle will result in acute intense pain.

In effect, the muscle now thinks it is already lengthened and any attempt to increase its length will result in considerable neural loading, resulting in pain. This tissue damage leads to the release of chemical substances such as prostaglandins, thromboxanes, leukotrienes, phosphate, neurotoxins, and monohydroxy fatty acids. These in turn promote the inflammatory response with consequential hyperalgesia, resulting in vasoconstriction. The local environment now floods with leukocytes, complement activators, and pain-producing neuropeptides including histamines, serotonin, and bradykinins.

PR methods ensure a relaxation of the local tissues at the site of the insult or injury. Removal of excessive tension leads to an improvement in blood supply at the specific local level, while providing the opportunity to reset the neuromuscular feedback mechanisms by placing them in a neurological sleep. Increased nutrient blood supply and improved interstitial circulation help to remove the chemical soup of noxious stimulators and mediators of inflammation. The resulting reduction in tissue tension and guarding reflexes contributes to additional decreases in the release of such substances.

PR and SCS techniques are wonderfully simple in their delivery and have amazing potential for restoring pain-free ROM.

An individual segment of the spinal cord can become inundated with neural activity. Neural researchers have found that if the volume or amplitude of impulses from proprioceptors, nociceptors, and higher centers channeled to a specific segment exceeds the capacity of the normal routing pathway, the electrochemical discharges may begin to affect collateral pathways. This is termed *spillover*.

Spillover of neural activity can be exerted ipsilaterally, contralaterally, or vertically. Impulses arising from any tissue feedback into the local segment can reach a threshold that once surpassed begins to be misinterpreted by the CNS. For example, efferent impulses intended to register as pain in the gallbladder could be felt as pain in the shoulder.

As stated previously, the simple reflex arc (see figure 3.12) is the foundation of many pain syndromes that will not resolve without the hands-on intervention of a qualified physical therapist. Spillover from excessive discharge due to irritated muscle-spindle activity and other receptors provides the self-perpetuating source of irritation and pain. PR and SCS provide a damping effect on the level of neural excitability within a specific segment, allowing the possibility of a return to homeostasis.

In my early years, Leon Chaitow emphasized the need to understand numerous variations of PR and SCS to meet the various needs of patients in different settings. In PR/SCS, neuromuscular therapists generally use verbal feedback from the patient (if the patient cannot give verbal feedback, other methods can be employed, such as visually indicating the level with one, two, or more fingers as appropriate) as to the level or intensity of pain and/or tenderness of a pain point, located with the use of finger or thumb neuromuscular techniques. This may or may not be a MTrP—it may simply be a painful point in a muscle or tissue. The therapist uses this verbal feedback to act as a monitor as they guide the body part or limb into a position of reduced pain and/or ease.

Other methods employed by the neuromuscular therapist do not necessarily rely on verbal feedback but rather the therapist must "plug into" the tissues, palpating, seeking, listening, and recognizing a position of ease, with their "listening" hands or fingers becoming an intelligent extension of their brain. Palpatory skill development is the key to accurate assessment of myofascial involvement. Palpation pressure must be consistent throughout the treatment and is useful for assessment of tender or pain points, but is not required during the release or after 16 seconds.

It is not always necessary to have a pain point, such as in PR variations. PR involves the positioning of a patient's limb(s), muscle, fascia, or body part into a position where inappropriately tense, hypertonic, short, indurated (spastic), or contractured tissue is placed in a position of comfort (ease) and away from resistance barriers (bind). This provides the potential for a return of normal neurovascular activity. Achieving this therapeutic response requires expert knowledge of anatomy and palpation skills, coupled with knowledge of neurophysiology and circulation dynamics. One must appreciate the subtle differences of PR/SCS to individualize a treatment strategy unique to the patient's circumstances and needs.

This book will not include the many variations of PR/SCS, such as mobilization with movement, PR taping, and so on (Chaitow 2006).

When a sudden unaccustomed increase in muscle length occurs, a combination of neurological and circulatory changes can take place. Due to instant proprioceptive reactions, a change to the resting length of the muscles opposite those that were actively contracting at the time of perceived pain might occur. The resulting muscular spasm is known as the *primary afferent muscle spindle response*. The result is contradictory proprioceptive feedback.

The muscle's proprioceptors now reset their parameters, recording the new short status of the muscle as being lengthened. Any attempt to lengthen the now spastic muscle results in a protective reflexive contraction and pain. This spasm creates an ischemic environment—depriving the fibers of sufficient oxygen—resulting in hypoxia. Over time, this can lead to the formation of MTrPs. Vasoneuroactive substances, including bradykinins, phosphates, prostaglandins, and others, create neural sensitization (both spinal-segmental and local) by means of a process known as *facilitation*. Coupled with high levels of inorganic phosphates and lactates, the muscle's acidity rises, causing further hypersensitivity to touch. I refer to this as the "production versus removal dilemma," meaning that when production of certain chemicals far exceeds their removal from a specific site, there is a potential for increased sensitivity.

The longer this status is allowed to continue, the greater the risk of neural overload, entrapment, and *crosstalk*. Crosstalk involves axons overloading and passing impulses directly to one another. The result can be spasm, vasomotion, pain impulses, reflex mechanisms, and disturbances in sympathetic activity, which requires a local and global rehabilitation approach. The local approach may involve the use of PR intervention, MET, MTrP therapy, or a gentle combination or synergy of each. In fascia-focused therapy, we refer to this as *integrated neuromuscular inhibition technique* (INIT).

There are various ways to help you perform quality touch:

- Take time to position yourself for maximum ease and transference of forces from you to the patient.
- Keep as straight as you can during motion, ensuring your pelvis and shoulders are in alignment to your direction of force.
- Place your hands or fingers gently and search slowly. Keep listening with your hands and fingers.
- Avoid poking or shoving the tissue.
- Ask the patient for movement when applying elbow or digital ischemic pressure, to provide additional neural involvement (direct technique).
- A softening or viscosity may occur in the tissues you are working on. Avoid rushing at this stage and watch out for autonomic cues such as a deep breath, blinking, sighing, and so on.
- Spend time releasing the tissues around the bony margins, as the deep and superficial fascia merge there.
- Keep a close eye on your patient's reactions and breathing. Working slowly will lead to you synchronizing your work with your patient's breath.
- Position your patient using pillows and bolsters to achieve a sense of floating.

This will reduce the amount of force needed to access the deep tissues.
- Visualize the anatomical structures beneath the skin that you are working on. This requires excellent knowledge of human anatomy.
- Always apply warm hands and fingers. Avoid cold touch.

Uniform Guidelines for PR

1. Start with the recommended investigation and assessments, including special tests.
2. Always ask the patient to first show you or demonstrate their present ROM of the target muscles.
3. Evaluate for relative shortness and/or onset of pain.
4. Investigate the muscle for a point of pain (this may be a MTrP or simply a painful point).
5. Apply ischemic pressure. Ask the patient to report when they feel the level of pain reaches 8 out of 10 (remember the VAS scale).
6. Hold the ischemic pressure for a series of five seconds (part 1), with release of the pressure for two seconds (part 2).
7. Continue this two-part cycle until the patient feels their pain level is diminishing. This may involve several cycles, so please be patient.
8. Apply ischemic pressure to produce a level of pain between 5 and 8 out of 10 (patient feedback).
9. Slowly, and with great sensitivity, begin to passively move the target muscle/limb into a shortened or crowded position.
10. Move the muscle/limb toward a position of ease, avoiding or backing off any feeling of

bind or restriction. Combining palpatory excellence (a listening hand) with patient feedback will lead you to positioning the target muscle into a position of greatest ease or least pain (this is usually in the order of a 75 percent reduction).

11. Hold this position with continued ischemic pressure for sixteen seconds or without ischemic pressure for ninety seconds.

12. Passively return the target muscle/limb to the starting position.

13. If appropriate, introduce a mild neuromuscular stretch.

Ten General Rules of PR

- Follow ease of motion.
- Move away from pain.
- Approximate origin and insertion of muscle.
- Move away from bind or barrier.
- Recreate the original position of injury or insult.
- Ensure the patient avoids contracting the target tissue.
- Palpate for softening of tissues (a listening finger).
- Find dynamic neutral.
- Return to the starting position slowly (passive).
- Incorporate MET as appropriate.

Patient Advice

Patients need to be informed that following any treatment including PR/SCS, a period of altered function may occur, with physiological adaptations that can lead to post-treatment soreness. This soreness can last from hours to days. An application of cold water from a shower for three to six minutes should be all the intervention needed to reduce any soreness or discomfort.

Guidelines Concerning Use of Tender Points

Anterior tender points require flexion, lateral flexion, and rotation toward the tender point. Posterior tender points require extension, lateral flexion, and rotation away from the tender point. Choose tender points most proximal and medial and those that seem most painful for primary attention. The most medial tender points require less lateral flexion and rotation. Posterior tender points may need side bending away from the side of the palpated pain point.

Variations

Within fascia-focused therapy, we use the terms *bind* and *ease*. *Bind* is the first sign of resistance or undue tension, and *ease* refers to a lack of antagonistic tension, or restriction, within a ROM.

Two separate procedures involve direct and indirect techniques. *Direct* refers to going against the restrictive barrier or bind, or going *into* the tissue restriction, while *indirect* involves going away from the restrictive barrier or shortening the tissues.

Exaggeration of the Distortion

This variation is typically used in the acute stage of muscle or soft-tissue insults, such as a spasm, whereby a limb is forced into a position of flexion (or extension). Attempts to extend the limb or body part may result in severe pain. In this situation a pain point is not required. This variation requires moving the patient into an exaggeration of the distortion, with fine-tuning using rotation in one direction or another, until the patient reports a significant reduction of pain, usually in the order of 70 to 75 percent. If the perceived pain reduces by only 50 percent, the therapist may provide additional vectors such as distraction, compression, cold therapy, gentle rocking, or oscillations. At this phase, breath holding in the active or passive phase of respiration, for a maximum of three seconds, may prove helpful.

The therapist, who should be using gravitational forces or bolstering effectively, holds the target muscle/limb in this exaggerated position. The patient can be instructed on how to take a limb or muscle into a passive position utilizing bolsters, cushions, or pillows as part of home care. The position can be held for an appropriate period of time, in some cases lasting from ninety seconds to several minutes or even longer.

An addition to this variation is to provide RI to the target tissues. To do this, the therapist offers gentle resistance (in the order of 50 percent of available strength) to the patient's opposing muscles (i.e., opposing the target muscle) on returning the affected body part to the neutral position. This approach will contract the opposing muscles and provide the best possible chance of the target tissues returning to normal resting length, as muscle spindle activity is dulled throughout the ROM.

This variation on muscle inhibition allows a greater muscular effort than the 25 to 30 percent of effort recommended when contracting the target muscle, ensuring we target specific type 1 fibers. Here, we are contracting the muscle opposite the target muscle, and can therefore use a greater effort to encourage a response that is in proportion to the effort. This is another example of a specific adaptation to an imposed demand.

Replication of the Position of Strain

This is a perfect example of the subtle nature of differentiation within PR. Should the patient remember what they were doing at the time they were injured or felt pain, then this variation may offer the therapeutic intervention required.

Imagine your patient was watching their child playing football. Their right foot was placed on a large rock at the level of their left knee and their right forearm was resting on the front of their thigh, supporting their weight as they leaned on their right leg. Their child suddenly scores a goal, and in the excitement, they throw their arms and body up and back as their foot slips from the rock and travels at speed toward the ground. The result is a spasm in the hip flexors (figure 5.9).

This patient will find that they can move further into flexion with ease. Any attempt to move into extension will result in severe pain, usually felt across the lower back. Replicating the position they were in at the time the injury occurred (forward flexion), and holding that position with perhaps some fine-tuning, should result in a beneficial therapeutic outcome, returning the tissues to normal or near normal neural activity. The therapist must passively assist the patient's right leg to the floor, and in this scenario, the patient can actively extend their torso, contracting gluteus maximus and the erector spinae (among others), offering RI to the target muscles.

Contrary Points Methodology

In this approach, the therapist is encouraged to seek pain points in muscles or tissues opposite those that are "active" when pain or restriction is noted. Of course, this variation will work only if the patient can remember what they were doing when the injury occurred. It is worth emphasizing that the pain point is not located in muscles opposite those where pain is noted. So, for example, in the case of the biceps brachii, pain would be noted in the elbow, and tender points for treatment would be sought in the triceps brachii (the muscle opposite the one contracting; figure 5.10).

In one simplified example, I had a right-handed patient who presented with a pain

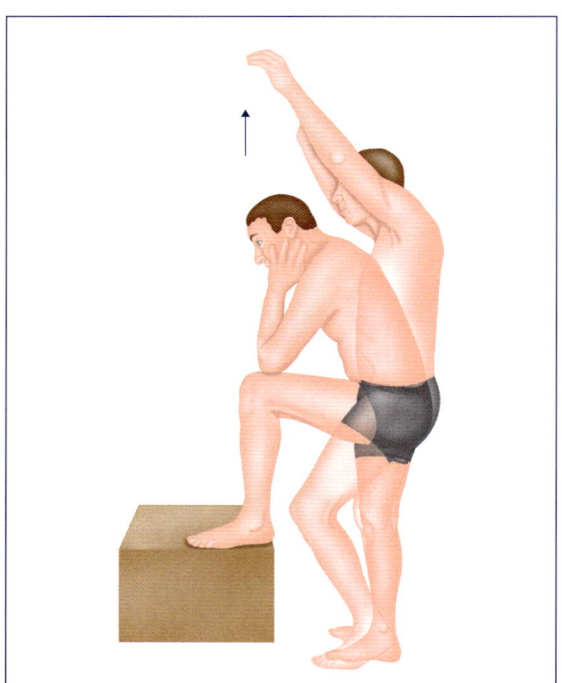

Figure 5.9. Sudden movement causing muscle spasm in psoas and referred pain to the lower back.

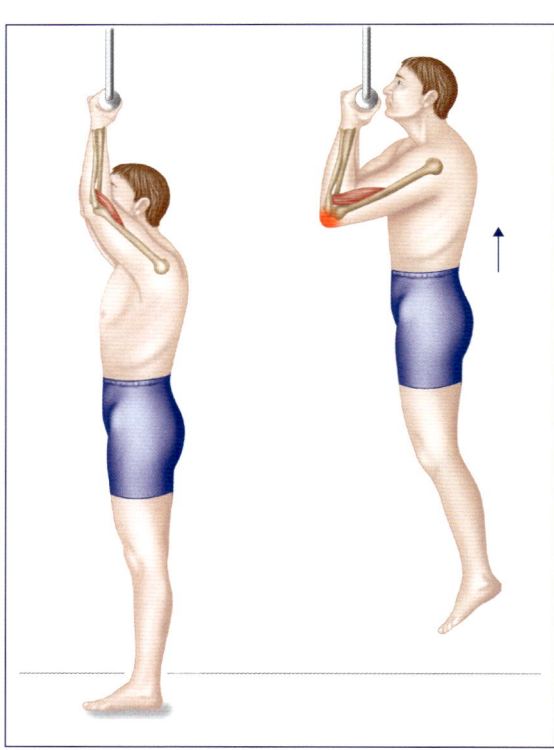

Figure 5.10. Contrary points methodology. In this example, pain is experienced in the elbow as the biceps brachii contract. Tender points for treatment would be sought in the triceps brachii (the muscle opposite the one contracting).

in his *left* shoulder and neck, significantly reduced ROM, and change of sensation down his arm into his third, fourth, and little fingers. He also complained of pain in his deltoid. When asked during the initial stage of assessment if he could pinpoint a time and place when the pain problems began, he said it had been four and a half years previously.

This important input from the patient was the foundation to restoring homeostasis to his muscles. The patient described how he was throwing a tennis ball upward in a serving action with his left arm, and while still holding the tennis ball (this was vital information) he felt immediate sharp pain in his neck. He lowered his arm, waited a moment or so, and repeated the motion, this time completing the serve. His problems became more intense over the following days. Over the next four and a half years his pain manifested itself in what seemed a complicated, illogical pattern.

In this case, the muscles opposite those that were contracting at the time the pain was experienced included latissimus dorsi, teres major, lower trapezius (ipsilateral to the arm holding the ball), and upper trapezius and quadratus lumborum (contralateral to the arm holding the ball). Latissimus dorsi was initially treated, which resulted in almost complete restoration of ROM and removal of pain. Subsequent treatments and a medical exercise program helped this patient to return to playing tennis.

Stacking (Functional or Facilitated Technique)

This wonderful technique requires knowledge of planes of motion and excellent palpatory skills. The therapist engages in a subtle evaluation concerning the quality and ROM in the target tissues or limb. The focus here is to take the target limb or tissue into what I call *dynamic neutral* (DN), or a *combined position of ease*. This position is then held and supported by the therapist for an appropriate period of time. This can range from ninety seconds to several minutes. In fact, the DN position could be taped in place and left passively supported for several hours with supportive taping or strapping.

An example of when to use this might be with a patient who has restricted movement in the right glenohumeral joint. The therapist, standing slightly behind and to the right of the patient, places a listening left hand draped across the shoulder joint, covering as much surface as possible.

The right hand passively moves the arm in the frontal plane, assessing changes in tissue tone and feeling for the first sense of bind in both abduction and adduction, until the point of least restriction is found. This point now represents the starting position for the next plane of motion—for instance, flexion and extension in the sagittal plane. Once again, the therapist moves the arm passively and slowly, and stops and holds the position of greatest ease or least restriction.

Once more the therapist will move the limb through the next plane, offering rotation on the transverse plane. Once the new position of ease has been identified, this can be held for an appropriate period (e.g., ninety seconds). Additional factors such as compression or distraction can be applied. Stacking one plane of motion on top of another brings us to the DN position. This position of ease is held for an appropriate period. This variation can be used in a similar fashion at other joints throughout the body.

Induration Technique

Following a detailed investigation and assessment (if appropriate, using thumb or finger techniques and/or skin drag assessment), the therapist can identify tissues with increased hidrosis. Hidrosis (sweating) is a physiological response to increased sympathetic activity, including MTrP activity in the tissues overlying the area of the transverse processes. With the patient lying prone, the therapist stands on the side contralateral to the muscles in which pain has been identified. One hand is used to apply pressure to a pain or MTrP slightly lateral to the laminar groove, to a point where the patient scores the pain no more than 8 out of 10.

The therapist then places the soft thenar eminence of their opposite hand lateral to the opposite spinous process most adjacent to the MTrP. Direct pressure toward the pain allows a slackening of the target tissue, and pain should begin to reduce. As with most PR/SCS methodologies, fine-tuning can be introduced to lower the perceived pain by the recommended minimum of 70 to 75 percent or more.

A Note on Ischemic Pressure

Applying pressure to a tissue can significantly reduce the blood supply to the tissues directly beneath your finger or thumb. When the pressure is removed, an increase in fresh, nutrient-rich blood is the desired therapeutic outcome. When you use ischemic pressure to create pain as a feedback mechanism, I recommend you hold the pressure for no longer than sixteen seconds. If you choose to hold the tissues in the shortened state for longer, remove the ischemic pressure, and if you wish, leave your finger or thumb over the tissue to "listen" and record any changes or reduction in spastic activity.

Ischemic pressure is not always required, and in some circumstances is contraindicated, especially if the patient cannot provide feedback. If your patient complains of intensely painful tissues, or if they are very sensitive or fragile, ischemic pressure should be avoided.

Integrated Neuromuscular Inhibition Technique (INIT)

1. Identify an MTrP (or simply a pain point) utilizing TNTq and ischemic pressure, if appropriate, within a target muscle.
2. Find dynamic neutral, with (if appropriate) the patient reporting a reduction in pain and holding this position of ease for a period of ninety seconds.
3. Ask the patient to provide an isometric contraction (25 to 30 percent) of the target muscle(s) at the specific joint angle (DN)

and hold the contraction for eight to ten seconds. Breath holding is often seen at this stage. Breath holding is of little consequence in young people or patients with no medical history. Be cautious, however, to encourage patients with conditions such as high or low blood pressure to avoid holding their breath when contracting muscles or exerting an effort.

4. Passively move the target muscle(s) into a gentle stretch.

5. To finish, following a gentle stretch, return the muscle(s) to the resting position. The tender point can now be reassessed for comparison and the patient can be instructed to move the limb or body part by gently contracting the targeted muscle(s) a few times. Ask for patient feedback with the aim of increasing/ improving pain-free unrestricted ROM.

Osseofascial Technique

Bones are considered a harder type of fascia. Osseofascial tissues are composed of a network of collagen fibers, hydroxyapatite, and other proteins, providing the pliable and malleable characteristic expression of healthy bone. Osseofascial insults may occur whereby bone shortens or lengthens (i.e., shape changes) but does not fracture, resulting in severe chronic pain for the patient. Typically, such insults do not show up on medical imaging and can, as a result, go undiagnosed.

There are numerous precisely controlled interventions using specific force transfer applications; however, the following description is the most common approach in the fascia therapy setting. Indications for treatment, following appropriate investigation and taking account of the history provided by the patient, include unremitting pain, loss of function, and no obvious traditional explanation for the root of pain. Having ruled out other possible sources, the fascia-focused therapist may suspect osseofascial involvement is central to the patient's pain complaint.

There are many variations on the osseofascial technique, with different hand positioning, degree of force, compression, distraction, rotation, opposition, duration, breath, and repetition.

When treating cylindrical long or short bones, if possible have the patient seated with both feet firmly on the floor during the therapeutic intervention. Engaging the feet to the floor ensures a bottom-up frequency-specific activation of the fascial net. This should be a gentle engagement and not at all forceful. Ask the patient to consciously feel the ground reaction force engage their fascia network from the sole of the feet to the head.

In this case, I will use the humerus as an example. Having assessed and identified the target tissue, position yourself to the patient's side, taking a seated or standing position as appropriate. If targeting the patient's right humerus, place the palm of your left hand over the patient's right acromion process, and the palm of your right hand directly over the olecranon process of the ulna. Gently engaging the bone between your hands, apply a gentle compressive force, seeking feedback from the patient. If decreased pain or discomfort is noted, you can offer rotation either from each hand individually, while the other hand stays still, providing stability, or boths hands together at the same time (figure 5.11).

The hands may rotate in the same or opposite directions, looking for the patient to report a reduction in pain or altered sensation. If compression increases the patient's pain, you can gently grasp the proximal and/or distal ends of the humerus utilizing the spatulae and tips of the digits to provide a distraction in the sagittal plane. Once again, rotation can be staked or added in the direction of reduced pain on the VAS or reduced alteration in sensation. A reduction of 70 percent or more is optimal. Once a position of dynamic neutral has been achieved, hold this position for ninety seconds.

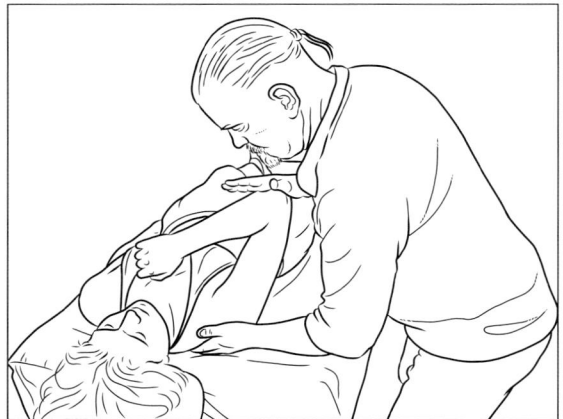

Figure 5.11. The osseofascial technique is an ideal intervention for unresolved deep, boring pain and requires engaging a bone from its proximal and distal ends—here, placing the ends of the humerus into the palms of the hands. The therapist applies a compressive force, approximating or bringing both hands closer together. Alternatively, one hand can provide a foundation while the other hand compresses in one direction, proximal to distal or vice versa, until a reduction in pain is reported by the patient.

Endless Variations

Once you have gained clinical experience, you can begin to mix and mingle variations as you deem appropriate. Allow yourself to listen to your patient's tissues, and they will prompt you as to what they need. This is an intuitive skill, based on excellent knowledge of anatomy, neurophysiology, and palpatory literacy. Increased pain is considered a contraindication.

Active Cryotherapy Techniques (ACTs)

Caution: Stretch and spray is not always appropriate. Certain muscles or tissues are more suited than others for the application of this powerful technique. Some patients have adverse reactions to sprays, and this should be identified in the screening stage. Care should be taken to ensure that the patient and therapist cover their mouths and do not inhale the spray, which should not be used without the correct training. It is also possible for patients to have an allergic reaction to creams and oils. This should be discussed beforehand with the patient. It is advised to perform a skin test in advance of application of creams, oils, and sprays or ACTs. Cold spray over the area of the carotid artery and thyroid gland should be avoided. It is strongly recommended that therapists should have appropriate knowledge of emergency first aid and a system in place for effectively dealing with such an event.

Slow twitch type 1 muscle (oxidative or aerobic) fibers contain large numbers of muscle spindles that are sensitive and respond to muscle lengthening. Fast twitch type 2 (glycolytic or anaerobic) fibers, such as gluteus maximus, contain far fewer muscle spindles and therefore have less of a tendency to shorten because of neuromuscular influences manipulated by muscle spindle activity. Having carried out special tests to identify short or spastic muscles, this technique can offer another important option in your treatment of pain and change in sensation.

ACTs aim to irritate the spindles, initially, by placing the target muscle into a lengthened position. The patient will feel some discomfort but should not feel inappropriate pain. This stretching will result in the muscle contracting in response to the muscle spindle activity (i.e., a monosynaptic reflex arc). At this stage, the therapist provides an application of cold spray over the skin in the direction of the lengthened fibers from origin to insertion, and further up and down the kinetic system if deemed appropriate (appropriate care must be taken to avoid damaging the skin or causing an ice burn).

Following the application of the cold spray, the therapist must passively bring the target muscle back to the starting or resting position. A variation could include passively shortening the target muscle beyond its anatomical resting position and holding this position for one or two seconds. Next, the therapist must wipe the skin and dry the area well. This area can now be actively moved, slowly, by the patient to help restore normal neuromuscular parameters.

My stretch and spray technique has proven to be excellent at disassociating adhered tissues, but it must be noted that the patient will often feel muscle soreness the following day and

possibly for some days later. I first introduced this stretching technique at a fitness instructor conference in the UK in 1986. At the time, it caused quite a stir. After nearly forty years of clinical experience, I recommend it more than ever, having witnessed the therapeutic results.

A wet ice cube can be used as an alternative, moving it up and down the targeted muscle while under stretch. Ice should never be applied directly to skin in the first instance. Avoid static application of the ice in this specific situation. By wetting the ice cube, therefore allowing it to melt a little, the risk of an ice burn is avoided. The therapist should use tissue paper to hold the ice between their fingers rather than holding it directly, to avoid the risk of damage.

Connective Tissue Release (CTR)

This is a wonderful and versatile technique with many variations on the theme. As discussed previously, critical fiber distance (CFD) needs to be maintained to ensure full ROM and ease of movement without restriction. CTR, also known as *soft tissue release* (STR), requires knowledge of a muscle's origin, insertion, tendon type (or aponeurosis), and muscle fiber direction. Muscle fibers can become adhered to one another, and muscles can, in turn, adhere to neighboring muscles, structures, or fascia.

CTR aims to trap a portion of tissue (connective tissue lock) and move the remaining tissue below—including any fibers contained within the tissue—into a stretch position (figure 5.12). The application of the spatula portion (or indeed any other portion) of a thumb, finger, or elbow into a muscle, locking down the tissue directly

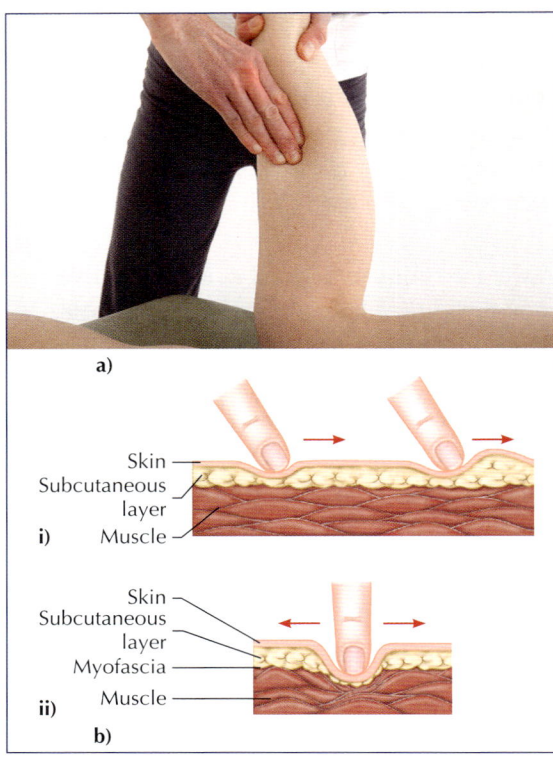

a)

b)

Figure 5.12. Connective tissue lock. (a) Fingers are used to delve between the tissues of gastrocnemius and soleus; (b) myofascial release lock: (i) superficial fascia (subcutaneous layer); (ii) myofascial mobilization into the fascial layer of muscle.

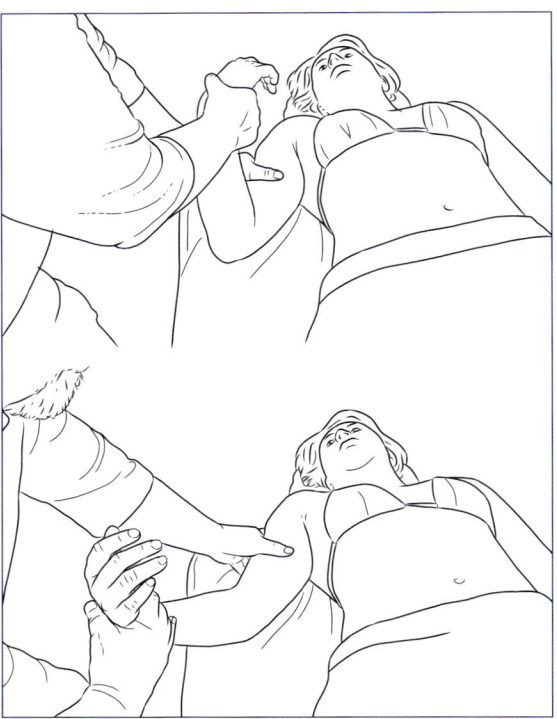

Figure 5.13. Application of CTR on biceps brachii and associated myofascial structures. The patient is best positioned supine, with the therapist standing on the same side as the limb being treated. For right-limb treatments, the therapist should hold the patient's wrist with their left hand and apply the connective tissue lock with their right hand. Having assessed the muscle, the therapist will flex the upper limb at the elbow to shorten the target tissues.

A specific small group of fibers can be targeted using a single digit (e.g., spatula of thumb), or a broader fascia-focused application can be applied using a full palmar compression and soft tissue lock.

beneath, ensures a specific point from where the application of ischemic pressure can be combined with a lengthening force, either passively (therapist) or actively (patient moves the limb or body part). See figures 5.12–5.15.

Starting superficially and working deeper, the therapist repeats the application of connective tissue lock and lengthening movement, providing a unique rhythm, or pace, that meets and matches that of the adhered tissue beneath the listening finger or elbow. This application aims to improve range and quality of motion by breaking up the adhesive relationships of

once-autonomous fibers or tissues. By its very nature, CTR leads to minor tissue damage and inflammation. Patients must be informed that following this treatment, typically within twelve to twenty hours, muscles will be sore. This is temporary and will reduce and subside within a day or so.

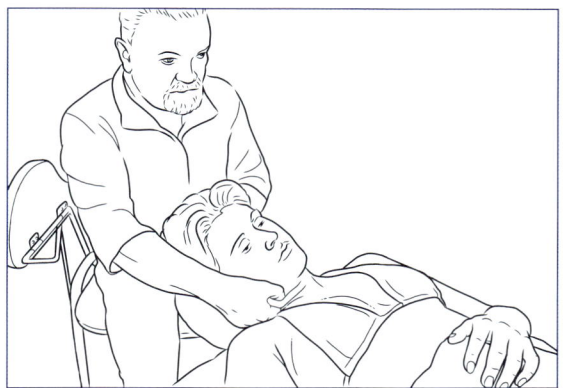

Figure 5.14. A pincer grip is applied to the belly of sternocleidomastoid, whereby the flat surface of the spatula of the thumb is positioned on the anterior fibers, while the first and second digits lie against the posterior fibers, using a mild compression to soften the tissues.

CTR is complemented by gently providing effleurage to the target muscles either before or after treatment. The use of oil or cream is optional, and the therapist may find they can engage, grip, or lock into the tissue more effectively through a light towel or directly to the skin by reducing the amount of lubricant used.

A wonderful variation on this technique is the application of broad-based pressure applied by anterior surfaces of the distal phalanges to encourage a broadening of the muscle fibers during the concentric contraction phase of muscular activity. The simplest example is where the patient is sitting on the end of a massage table (plinth). The therapist places the anterior aspect of the distal phalanges (one or both hands, preferably both) onto the patient's quadriceps, with their thumbs touching, applying gentle pressure with the knee in flexion. On command, the patient extends the leg at the knee joint while the therapist rotates their arms into outward rotation. The muscle fibers will move apart as the muscle contracts.

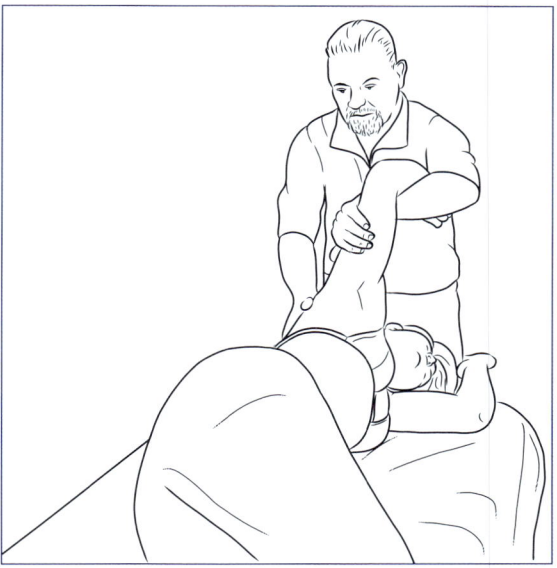

Figure 5.15. This technique provides the opportunity to target specific small/deep soft tissue or broader and more superficial tissues by the application of digital or full palmar connective tissue lock, using a compression hold while moving the associated limb or body part through a specific range of movement.

Gentle assistance from the therapist is a powerful additional intervention to encourage critical fiber distance. Fingers, thumbs, and elbows can be used in different body regions in targeting more precise, or smaller numbers of fibers.

Contraindications will include any bone pathology, muscle tears, or open skin.

Mechanotherapy (Body Mobilization or Harmonic Technique)

This involves controlled passive oscillations and gentle vibrations (provided by the therapist) through the connective tissue elements and joints. This provides the opportunity for a patient with high sympathetic tone to "let go," similar to how one would gently shake free a bundle of electrical wires that had become wrapped up in one another, with cyclical rhythmic resonant motion.

Mechanotherapy offers a gentle unwinding of muscle fibers. The therapist must move the body part or structure starting slowly and building up to a rhythmic motion and resonance that is dictated by, and in tune with, the patient's own frequency-specific resonance. This technique can be used as a diagnostic tool for identifying areas of excessive tissue tension and restrictions.

By placing one hand on the patient's sacrum while they are in the prone position, the therapist can offer a full-body rocking, gently allowing the soft tissues to "wobble" on the osseous tissues. The therapist places their other hand over the moving tissues, "listening" and comparing freedom and quality of movement of left to right. They can confirm their findings visually. A slight change in position of a limb, such as internal or external rotation or the introduction of a bolster strategically placed or wedged beneath a joint, can provide the correct intervention, allowing unrestricted flow of the energy provided by the oscillations.

Interoception and Central Sensitization

Interoception and central sensitization are two concepts related to the processing of sensory information in the body. *Interoception*

refers to the ability to perceive internal bodily sensations, such as hunger, thirst, and pain. *Central sensitization*, on the other hand, refers to a process by which the CNS becomes more responsive to incoming sensory signals, leading to heightened sensitivity and possible increased pain perception.

Other than interoception, *exteroception* is the other main sensory modality providing information concerning the internal and external environment. *Exteroception* refers to the perception of external stimuli, such as touch, vision, and hearing.

These processes can interact and influence one another in complex ways., as chronic pain conditions can lead to central sensitization, which can increase the perception of internal bodily sensations. This, in turn, can influence exteroceptive processing by altering attentional and cognitive processes in the brain related to pain. Additionally, pain can trigger changes in the autonomic nervous system, which can further affect interoceptive and exteroceptive processing, leading to hypersensitivity.

Understanding the interrelationships among these sensory modalities is important for the development of effective pain-management strategies. For example, focusing on improving interoceptive awareness or reducing attentional bias toward pain-related stimuli may be helpful for managing chronic pain. Similarly, interventions that target exteroceptive processing, such as PR techniques, relaxation, mindfulness strategies, and environmental modifications, may also be effective in reducing pain perception.

PART III

REVIEW OF THE MAJOR SKELETAL MUSCLES AND REFERRED PAIN PATTERNS

Muscles of the Face, Head, and Neck

OCCIPITOFRONTALIS

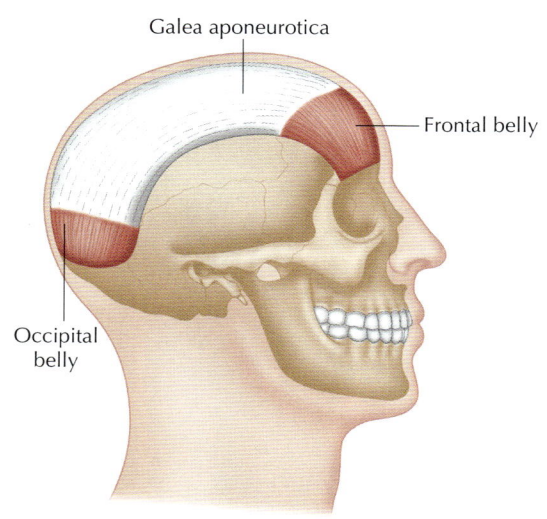

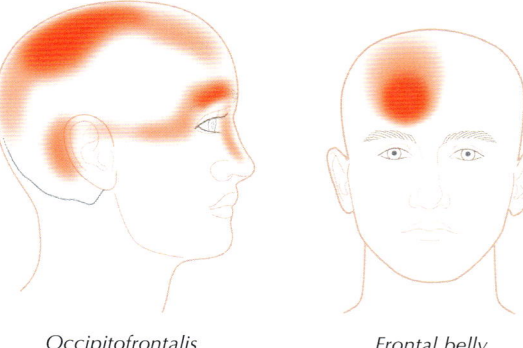

Occipitofrontalis   *Frontal belly*

Latin, *occiput*, back of the head; *frons*, forehead, front of the head.

Origin

Occipital belly: Lateral two-thirds of the superior nuchal line of the occipital bone, and mastoid process of the temporal bone.
Frontal belly: Galea aponeurotica.

Insertion

Occipital belly: Galea aponeurotica.
Frontal belly: Fascia and skin above the eyes and nose.

Nerve

Facial VII nerve.

Action

Occipital belly: Moves the scalp backward. Assists the frontal belly to raise the eyebrows and wrinkle the forehead.
Frontal belly: Moves the scalp forward and wrinkles the skin of the forehead horizontally.

Kinetic System Comment

Occipitofrontalis is essentially two muscle bellies with a strong fascial connection between them, the "galea aponeurotica." Spasm in muscles such as the hamstrings (e.g., biceps femoris) or the plantar fascia can cause tightness through this area, ultimately causing tension in the head and neck, or headaches.

Tension anywhere along the posterior backline kinetic system can lead to shortening of the galea aponeurotica, resulting in tension headaches and a hyperextended cervical spine. This can result in a posteriorly tilted pelvis to provide a level eye view when walking or running and is a recipe for myofascial trigger point formation.

Myofascial Trigger Point Comment

Pain is referred upward from the frontal belly over the forehead on the same side. The occipital belly can refer pain into the eyeball or behind the eye. Pain can travel down behind the ear and into the nose. Sensitivity to sound and light are reported, with a resulting increase in experienced pain. I have had patients who complained of severe pain "inside their head;" on investigation, myofascial trigger points in the occipital belly reproduced a recognizable pain.

TEMPORALIS

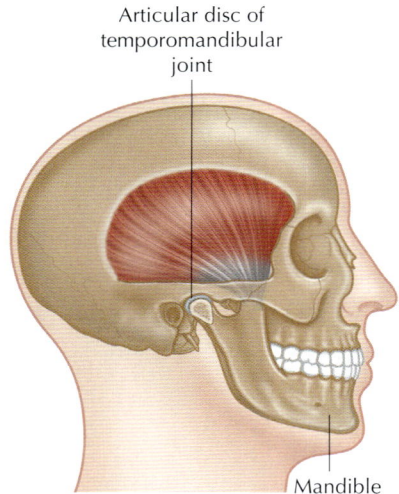

Articular disc of temporomandibular joint

Mandible

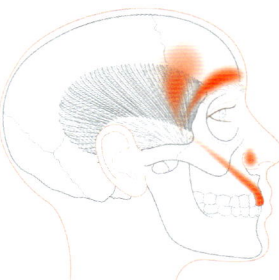

Lower front attachment TrP

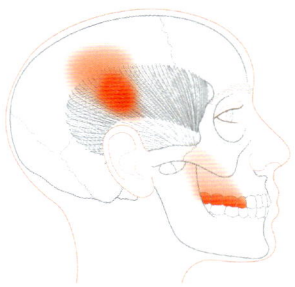

Lower rear attachment TrP (in front of ear area)

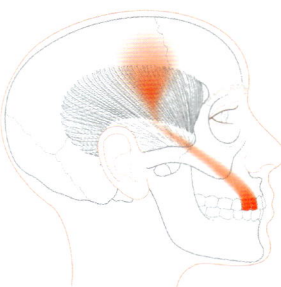

Lower center attachment TrP

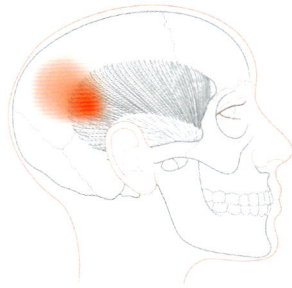

Central temporalis TrP (behind ear point)

Latin, *temporalis*, relating to the side of the head.

Origin

Deep surface of the temporal fascia, and the entire fossa. The floor of the fossa is made up of the zygomatic, frontal, parietal, sphenoid, and temporal bones.

Insertion

Medial/lateral apex and deep surfaces of the coronoid process of the mandible, and anterior border of the ramus of the mandible.

Nerve

Anterior and posterior deep temporal nerves from the trigeminal V nerve (mandibular division).

Action

Closes the jaw (elevates the mandible), assists side-to-side deviations of the mandible and clenching of the teeth. Pulls the ears up to create tension across the scalp.

Kinetic System Comment

Temporalis and masseter are synergists. An overdeveloped upper trapezius can be an overlooked contributor to problems associated with these muscles. A short temporalis leads to teeth clenching, which can damage the sensitive proprioceptive covering on the teeth. Temporal dysfunction can ensue, with loss of balance, vertigo, nausea, hearing difficulties, tinnitus, trigeminal neuralgia, and optical problems. The neck, face, and head muscles are as important to global muscle function as the core (lumbopelvic-hip complex). Habits such as chewing gum can cause repetitive stress and strain.

This is an important muscular link in the lateral chain, and spasm in this muscle can play havoc on the positioning of the temporomandibular joint. Short, spastic temporalis can reduce the normal ebb and flow of cerebrospinal fluid, inhibiting other muscles. Neuromuscular intervention is called for in this case.

Myofascial Trigger Point Comment

One must appreciate the chain effect that an inhibited masseter could have on this muscle. Temporalis and masseter may develop myofascial trigger points in an effort to provide much-needed tension. A forward-head posture is most likely the evident posture. Pain passes upward and over the forehead on the ipsilateral side. Pain spills over just above the ear and into the nuchal line of the occiput. Temporalis should be considered in all headache patients.

Pain in the upper or lower teeth and gums is the most common pain pattern with this muscle. A deep pain has also been reported over the eyebrow and occasionally into the same side and back of the head. The treatment of other muscles on the basis of their pain referral patterns, if associated with this area, should also be carried out as part of the myokinetic system.

MASSETER

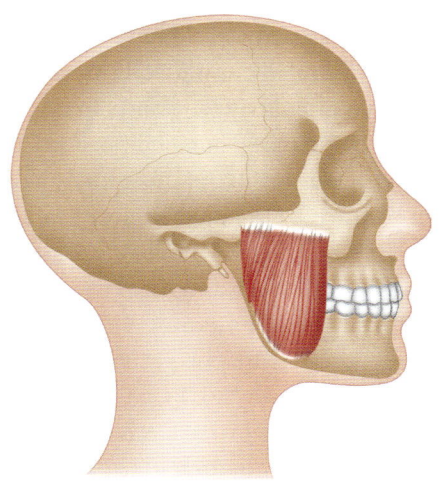

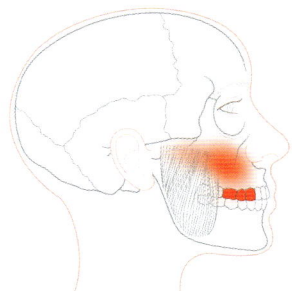

Superficial masseter upper attachment TrPs

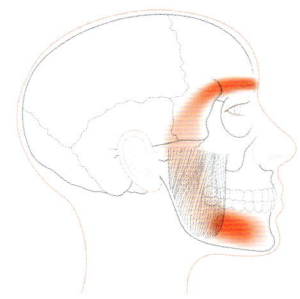

Superficial masseter lower attachment TrPs

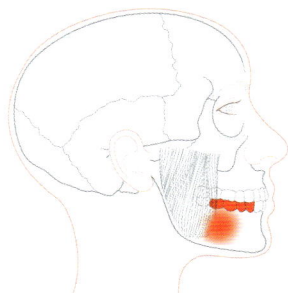

Superficial masseter central TrPs

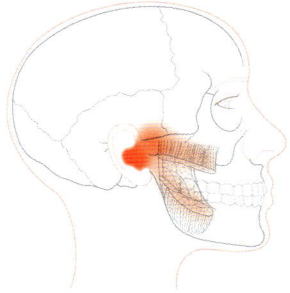

Deep masseter upper posterior TrPs

Greek, *maseter*, chewer.

Origin
Superficial portion: Zygomatic process of the maxilla, and anterior two-thirds of the zygomatic arch.
Deep portion: Surface of the zygomatic arch.

Insertion
Angle of the mandible, and outer surface of the ramus (superficial) and coronoid process of the mandible.

Nerve
Trigeminal V nerve (mandibular division).

Action
Closes the jaw. Elevation of the mandible and slight protraction of the jaw.

Kinetic System Comment
A forward-head posture places the mandible in a position that puts the masseter under undue stress. Antagonist muscles, such as

the geniohyoid, omohyoid, and digastric, can all become spastic due to overtraining of the abdominal muscles using poor technique. This in turn may inhibit the masseter, with resulting myofascial trigger point formation to provide stiffness or tension within the muscle.

Changes in associated suboccipital muscles lead to changes in homeostasis of the head and face muscles. A change in the positioning of the temporomandibular joint will also affect the position of the cervical spine. Correct alignment of the temporomandibular joint requires treatment of the masseter and pterygoids at the local level, with attention to core efficiency at the global level.

The ideal solution is the combination of fascia-focused therapy supported with appropriate, graded medical exercise.

Myofascial Trigger Point Comment

Masseter is a complex muscle, and pain is referred into the eyebrow, maxilla, mandible (anterior), and upper and lower molar teeth. Any person with a toothache will rightly go to a dentist. With no obvious pathology presenting, it is in the patient's best interests to rule out the possibility of referred pain from myofascial trigger points being at the root of the pain.

Other related sensations include hypersensitivity to pressure and temperature changes, e.g., during flights. Pain and changes in sensations can also refer into the temporomandibular joint and inner ear. Remember, it is not always about pain. Masseter myofascial trigger points are significant contributors to headaches.

PTERYGOIDS

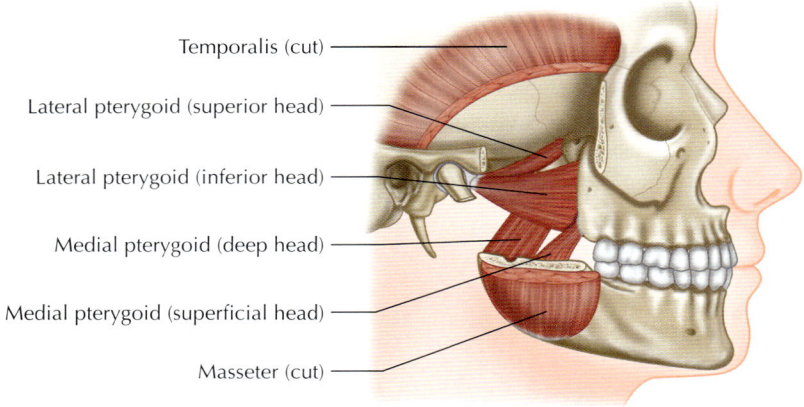

Temporalis (cut)
Lateral pterygoid (superior head)
Lateral pterygoid (inferior head)
Medial pterygoid (deep head)
Medial pterygoid (superficial head)
Masseter (cut)

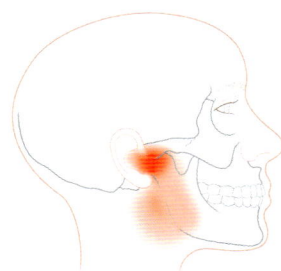

*Medial pterygoid
referred pain pattern*

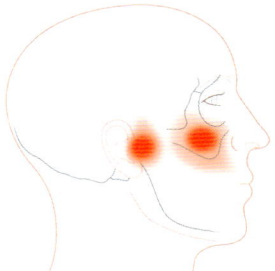

*Lateral pterygoid
referred pain pattern*

Greek, *pterygoeides*, wing-like. **Latin**, *medialis*, relating to the middle, *lateralis*, relating to the side.

Origin
Medial pterygoid
Deep head: Medial side of the lateral pterygoid plate, behind the upper teeth.
Superficial head: Maxillary tuberosity.
Lateral pterygoid
Superior head: Lateral surface of the greater wing of the sphenoid.

Inferior head: Lateral surface of the lateral pterygoid plate of the sphenoid.

Insertion
Medial pterygoid
Medial (fovea) angle of the mandible.
Lateral pterygoid
Capsule and articular disc of the temporomandibular joint, and neck of the mandible.

Nerve
Trigeminal V nerve (mandibular division).

Action

Medial pterygoid

Acts to elevate the mandible and close the jaw and helps the pterygoid lateralis in moving the jaw from side to side.

Lateral pterygoid

Opens the mouth, protrudes the mandible, and provides side-to-side movement.

Kinetic System Comment

Lower limb length inequalities cause mechanical stress which has been associated with myofascial trigger point formation in the neck muscles, especially sternocleidomastoid. Sternocleidomastoid in turn can be the site of mom or dad myofascial trigger points that form baby or satellite myofascial trigger points in the pterygoids. I do not encourage efforts to strengthen this muscle with resisted protrusion and static stretching; that, I believe, can offer short-term removal of symptoms but long-term reinforcement of the problems. A focus on removing myofascial trigger points is vital but must be followed by a program of appropriate physical activity involving full-body kinetic system movement.

Myofascial Trigger Point Comment

Pain is referred deep into the temporo-mandibular joint and maxillary sinus. These myofascial trigger points are most often mistaken for arthritis or sinusitis. Pain has also been reported to be a causative factor in tinnitus. Pain can also be experienced in the tongue and the back of the mouth, with difficulty swallowing.

PLATYSMA

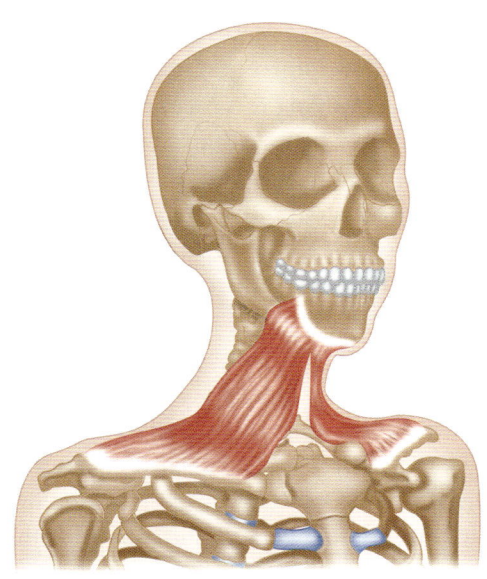

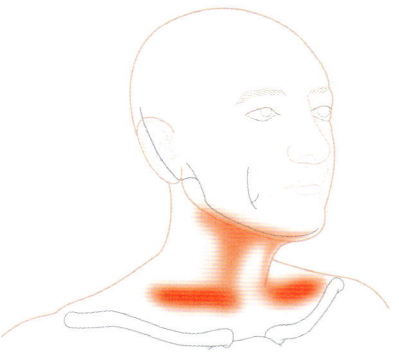

Greek, *platys*, broad, flat.

Origin
Skin and superficial fascia of the neck and upper quarter of the chest, and sometimes out to the shoulder.

Insertion
Subcutaneous fascia of the chin and jaw, including the associated muscles.

Nerve
Facial nerve VII (cervical branch).

Action
Assists in opening the mouth and produces an expression of effort or horror. Pulls the lower lip from the corner of the mouth down and out to the side.

Kinetic System Comment
Platysma is a muscle of the integumentary system and is used by horses to shake off irritating insects. Hypertension in this muscle pulls the mouth downward and the thoracic skin forward. It is considered that tissues overlying the thyroid gland might have an influence on glandular function, and so should be examined when glandular dysfunctions are noted. Referral is recommended. This muscle is often punished when exerting fatigue sets in, because of neuromuscular inefficiency or lack of fitness, leading to strain being placed on platysma. A short, tight masseter can inhibit platysma, resulting in teeth grinding, especially during sleep.

Myofascial Trigger Point Comment
A hot prickling pain in the upper chest and under the jawbone can be the result of myofascial trigger points in this integumentary muscle. The fibers of platysma blend into the associated muscles of the face and upper chest wall, such as orbicularis oris (mouth), subclavius, and pectorals. Myofascial trigger points can develop, provoking anterior throat stiffness and increased blinking of the eyelids.

HYOIDS

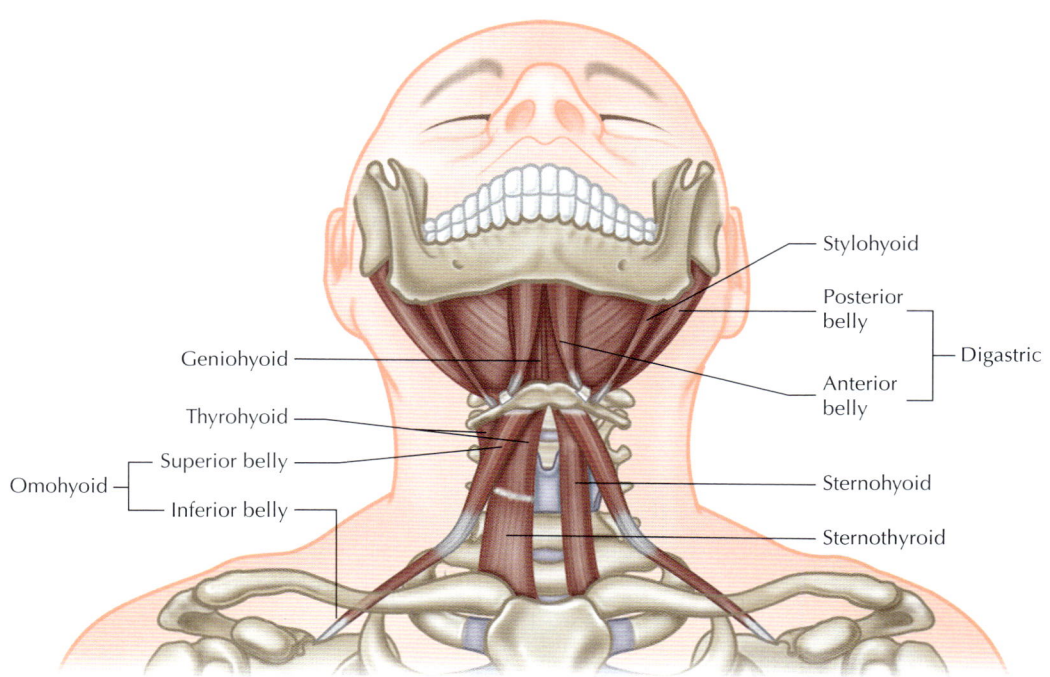

Greek, *hyoeides*, shaped like the Greek letter upsilon (υ), *omos*, shoulder; *hyoeides*, shaped like the Greek letter upsilon (υ).

Origin

The many muscles of the hyoid group have attachments to the mandible, the temporal bone, the manubrium, the clavicle, the costal cartilage of the first rib, and the thyroid cartilage.

Omohyoid

Posterior belly: Mastoid notch on the mastoid process of the temporal bone.

Anterior belly: Inferior border of the mandible.

Insertion

Hyoid bone.

Nerve

Ansa cervicalis nerve C1–3.

Action

These muscles affect the positioning of the hyoid bone. They particularly offer stiffness to stabilize the hyoid when other muscles are carrying out some function. Omohyoid depresses the hyoid bone.

Kinetic System Comment

Mylohyoid, sternohyoid, omohyoid, geniohyoid, sternothyrohyoid, thyrohyoid, stylohyoid, and digastric (indirect attachment) all contract to hold the hyoid in place when performing supine sit-ups. They can only

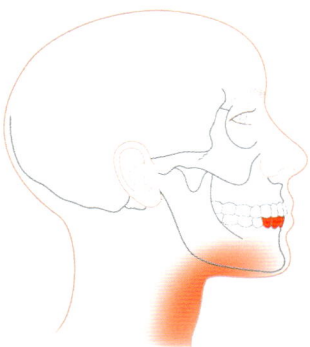

Hyoids referred pain pattern

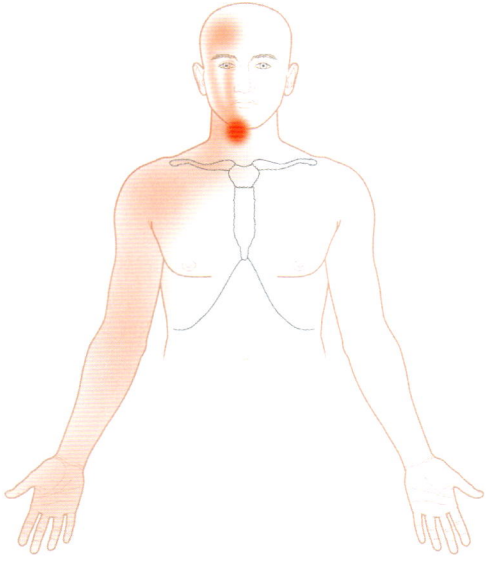

Right omohyoid referral pattern

do this effectively if the tongue, which also attaches to the hyoid, is held in its physiological resting position in the roof of the mouth.

Omohyoid can literally pick up the lungs, as its superior transverse ligament has a fascial connection to the apex of that organ. The hyoids are important muscles in forced inspiration. If they cannot provide

the necessary forces, it is easy to assume an individual would have difficulty improving their aerobic fitness or have difficulty breathing when under stress or increased intensity because of physical activity.

Omohyoid eccentrically decelerates the tilting of the head to the contralateral side and the depression of the scapula.

Myofascial Trigger Point Comment

Myofascial trigger points can form in the hyoids, referring pain into the lower front teeth and throughout the cervical spine, mostly as anterior neck pain. I suggest that myofascial trigger points can develop in these muscles because of inhibited transversus abdominis and obliquus internus abdominis, coupled with spastic sternocleidomastoid and suboccipital muscles, caused by faulty training.

Relating to omohyoid, patients often complain of sore throats and difficulty swallowing. My experience has been that this muscle can send pain into the shoulder and up into the head on the same side. Tenderness on the hyoid bone itself is noted. Pain in the shoulder, neck, arm, and hand, as well as in the scapular, supraclavicular, mandibular, and temporal regions, may be caused by the omohyoid. The pain may be primary, caused by vomiting or by some other intense use of the muscle.

Caution: Myofascial trigger points may be secondary, occurring due to rheumatoid myositis, ankylosing spondylitis, non-ankylosing rheumatoid spondylitis, gouty myositis, or other disorders, which should be ruled out in the first instance.

DIGASTRICUS

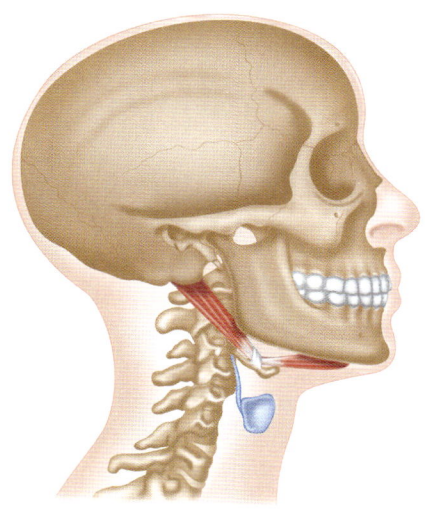

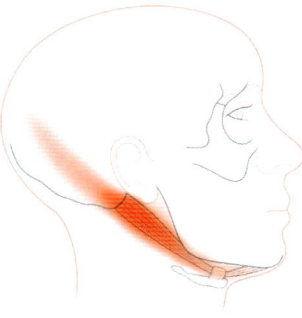
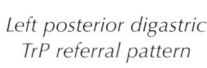

*Left posterior digastric
TrP referral pattern*

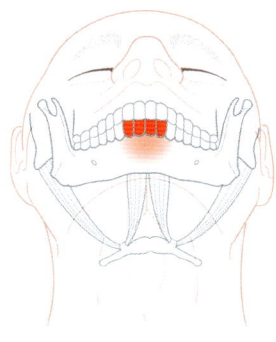

*Anterior digastric
TrP referral pattern*

Latin, *digastricus*, having two (muscle) bellies.

Along with stylohyoid, mylohyoid, and geniohyoid, a suprahyoid muscle (therefore lying above the hyoid bone).

Origin
Anterior belly: Digastric fossa on the inner side of the lower border of the mandible, close to the symphysis.

Posterior belly: Mastoid notch of temporal bone.

Insertion
Body of the hyoid bone, by means of a fascial sling over its intermediate tendon.

Nerve
Anterior belly: Mylohyoid nerve, from trigeminal V nerve (mandibular division).

Posterior belly: Facial (VII) nerve.

Action
Raises the hyoid bone. Depresses and retracts the mandible.

Kinetic System Comment
Digastricus must be allowed to create appropriate tension during movements such as crunches or sit-ups. When the tongue is not placed in its physiological resting position, digastricus cannot create this tension, causing sternocleidomastoid to stiffen and shorten—resulting in a forward-head posture—leading to myofascial trigger points down the kinetic system.

Myofascial Trigger Point Comment
Pain is experienced in the front teeth and anterior jawbone, and into the upper part of sternocleidomastoid (occasionally onto the base of the occiput) and into the throat under the chin. Digastric myofascial trigger points have been reported to be responsible for satellite myofascial trigger points in occipitofrontalis and for referring pain into the ear.

LONGUS COLLI

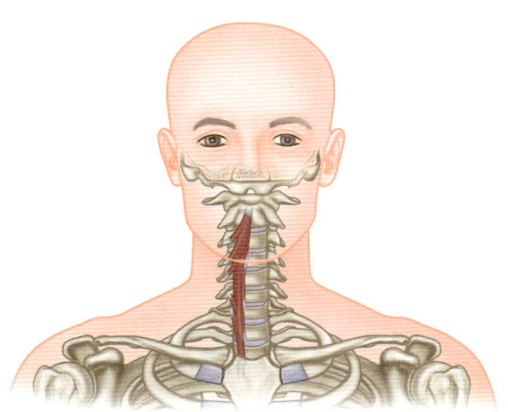

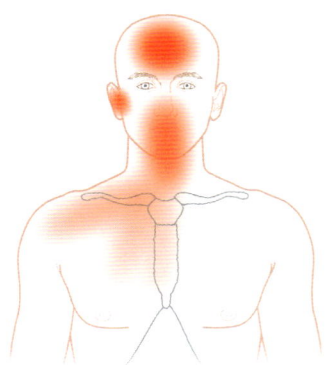

Latin, *longus*, long; *colli*, of the neck.

Origin
Longus colli has three specific parts—superior oblique, inferior oblique, vertical—lying on the anterior lateral aspect of both the upper cervical and thoracic vertebrae. The origin ranges from the transverse processes of C3–5 with attachments to the anterior aspects of C1–2 and including the anterior surface of the T1–3.

Insertion
Anterior tubercle of the atlas, and anterior tubercles of the transverse processes C5, C6.

Nerve
Ventral rami of cervical nerves C2–7.

Action
Bilaterally flexes the cervical spine, while unilateral contraction assists in rotation to the opposite side and lateral neck flexion.

Kinetic System Comment
Longus colli becomes short and tight because of inappropriate neck movements resulting in short scalenes as well as a short, tight psoas, which in turn affects the action of the diaphragm, thereby leading to myofascial trigger point formations that cause neck, upper back, and lower back pain. Longus colli bilaterally decelerates extension of the neck, and unilaterally decelerates ipsilateral rotation and lateral neck extension.

Myofascial Trigger Point Comment
Common symptoms are problems with swallowing, pain in the anterior neck, mouth, ear, and head, and a feeling of a lump in the throat. Patients may complain of a sore throat. I have experienced myofascial trigger points that refer pain across the upper chest on the affected side to the ipsilateral deltoid and produce a feeling of tightness across the chest. Patients also report pain across the anterior clavicle and into the tongue.

A short spastic psoas can have a significant effect on the development of myofascial trigger points in longus colli and associated muscles of the neck. Local pain is reported as a deep, thin, and acute sensation at the vertebral level, rising to the eye on the ipsilateral side. Longus colli can be the true source of sternocleidomastoid pain and is worth considering for treatment in sternocleidomastoid pain issues.

LONGUS CAPITIS

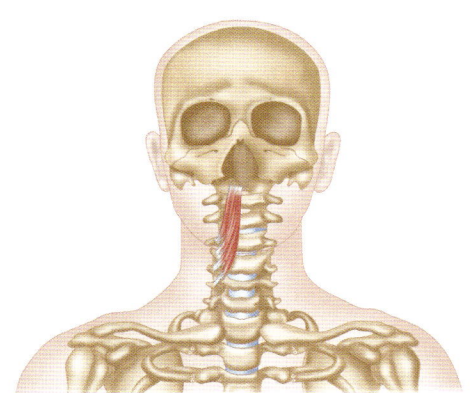

Latin, *longus*, long; *capitis*, of the head.

Origin
Anterior tubercles of the transverse processes of C3–6.

Insertion
Inferior surface of the basilar portion of the occiput.

Nerve
Ventral rami of cervical nerves C1–4.

Action
Flexes the neck and superior portion of the cervical spine.

Kinetic System Comment
Longus capitis decelerates neck extension. It may be worth treating short psoas muscles as part of the treatment of longus capitis since myofascial trigger points can be formed as a response to spasm in the lower chain muscles.

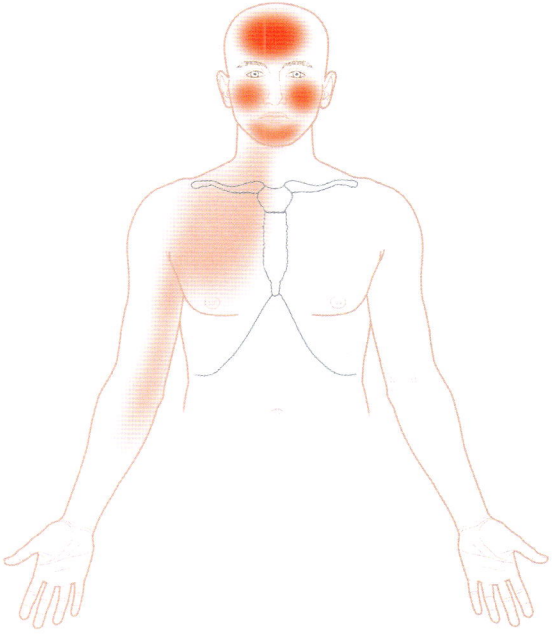

Myofascial Trigger Point Comment
Longus capitis can contribute to general pain in the head, face, teeth, and jaw while referring pain down the arm and chest wall. Patients experience pain in the front of the throat and complain of difficulty swallowing. A feeling of a lump in the throat and sinus-type pain is reported.

RECTUS CAPITIS (ANTERIOR, LATERALIS)

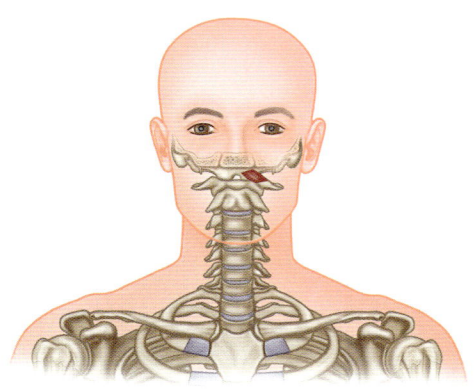

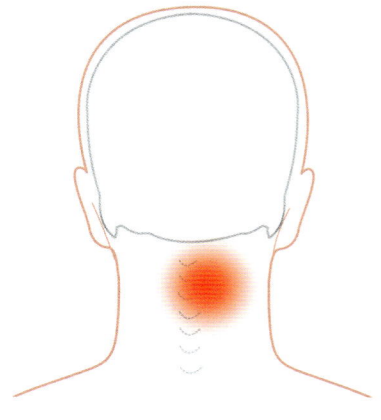

Rectus capitis anterior

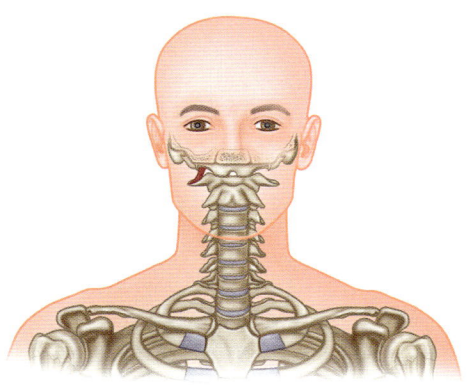

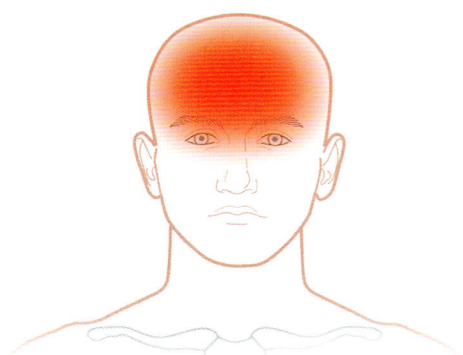

Rectus capitis lateralis

Latin, *rectus*, straight; *capitis*, of the head; *anterior*, at the front; *lateral*, relating to the side.

Origin
Anterior: Anterior surface of the lateral mass of the atlas.
Lateralis: Transverse process of the atlas.

Insertion
Anterior: Basilar portion.
Lateralis: Jugular process.

Nerve
Loop between the ventral rami of cervical nerves C1, C2.

Action
Anterior: Flexes the head.
Lateralis: Lateral flexion to the same side.

Kinetic System Comment
Rectus capitis decelerates the head during extension and contralateral flexion. Spasm or shortness in this muscle can set up the

foundation for retarded proprioceptive facilitation and a tendency to collide with objects, get timing wrong, and reduce accuracy. Attention should be paid to the sternocleidomastoid and head position, in conjunction with a focus on the posterior myofascial chain.

Remember, from a kinetic system viewpoint, the true source of rectus capitis dysfunction could be as far away as the plantar fascia.

Myofascial Trigger Point Comment

Myofascial trigger points in this muscle can feel like severe migraine-type pain everywhere inside the head. Patients may say they cannot pinpoint the pain but feel it widespread throughout the cranium. As in other posterior neck muscles, these myofascial trigger points can contribute to painful tension-like or cervicogenic headaches; the eyes become sensitive to bright light, and patients experience difficulty concentrating.

Changes in sensations can include numbness, tingling, and burning in the scalp. Myofascial trigger points can reduce or retard blood flow and impede nerve tissue.

SCALENES

Scalene anterior
Scalene minimus
Subclavian artery
Lung

Scalene medius
Scalene anterior
Scalene posterior

Greek, *skalenos*, uneven.

Origin
Transverse processes of all cervical vertebrae.

Insertion
First rib and/or suprapleural membrane. Posterior portion may attach to the first two ribs.

Nerve
Ventral rami of cervical nerves C3–8.

Action
Elevates the ribs for respiration if the ribs are fixed. Rotates to the side opposite to the muscle contracting. Laterally flexes to the contracted side. Bilaterally flexes the neck.

Kinetic System Comment
Myofascial trigger points causing short psoas muscles can lead to adaptations in scalenes, resulting in a short, contracted state, thereby pulling up the ribcage and affecting respiratory efficiency.

Myofascial Trigger Point Comment
Pain and numbness can be experienced in the anterior chest, the upper back, and the lateroanterior shoulder down the arm, radiating into the thumb and second digit. These are a complex group of muscles with varying muscle fiber lengths, and therefore demonstrate the potential for many myofascial trigger points. Excellent palpatory skills will be required to successfully locate such myofascial trigger points.

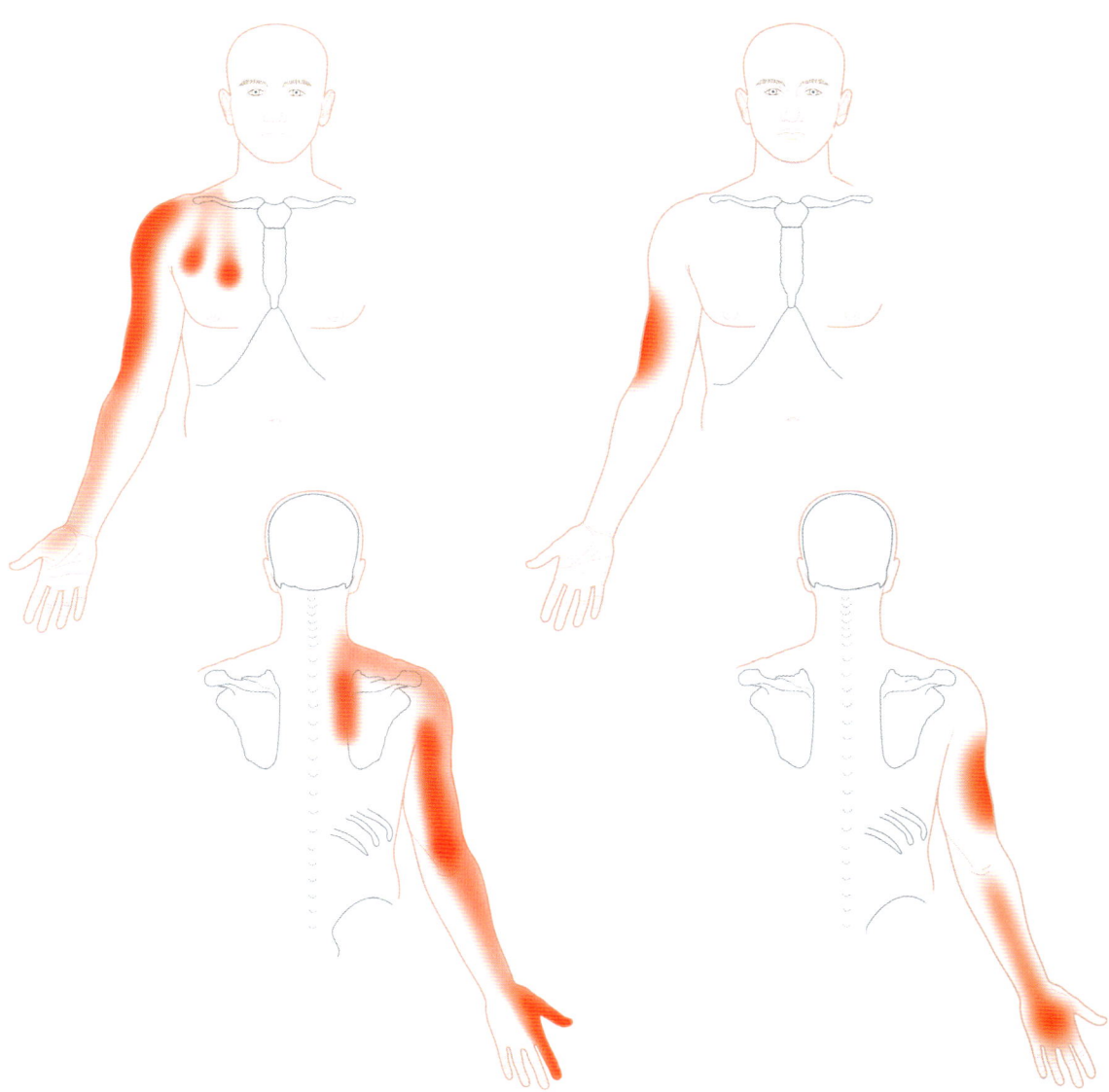

Combined referral pattern for scalenes medius, anterior, and posterior, which, together, are called the scalene major

Combined referral pattern for scalene minimus

STERNOCLEIDOMASTOID

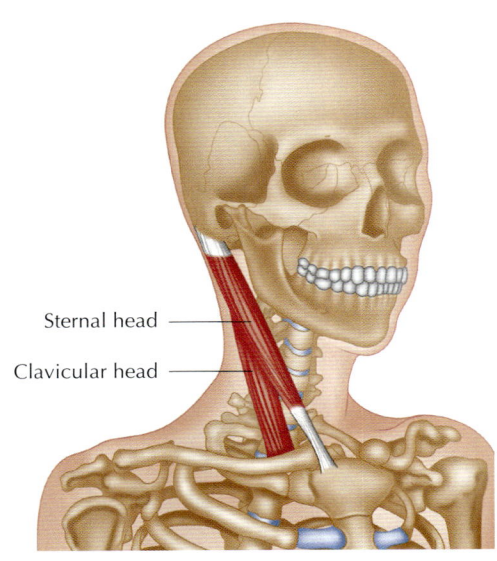

Sternal head

Clavicular head

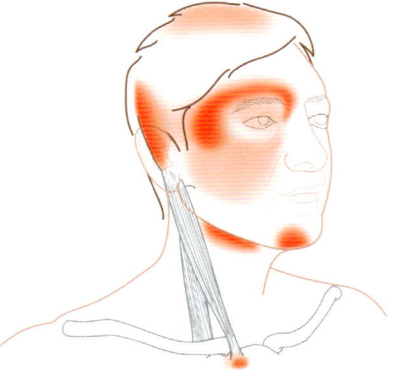

Sternal division

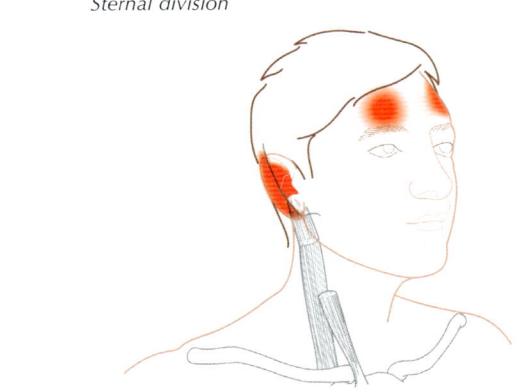

Clavicular division

Greek, *sternon*, chest; *kleis*, key; *mastoeides*, breast shaped.

Origin
Manubrium of the sternum and medial portion of the clavicle (two heads).

Insertion
Mastoid process of the temporal bone.

Nerve
Accessory XI nerve, with sensory supply for proprioception from cervical nerves C2, C3.

Action
Rotates head to the side opposite that contracting and laterally flexes to the contracted side. Bilaterally flexes the cervical spine (neck).

Kinetic System Comment
Generally, sternocleidomastoid is the muscle that most people feel hurting or tense when performing sit-ups. When short, it changes the position of the head on the neck, resulting in a forward-head posture; this sets up the foundation for kinetic system pain and postural changes, leading to compensation, change of gait, and decompensation. Rounded shoulders often have their roots in a short sternocleidomastoid.

Myofascial Trigger Point Comment
Sternocleidomastoid symptoms include problems with balance, visual difficulties, and headache. Because of their anatomical position, myofascial trigger points in this muscle can be mistaken for swollen glands.

Referred pain can be felt as a headache across the front of the brow, deep eye pain (involving decreased or blurred vision), pain on swallowing, and pain behind the ear (including a degree of deafness) and in the top (crown) of the head.

I have had patients with sternocleidomastoid myofascial trigger points who experienced pain similar to trigeminal neuralgia; such pain can be diagnosed as sinusitis. Rare pain referral can also include toothache in the back molars, and pain on the opposite side of the forehead. Pain in the manubrium of the sternum has also been reported. Pain is referred to the temples, tongue, and throat, and to the side of the neck in some patients.

SUBOCCIPITALS

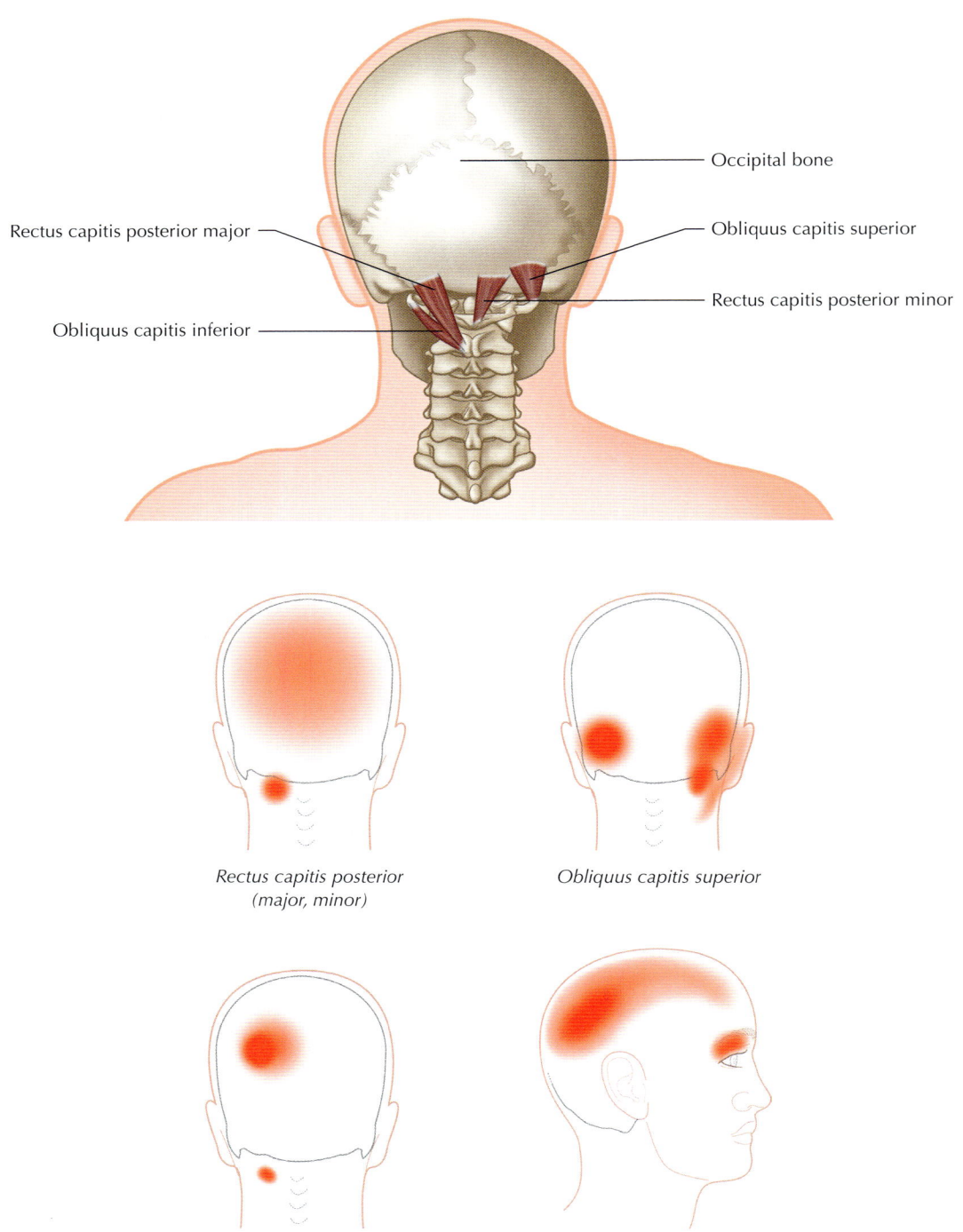

Occipital bone

Rectus capitis posterior major

Obliquus capitis superior

Rectus capitis posterior minor

Obliquus capitis inferior

*Rectus capitis posterior
(major, minor)*

Obliquus capitis superior

Obliquus capitis inferior

RECTUS CAPITIS POSTERIOR (MAJOR, MINOR)

Latin, *rectus*, straight; *capitis*, of the head; *posterior*, at the back; *major*, larger; *minor*, smaller.

Origin
Posterior process of the atlas (C1).

Insertion
Medial half of the inferior nuchal line.

Nerve
Suboccipital nerve (dorsal ramus of first cervical nerve C1).

Action
Extend and rotate the atlanto-occipital joint.

Kinetic System Comment
These muscles form part of the suboccipital group and are vital for reporting the position of the body in time and space. They are rich in muscle spindles, and their role is as much about sending information to the brain regarding head position, as it is about creating movement. With fascial attachments to the spinal cord and brain via the dura mater, these muscles are vital to spinal health and the healthy flow of cerebrospinal fluid.

Myofascial Trigger Point Comment
Mimicking migraine pain, these muscles often create what many patients refer to as "brain pain." A pain is felt deep in the head, but the patient cannot put their finger on exactly where the pain is. Migraine pain has often been attributed to these muscles.

OBLIQUUS CAPITIS INFERIOR

Latin, *obliquus*, diagonal, slanted; *capitis*, of the head; *inferior*, lower.

Origin
Spinous process of the axis (C2).

Insertion
Lateral mass of the atlas (C1).

Nerve
Suboccipital nerve (dorsal ramus of first cervical nerve C1).

Action
Rotates the atlanto-axial joint.

Kinetic System Comment
Any small change in head position will ultimately affect the status of this muscle.

Myofascial Trigger Point Comment
Pain shooting from the back of the head into the eye is a regular complaint of headache, particularly migraine, sufferers. As this is the pain referral of the obliquus capitis inferior, it should be included as part of any treatment plan for patients complaining of similar patterns.

OBLIQUUS CAPITIS SUPERIOR

Latin, *obliquus*, diagonal, slanting; *capitis*, of the head; *superior*, upper.

Origin
Lateral mass of the transverse process of the atlas (C1).

Insertion

Lateral half of the inferior nuchal line.

Nerve

Suboccipital nerve (dorsal ramus of first cervical nerve C1).

Action

Laterally flexes the atlanto-occipital joint.

Kinetic System Comment

Decelerates flexion and contralateral extension of the head at the neck. Obliquus capitis superior and inferior are enriched with muscle spindles, and their positioning is very important to achieving efficient posture.

Myofascial Trigger Point Comment

Obliquus capitis superior will cause dull, deep pain over the lateral aspects of the occipital bone, with diffuse pain radiating down the sides of the jawbone and into the ears.

Muscles of the Trunk

ERECTOR SPINAE (SACROSPINALIS)

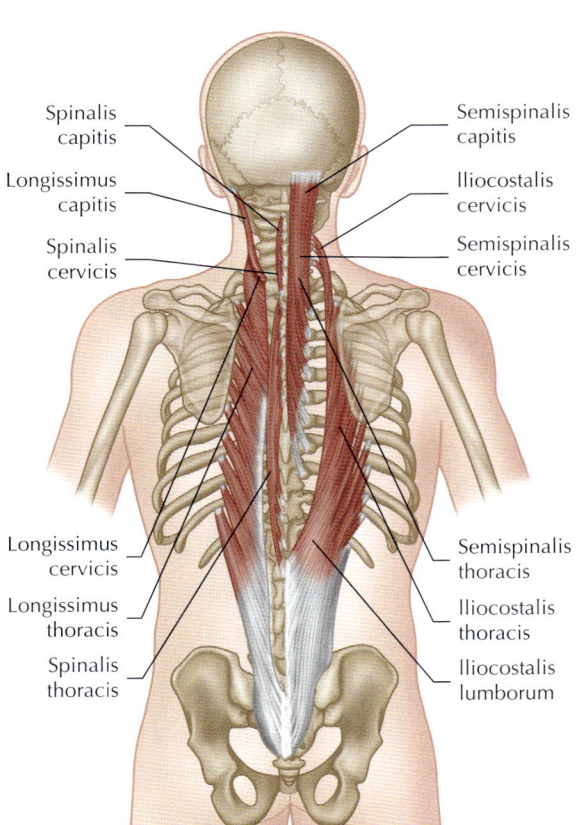

Spinalis
capitis

Longissimus
capitis

Spinalis
cervicis

Semispinalis
capitis

Iliocostalis
cervicis

Semispinalis
cervicis

Longissimus
cervicis

Longissimus
thoracis

Spinalis
thoracis

Semispinalis
thoracis

Iliocostalis
thoracis

Iliocostalis
lumborum

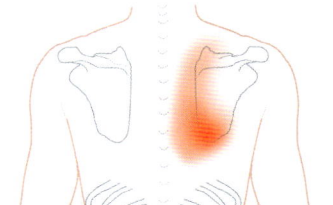

Upper iliocostalis posterior referral pattern

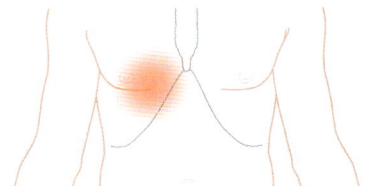

Upper iliocostalis anterior referral pattern

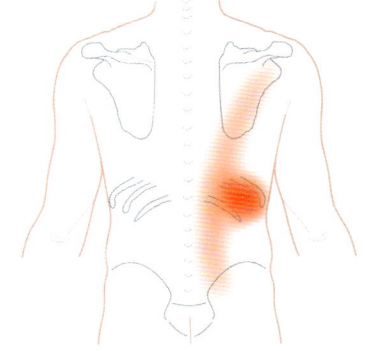

Posterior iliocostalis thoracis referral pattern

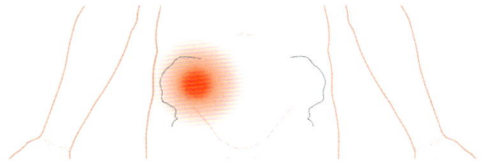

Anterior iliocostalis thoracis referral pattern

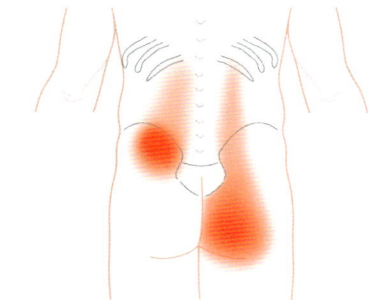

Lower thoracic longissimus thoracis referral pattern

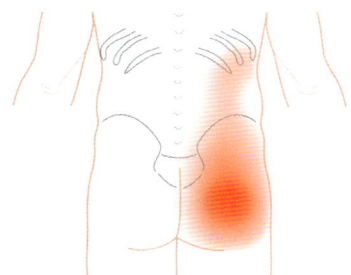

Iliocostalis lumborum referral pattern

Latin, *erigere*, to erect; *spinae*, of the spine; *sacrum*, sacred; *spinalis*, relating to the spine.

Origin
Each of the many erector spinae muscles conjoin with the thoracolumbar fascia that attaches at several different angles to the crest of the ilium and sacrum, and to the spinous processes of T11–12 and L1–5.

Insertion
Many different attachments to the posterior costal bones, the spinous and transverse processes of the thoracic and cervical vertebrae, and the mastoid process of the temporal bone.

Nerve
Dorsal rami of cervical, thoracic, and lumbar spinal nerves.

Action
Extends the vertebral column while the deep rotators and multifidi erectors rotate the spinal column to the opposite side. The semispinalis extends the vertebral column and the head.

Kinetic System Comment
This group includes the iliocostalis, longissimus, spinalis, and multifidi. Eccentrically, these muscles decelerate forward flexion, lateral flexion, and rotation. These muscles are the main stabilizers of the lumbar spine in normal gait.

Myofascial Trigger Point Comment
Refer pain from the lumbar erectors into the gluteal and sacral areas. As a loose rule, pain generally refers up and out, with myofascial trigger points in the suboccipitals, causing severe headaches. Mid-thoracic myofascial trigger points can refer pain into the anterior chest wall and abdomen. Pain experienced as rib pain can often be related to myofascial trigger points.

Myofascial trigger points in the cervical spine are often caused by repeated supine sit-ups or crunches performed on the floor, without first stabilizing the hyoid by means of correct tongue position. These in turn can perpetuate myofascial trigger points in the psoas, scalenes, and sternocleidomastoid, and down the chain into the plantars.

SPLENIUS CAPITIS

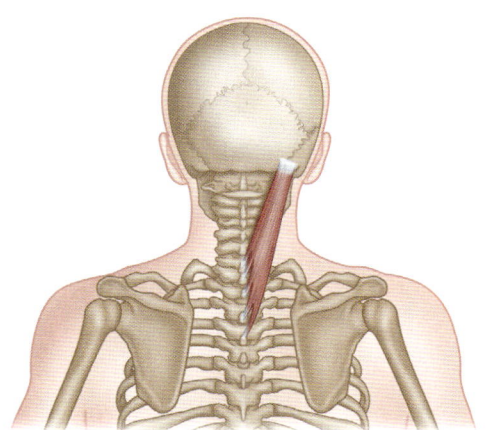

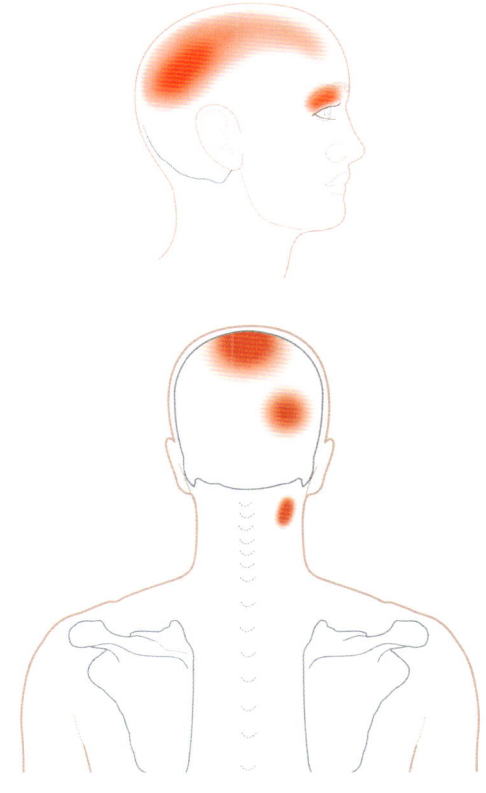

Greek, *splenion*, bandage. **Latin**, *capitis*, of the head.

Origin
Inferior aspect of the ligamentum nuchae, and spinous processes of C7 and T1–4.

Insertion
Mastoid process (posterior portion).

Nerve
Dorsal rami of middle and lower cervical nerves.

Action
Bilaterally extends the head and neck. Ipsilaterally flexes and rotates the neck.

Kinetic System Comment
Poor computer positioning or poor posture when reading can lead to stress of the splenius capitis. Eyes positioned below the level of a computer screen require the operator to look up, activating these muscles and over time creating a hyperextended cervical spine. This requires the pelvis to tilt anteriorly to flex the head so that the eyes can once again be level.

Myofascial Trigger Point Comment
All the muscles of the posterior cervical spine should be investigated when patients complain of tension-type headaches. Splenius capitis is yet another contributor of referred pain into the skull. Any head movement will involve this muscle in any one of a number of ways; it is therefore an important muscle in ensuring appropriate head positioning. Pain spreads up to the crown of the head and into the back of the ipsilateral eye (similarly to the sternocleidomastoid). Blurred vision and a headache with explosive pressure in the eye are often reported. Once serious eye pathologies have been ruled out, myofascial trigger points are the most likely cause of complaint.

SPLENIUS CERVICIS

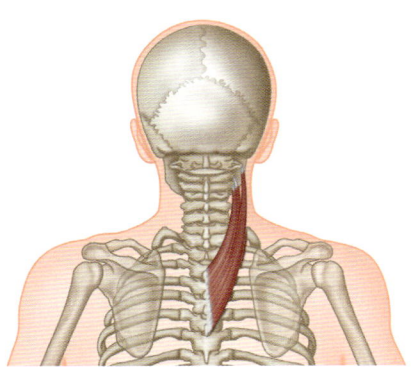

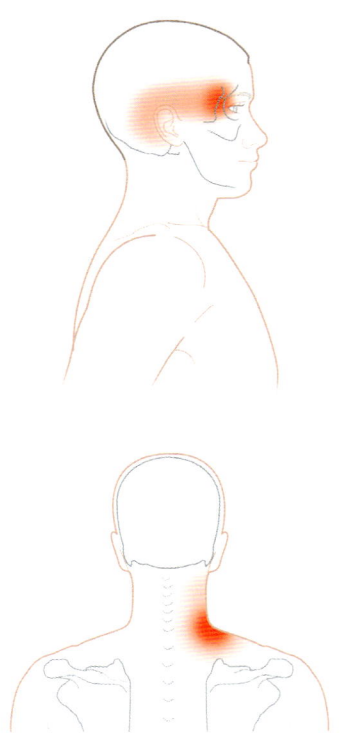

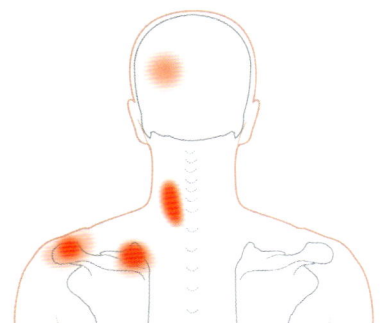

Greek, *splenion*, bandage. **Latin**, *cervicis*, of the neck.

Origin
Ligamentum nuchae, and spinous process of C7.

Insertion
Spinous process of C2 (axis).

Nerve
Dorsal rami of spinal nerves.

Action
Extends the vertebral column. Keeps the spine upright, giving lift when standing.

Kinetic System Comment
The cervical muscles—including splenius cervicis—are as important to full-body movement as they are to core musculature.

A short splenius cervicis can displace the cervical or thoracic vertebrae, thereby affecting fourth-layer muscles (splenii, semispinalis, multifidus, and rotatores) and the positioning of the thoracic ribs. Such changes result in postural adaptations up and down the kinetic system.

Myofascial Trigger Point Comment
Pain is referred down onto the superior angle of the scapula and anteriorly out to the acromion process. Myofascial trigger points in this muscle contribute to tension-type headaches, with pain felt over the temporal and occipital bones.

LONGISSIMUS CAPITIS

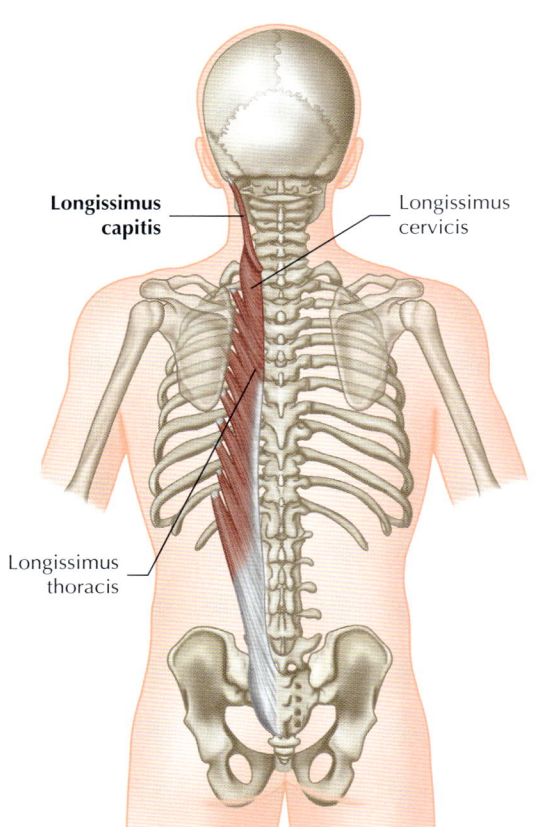

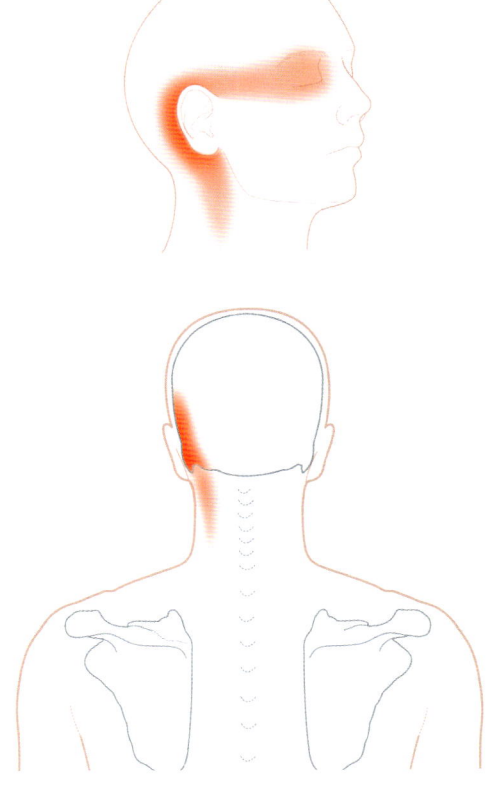

Latin, *longissimus*, longest; *capitis*, of the head.

Origin
Upper five transverse processes of the thoracic vertebrae and articular processes of C5–7.

Insertion
Posterior margin of the mastoid process.

Nerve
Dorsal rami of middle and lower cervical nerves.

Action
This deep neck muscle extends the head and rotates the face toward the ipsilateral side.

Kinetic System Comment
Because of its proximity to important neurovascular structures, longissimus capitis is an ideal muscle to use as an example of the need for differential diagnosis and of the necessity to work within a multidisciplinary context, referring when in any doubt.

Pain, referred or otherwise, in this area could be a result of the following: degenerative disc disease (segmental, subluxation, somatic dysfunction), C2/3 radiculopathy (bulging, prolapsed, herniated disc), fibromyalgia, osteoporosis, osteoarthritis, rheumatoid arthritis, intervertebral or vertebral stenosis, vertebral vascular disorder, cerebral aneurysm, cerebral neoplasm (brain cancer), military neck (absence of normal cervical spine lordosis), cervical spine hyperlordosis, thoracic spine hyperkyphosis, scoliosis, tension/cluster headaches, suboccipital articular dysfunction, mastoiditis, cervical arthritis, cervical syndrome, subacute meningitis, polymyalgia rheumatica, polymyositis, systemic lupus erythematosus, acceleration/deceleration injury (whiplash), eye strain, ocular disease, sinusitis, tetanus, systemic infections or inflammation, nutritional inadequacy, metabolic imbalance, or toxicity or side effects of medications.

Appropriate screening will provide you with the necessary information to decide when to refer. Remember, if in doubt, refer.

Myofascial Trigger Point Comment

Pain referred from this muscle travels to the posterior aspect of the ear. The pain can also extend somewhat across the neck and behind the eyes. Myofascial trigger points in this muscle contribute to headache pain, with tenderness reported at the occipital bone and upper neck, sometimes accompanied by numbness and tingling in the scalp.

MULTIFIDUS

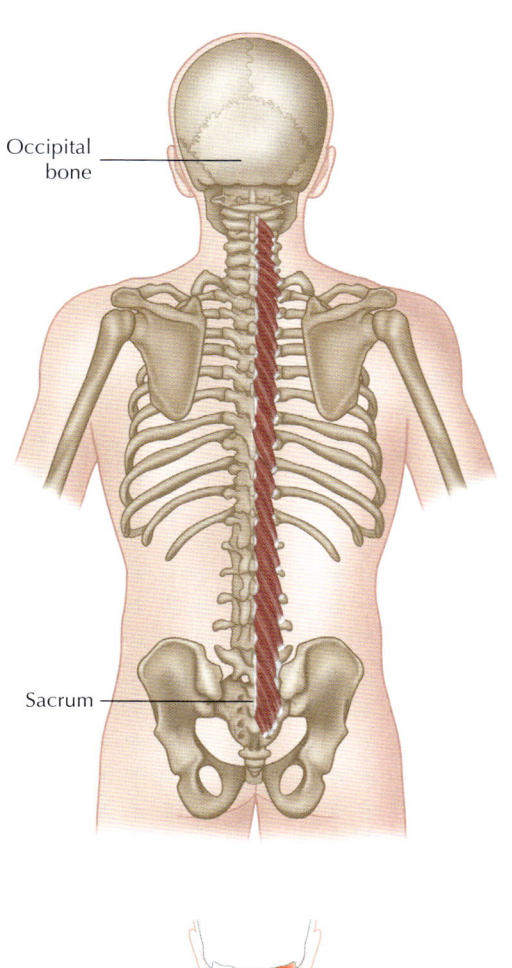

Occipital
bone

Sacrum

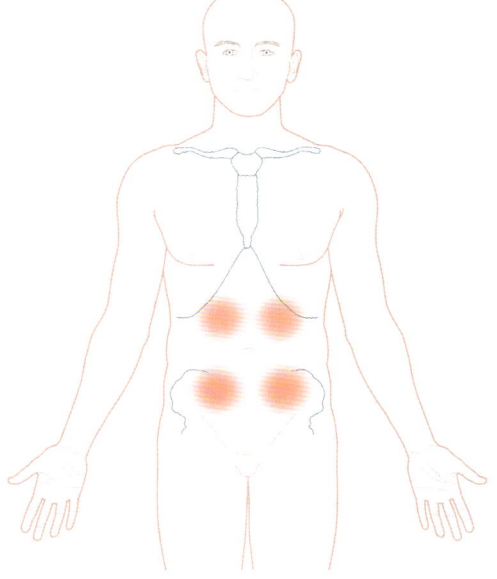

Anterior multifidi referral patterns

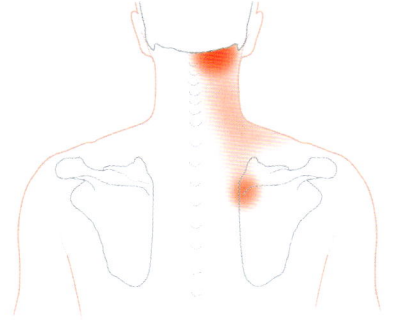

Cervical multifidi

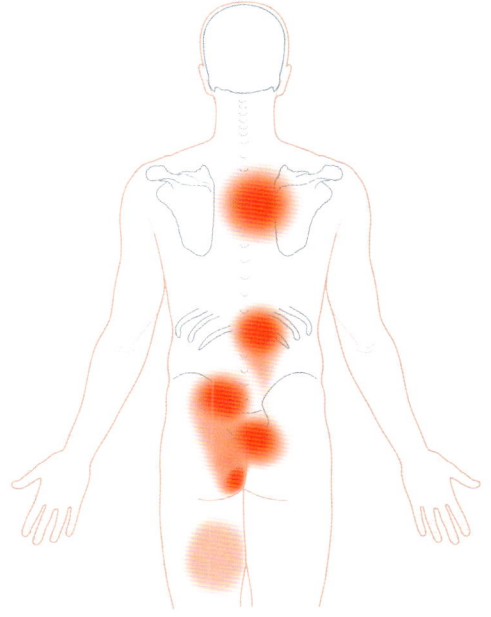

Thoracic and lumbar multifidi referral patterns

Latin, *multi*, many, much; *findere*, to split.

Origin

Posterior aspect of the iliac crest and sacrum, sacroiliac ligament, mammillary process of the lumbar vertebrae, and transverse processes of the thoracic vertebrae, including articular processes of C4–7.

Insertion

Spinous processes of superior vertebrae.

Nerve

Dorsal rami of spinal nerves.

Action

Extends, laterally flexes, and rotates the vertebral column, in addition to extending and laterally rotating the pelvis. A core fourth-layer muscle.

Kinetic System Comment

A major contributor to neuromuscular efficiency of the "core." The deep multifidus has a role in controlling intersegmental motion.

Note: Spinal integrity relies on the combined ability of all muscles; however, special consideration should be given to the transversus abdominis muscle in maintaining pelvic stability, and to the action of multifidus and rotatores in stabilizing the spinal structure.

Myofascial Trigger Point Comment

Pain is reported at the spinous processes of L1–5 and anterior to the abdomen. S1 projects pain down to the coccyx; this referral radiates laterally from the level of T4–5 to the inferior angle of the scapula. Myofascial trigger points located in the cervical region of the multifidus refer pain from the suboccipital region, down the posterior neck to the approximate segmental level of T3 and laterally to the rhomboids. There is also a lateral distribution at the base of the neck and upper back region.

ROTATORES

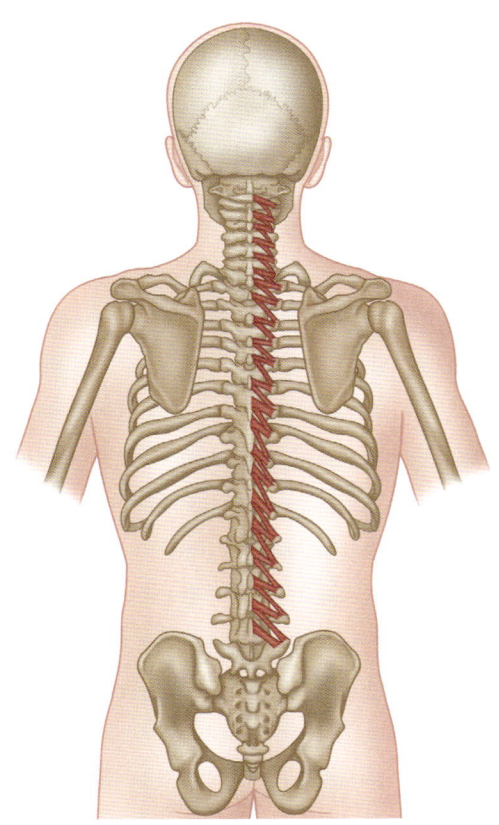

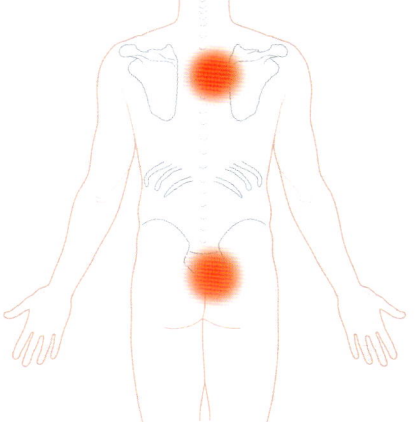

Latin, *rota*, wheel.

Origin
(Eleven pairs from the sacrum to C2).
Transverse process (inferior).

Insertion
Spinous process (superior).

Nerve
Posterior rami of the thoracic nerves.

Action
Extend and rotate the vertebrae.

Kinetic System Comment
A major muscle in neuromuscular efficiency of the "core."

Note: Spinal integrity relies on the combined ability of all muscles; however, special consideration should be given to the transversus abdominis muscle in maintaining pelvic stability, and to the action of multifidus and rotatores in stabilizing the spinal structure.

Myofascial Trigger Point Comment
In my years of human cadaver studies, I have seen no need to separate the rotatores from the multifidi when dealing with myofascial trigger points. These muscles are basal skull pain generators as well as neck and scapular pain generators.

Referral to a myofascial trigger point dry-needle expert may be called for, as these fourth-layer muscles are difficult to treat with fingers and thumbs without many years of experience.

INTERCOSTALS

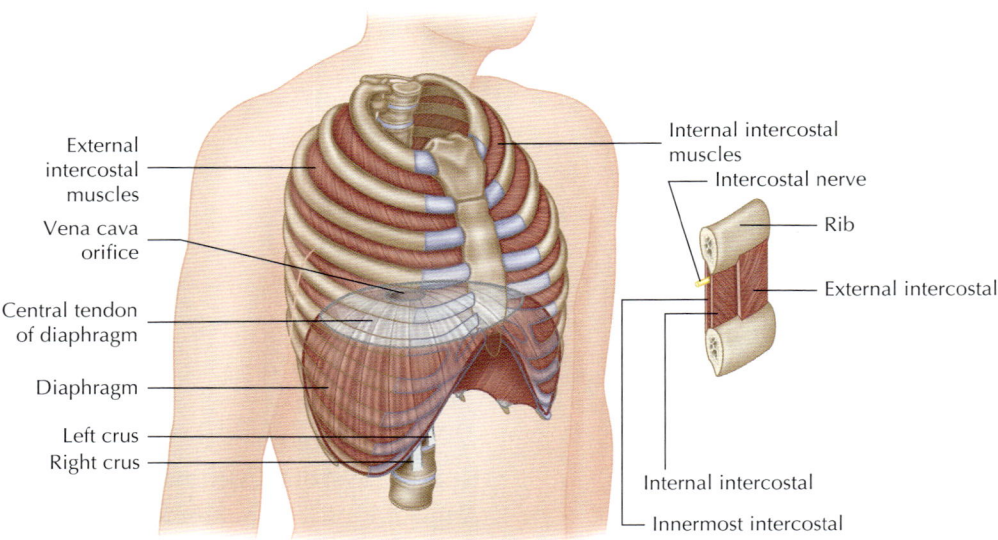

Latin, *inter*, between; *costa*, rib; *externi*, external; *interni*, internal.

Origin
Inferior border of the ribs, as far back as the posterior angles.

Insertion
Superior border of the ribs below, passing obliquely downward and backward.

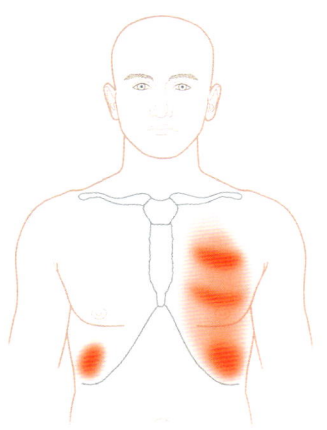

Nerve
Muscular collateral branches of intercostal nerves.

Action
Fix the intercostal spaces during respiration. Aid forced inspiration by elevating the ribs.

Kinetic System Comment
These are the principal muscles of respiration. Problems with these muscles can literally change the internal pH of the body. The intercostals draw the central tendon downward during resting respiration. These muscles will also affect frontal plane movement along the lateral line.

Myofascial Trigger Point Comment
Difficulty breathing is reported, with sharp pain felt, particularly on exhaling. Exercise- or activity-induced breathing difficulties can lead to myofascial trigger points being mistaken for exercise-induced asthma.

DIAPHRAGM

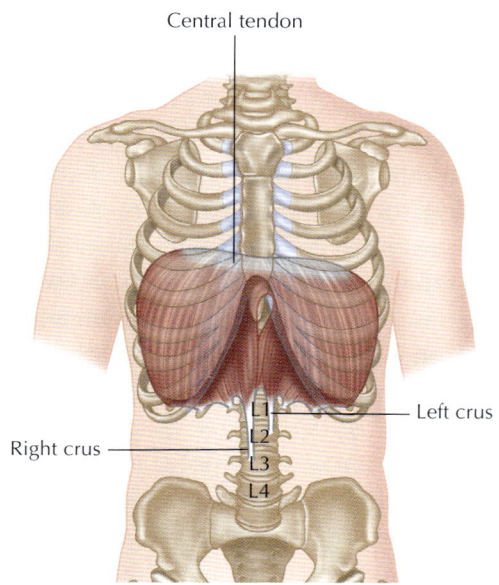
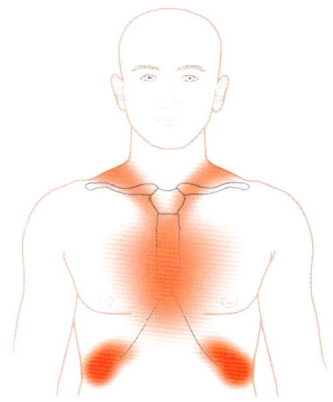

Greek, *dia*, across; *phragma*, partition, wall.

Origin
Sternal portion: Two slips from the posterior aspect of the xiphoid process.
Costal portion: Medial and lateral arcuate ligaments, inner aspect of the lower six ribs.
Lumbar portion: Crura from the bodies of L1–2 (left), L1–3 (right).

Insertion
Central tendon.

Nerve
Phrenic nerve (ventral rami) C3–5.

Action
Inspiration and assists in raising intra-abdominal pressure.

Kinetic System Comment
This dome-shaped musculofibrous muscle is penetrated by the aorta, the vena cava, and the esophagus. Fascial investments with the quadratus lumborum and psoas muscles highlight the importance of this structure, linking as it does the lower and upper quarters. The psoas and quadratus lumborum should be treated along with the diaphragm when dealing with respiratory dysfunction.

Myofascial Trigger Point Comment
Patients complain of chest pain, dyspnea, and not being able to take a full functional breath. A stitch in the side is common. Sudden increases in exercise intensity or physical activities can activate, or be the cause of, myofascial trigger point formation in the diaphragm.

INTERNAL OBLIQUE

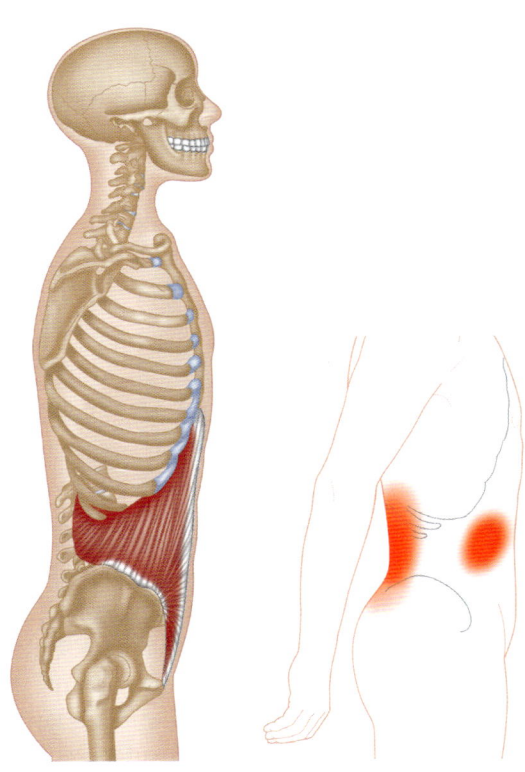

Latin, *obliquus*, diagonal, slanted; *internus*, internal; *abdominis*, of the belly/stomach.

Origin

Lumbar fascia. Anterior two-thirds of the iliac crest, and lateral two-thirds of the inguinal ligament.

Insertion

Costal margin, aponeurosis of the rectus sheath (anterior and posterior), and conjoint tendon to the pubic crest and pectineal line.

Nerve

Ventral rami of thoracic nerves T7–12, ilioinguinal and iliohypogastric nerves.

Action

Supports the abdominal wall, assists forced respiration, and aids in raising intra-abdominal pressure. Along with the muscles of the other side, obliquus internus abdominis abducts and rotates the trunk. The conjoint tendon supports the posterior wall of the inguinal canal.

Kinetic System Comment

The most common mistake in exercise programs is the attempt to isolate the internal obliques in relation to the other abdominal muscles, in the exclusion of efforts to train this muscle in the functional manner in which it operates. The internal obliques typically become inhibited when stressed, leading to muscular compensations and changes in pelvic positioning.

Myofascial Trigger Point Comment

Any abdominal pain should be treated with caution. Any suspicion concerning the type of pain or symptoms should be the cue for referral to a doctor. Internal oblique myofascial trigger points refer pain in many directions in the abdomen, including the lower back. Pain across the midline is possible. Patients can complain of burning, bloatedness, and stomach swelling.

EXTERNAL OBLIQUE

Latin, *obliquus*, diagonal, slanted; *externus*, external; *abdominis*, of the belly/stomach.

Origin
Anterior angles of the lower eight ribs.

Insertion
Outer anterior half of the iliac crest, inguinal ligament, pubic tubercle and crest, and aponeurosis of the anterior rectus sheath.

Nerve
Ventral rami of thoracic nerves T5–12.

Action
Supports the abdominal wall, assists forced expiration, and aids in raising intra-abdominal pressure. Along with the muscles of the opposite side, the obliquus externus abdominis abducts and rotates the trunk.

Kinetic System Comment
When considering physical activities to improve the function of the external obliques, one should try to include both open- and closed-kinetic-system movements. The feet should be placed on and taken off the floor. Movements such as those seen during swimming involve the external obliques in a way that can be trained with dry training, but this requires imagination.

Myofascial Trigger Point Comment
Pain can refer down into the groin and sometimes to the testicles. Similar to the other abdominal muscles, external oblique myofascial trigger points can refer pain anywhere locally throughout the abdominal region. This pain is often exacerbated during the menstrual cycle.

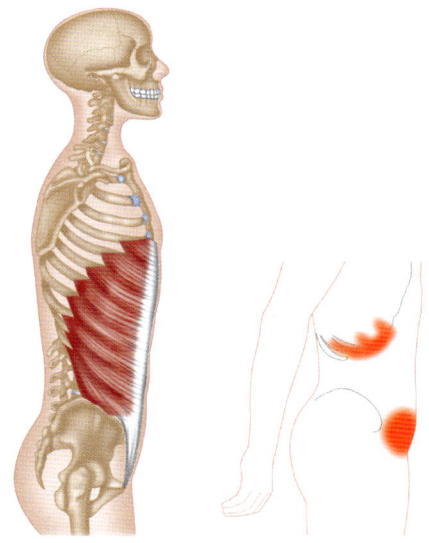

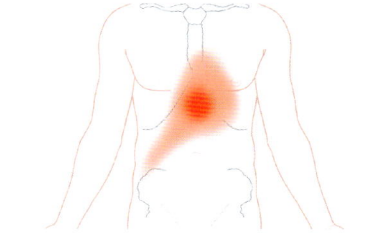

Abdominal oblique ᵀrP referral pattern can vary considerably from patient to patient

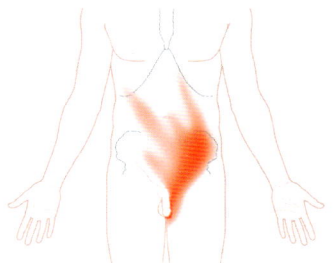

Lateral lower abdominal wall

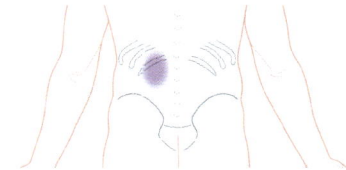

Belch button, posterior lower abdominal wall

TRANSVERSUS ABDOMINIS

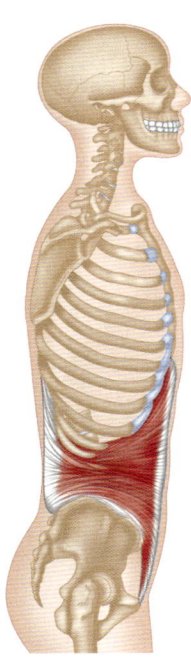

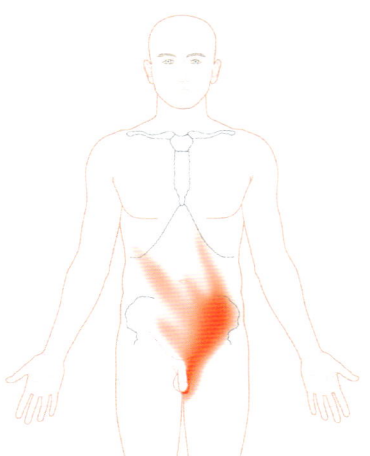

Latin, *transversus*, across, crosswise; *abdominis*, of the belly/stomach.

Origin
Costal margin, lumbar fascia, anterior two-thirds of the iliac crest, and lateral half of the inguinal ligament.

Insertion
Aponeurosis of the posterior and anterior rectus sheath, and conjoined tendon to the pubic crest and pectineal line.

Nerve
Ventral rami of thoracic nerves T7–12, ilioinguinal and iliohypogastric nerves.

Action
Supports the abdominal wall, and aids forced expiration and in raising intra-abdominal pressure. The conjoint tendon supports the posterior wall of the inguinal canal.

Kinetic System Comment
All abdominal muscles work on a moment-to-moment basis as we move, providing the tension required to translate forces from the lower limbs to the upper limbs. The transversus abdominis is the deepest of these muscles, and each one (right and left) wraps up the organs horizontally. Transversus abdominis fascial attachments include the lumbar vertebrae, ribcage, iliac crest, and inguinal ligament. The muscle also connects directly into the linea alba, furnishing a link between the xiphoid process, pyramidalis, and pubic bone. Transversus abdominis therefore provides essential support for the internal organs, as well as tensional support and lift for L2–3.

Myofascial Trigger Point Comment
Pain is experienced across the upper abdomen, with a focus on the xiphoid process. Patients can also experience a marked enthesitis along the inferior costal margin. Coughing is especially distressing.

RECTUS ABDOMINIS

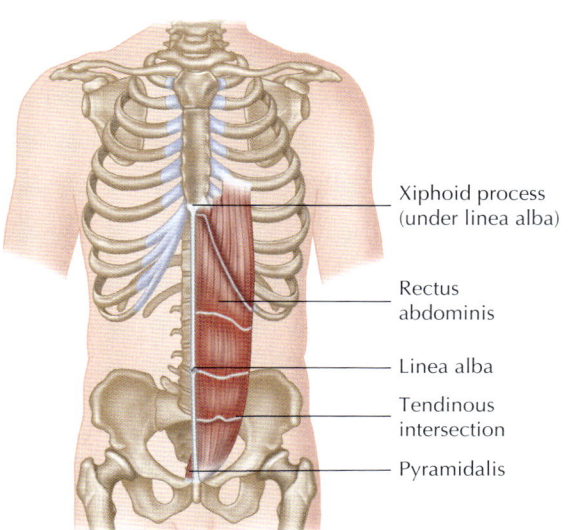

- Xiphoid process (under linea alba)
- Rectus abdominis
- Linea alba
- Tendinous intersection
- Pyramidalis

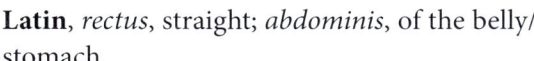

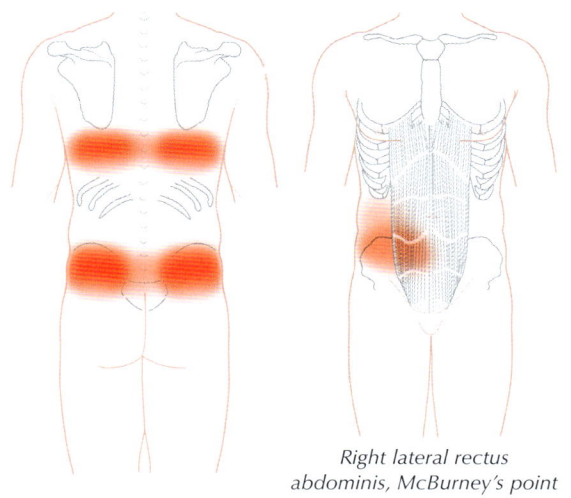

Right lateral rectus abdominis, McBurney's point

Latin, *rectus*, straight; *abdominis*, of the belly/stomach.

Origin
Pubic crest and symphysis pubis via two tendons separated by the linea alba.

Insertion
Costal cartilages of the fifth to seventh ribs, and xiphoid process.

Nerve
Ventral rami of thoracic nerves T5–12.

Action
With the origin fixed, the chest wall will move toward the pelvis. With the insertion fixed, the pelvis will move toward the chest.

Kinetic System Comment
This muscle decelerates trunk extension through eccentric action. It is worth noting that the full range of motion cannot be achieved with conventional sit-ups performed on the floor, which can contribute to muscle imbalances and neuromuscular inefficiency of the core.

Myofascial Trigger Point Comment
Rectus abdominis has two distinct pain patterns—at the level of the xiphoid process, spreading bilaterally across the middle back—and at the level between the umbilicus and the inguinal ligament, spreading pain into the sacroiliac joint and lower back. Rectus abdominis myofascial trigger points can also cause chest pain, heartburn, belching, diarrhea, dysmenorrhea, and appendicitis (McBurney's point).

ILIOPSOAS GROUP

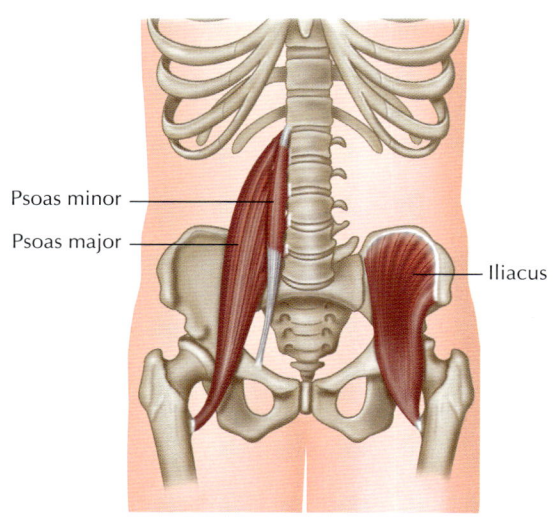

Psoas minor
Psoas major
Iliacus

Insertion

Middle surface of the lesser trochanter of the femur.

Nerve

Ventral rami of lumbar nerves L1–4.

Action

Flexes and medially rotates the hip.

Kinetic System Comment

Psoas major eccentrically decelerates hip extension and external rotation at the hip. This muscle is typically short, causing inhibition in the gluteal muscles, which sets up the foundation for kinetic system neuromuscular changes and the formation of myofascial trigger points.

Myofascial Trigger Point Comment

Prolonged sitting has been identified as a significant precursor to the formation of myofascial trigger points. Myofascial trigger points form in the psoas major due to primary myofascial trigger points in related muscles of the psoas functional unit. These muscles include the rectus femoris, pectineus, sartorius, tensor fascia latae, adductors, and gracilis. Pain is felt as a vertical pattern ipsilaterally along the lumbar spine, and downward over the sacroiliac joint and gluteal region. Pain can also be present in the groin and medial thigh. Psoas pain can be mistaken for lumbago and disc pathology.

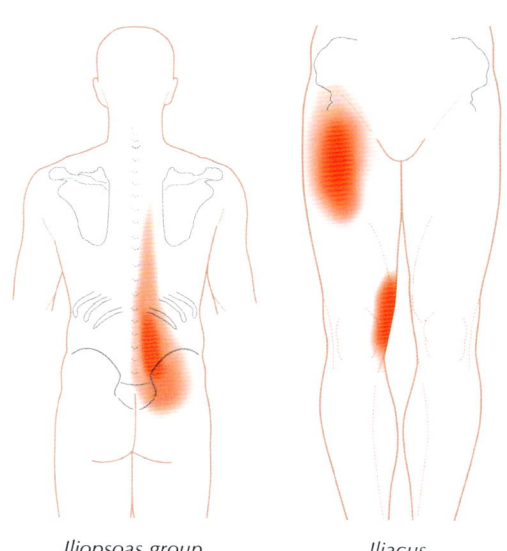

Iliopsoas group   *Iliacus*

PSOAS MAJOR

Greek, *psoa*, muscle of the loin. **Latin**, *major*, larger.

Origin

Transverse processes of L1–5, bodies of T12–L5, and intervertebral discs below bodies of T12–L4.

ILIACUS

Latin, *iliacus*, relating to the loin.

Origin

Iliac fossa by means of the superior two-thirds of the crest of the ilium, iliolumbar and anterior sacroiliac ligaments, and ala of the sacrum.

Insertion

Blends with the lateral aspect of the psoas major over the pelvic rim, slightly distal to the lesser trochanter of the femur, and a few fibers merging with the joint capsule of the hip.

Nerve

Femoral nerve L2–4.

Action

With its origin fixed, the iliacus will draw the femur forward in hip flexion, adduction, and internal rotation. With the insertion fixed, and acting bilaterally, the pelvis is drawn forward, thus tilting the pelvis, with flexion at the hip but with the trunk moving, thereby increasing lumbar lordosis. Unilaterally, the iliacus will assist in lateral flexion of the trunk toward the same side.

Kinetic System Comment

Iliacus and psoas major (including the psoas minor if one is evident) work together to provide a deceleration of internal rotation of the femur on heel-strike and slow hip extension. Bilateral contraction of this fleshy triangular muscle provides stability to the lumbar spine. These muscles are rich in muscle spindles and are therefore prone to shorten under stress. This in turn can cause inhibition in the gluteus maximus.

Myofascial Trigger Point Comment

Myofascial trigger points can form in the gaster of iliacus and the associated psoas

muscles, referring pain across the lower back and down into the buttock, anterior thigh, and groin. Difficulty breathing and urinating are often reported.

PSOAS MINOR

Greek, *psoa*, muscle of the loin. **Latin**, *minor*, smaller.

Origin

Bodies of T12 and L1 and intervening intervertebral disc.

Insertion

Fascia over the psoas major and iliacus.

Nerve

Anterior primary rami of L1, L2.

Action

Weak flexor of the trunk.

Kinetic System Comment

This muscle is present in only 50–60% of the population. Because of its unique relationship connecting the upper body and lower limb, any problems in this muscle result in full-body kinetic system adaptations and distortions. Areas of pain can include the neck, lower back, knee, and foot.

Myofascial Trigger Point Comment

A possible symptom of myofascial trigger points in this muscle is a posteriorly tilted pelvis, which causes a flat-back posture and compressed intervertebral discs. Lower back pain is the classical referral pattern, but pain can also be referred into the groin and thigh.

QUADRATUS LUMBORUM

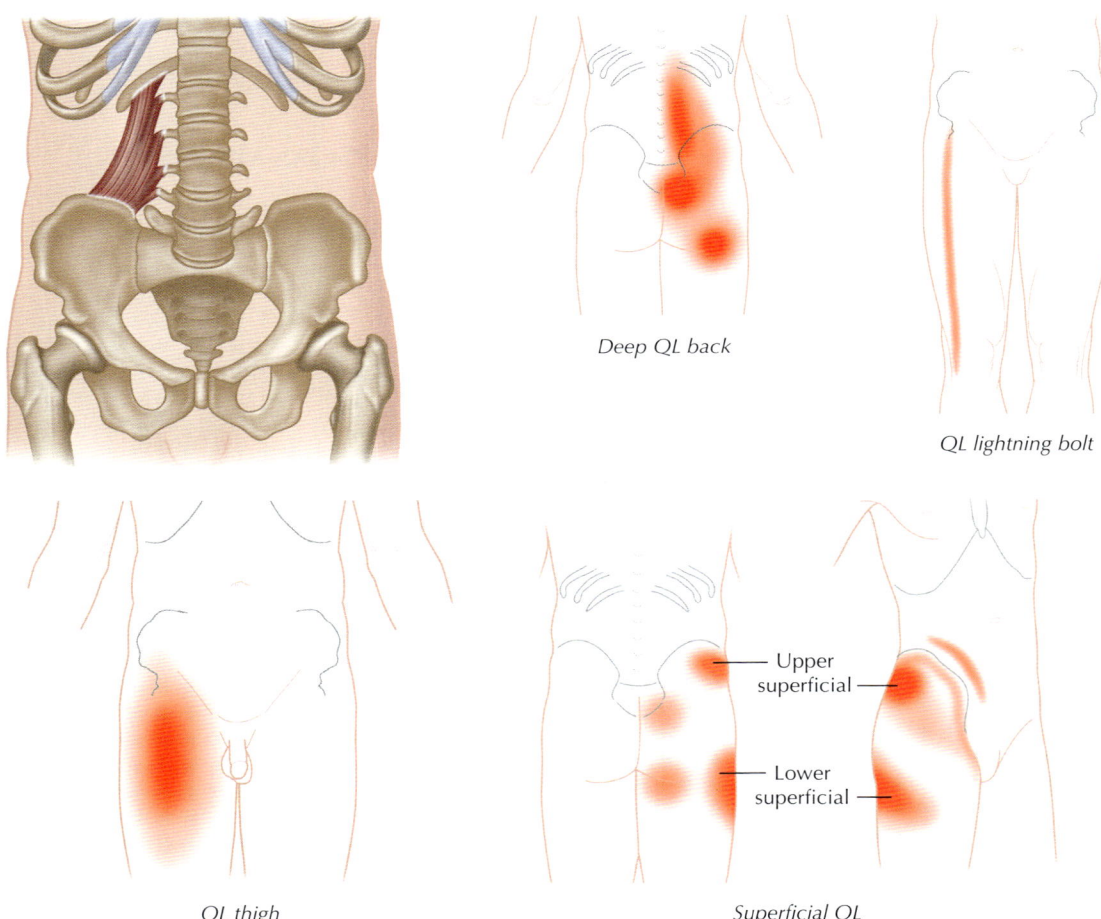

Deep QL back

QL lightning bolt

QL thigh

Upper superficial

Lower superficial

Superficial QL

Latin, *quadratus*, squared; *lumborum*, of the loins.

Origin
Inferior border of the twelfth rib.

Insertion
Apices of the transverse processes of L1–4, iliolumbar ligament, and posterior third of the iliac crest.

Nerve
Ventral rami of the subcostal nerve and upper three or four lumbar nerves T12, L1–3.

Action
Fixes the twelfth rib during respiration and laterally flexes the trunk.

Kinetic System Comment
A short quadratus lumborum leads to a functional short leg on the same side. This in turn leads to muscle adaptations, whereby

the contralateral adductors may shorten in an effort to pull the femur more posteriorly into the acetabulum. This can create the look of a short leg on the contralateral side and cause subluxation at the pubic symphysis and sacroiliac joint. Kinetic system problems continue both up and down the chain.

Myofascial Trigger Point Comment

Pain is experienced at the sacroiliac joint and into the gluteal muscles and the hip. Referred pain in the anterior thigh and groin can be very painful. Fear of coughing or sneezing because of intolerable pain in the lower back is common. As a result of pain on the affected side there may be difficulty sleeping. Myofascial trigger points in the quadratus lumborum can cause the hip to hike, which can lead to a scoliosis and subsequently an anatomical short leg.

Muscles of the Shoulder and Upper Arm

8

TRAPEZIUS

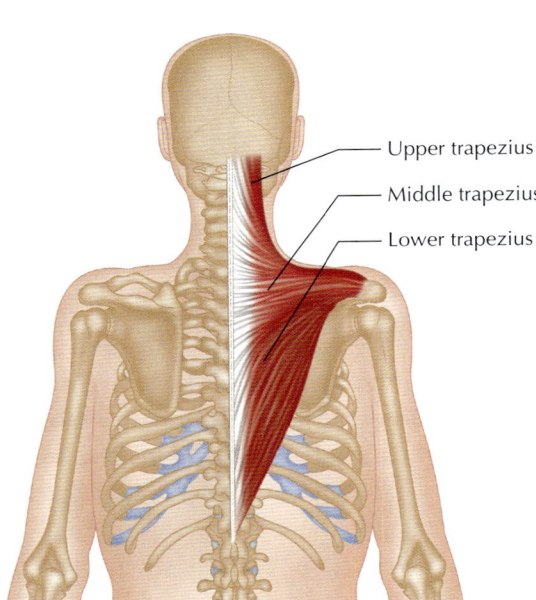

- Upper trapezius
- Middle trapezius
- Lower trapezius

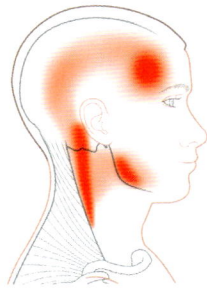

The referral pattern may be entire or in part, and usually results from TrPs in the most vertical upper trapezius fibers, occurring along the side of the neck between the collarbone attachment and the occipital attachment

Greek, *trapezoeides*, table shaped.

Origin

Medial third superior nuchal line, ligamentum nuchae, and spinous processes and supraspinous ligaments to T12.

Insertion

Upper fibers: Lateral third of the posterior border of the clavicle.
Lower fibers: Medial acromion, and superior lip of the spine of the scapula to the deltoid tubercle.

Nerve

Motor supply: Accessory XI nerve.
Sensory supply (proprioception): Ventral ramus of cervical nerves C2–4.

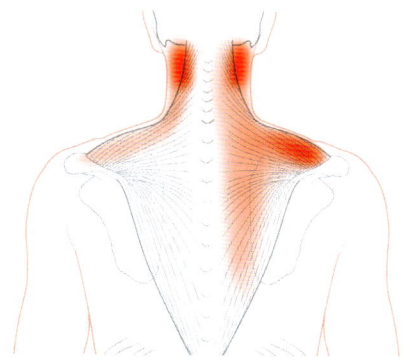

The referral pattern on the left of this figure is from TrPs found in the left most horizontal upper trapezius muscle fibers. The pattern on the right side is usually from TrPs found in the right lower trapezius, between the shoulder blade and the spine, fairly close to the shoulder blade

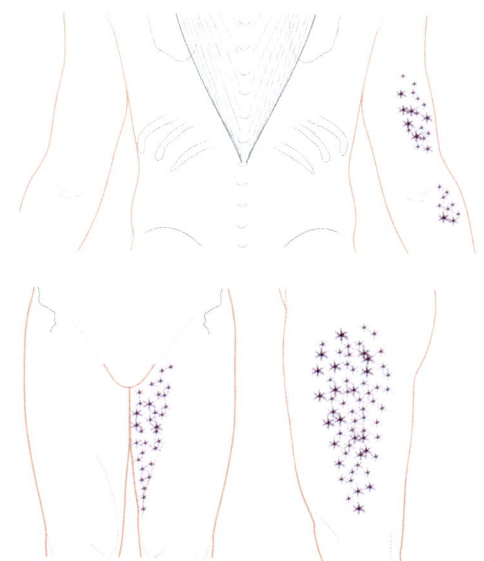

These figures represent patterns of gooseflesh rather than pain and vary with individuals. The TrPs producing them are often found in an oval trigger area above the upper inside edge of the shoulder blade triangle. Another area of TrPs can occur at the outer attachment area of the upper trapezius. TrPs in this area cause local pain

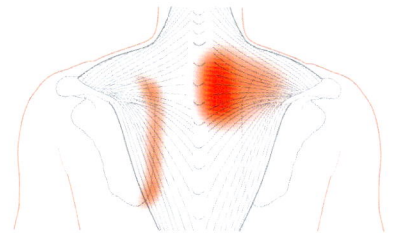

The referral pattern on the left side of this figure is usually from TrPs found in the left side, in the upper top corner attachment of the muscle covering the shoulder blade. The pattern on the right side of this figure is usually from TrPs found to the inside of the worst pain (deepest red) in the middle horizontal fibers of middle trapezius

Action

Laterally rotates, elevates, and retracts the scapula. Extends and laterally flexes the neck if the scapula is fixed.

Kinetic System Comment

As the trapezius is an important neck muscle, any spastic activity in the sternocleidomastoid, suboccipitals, scalenes, longus colli, levator scapulae, or many other muscles will affect its status. Many people hold emotional tension in the upper trapezius. The upper portion decelerates the head, the middle portion decelerates protraction, and the lower portion decelerates shoulder elevation.

Myofascial Trigger Point Comment

Myofascial trigger points here lead to tension headaches, with sharp pain felt in the temporal bone and into the masseter, behind the eye and ear (on the same side), and along the side of the neck. Occasionally, pain will travel to the back of the head, and a burning pain will be experienced down into the vertebral side of the scapula and middle back. Trapezius l myofascial trigger points can cause loss of balance and dizziness. Myofascial trigger points in this muscle are often mistaken for disc pathologies, neuralgia, spinal stenosis, shoulder bursitis, or arthritis.

RHOMBOIDS

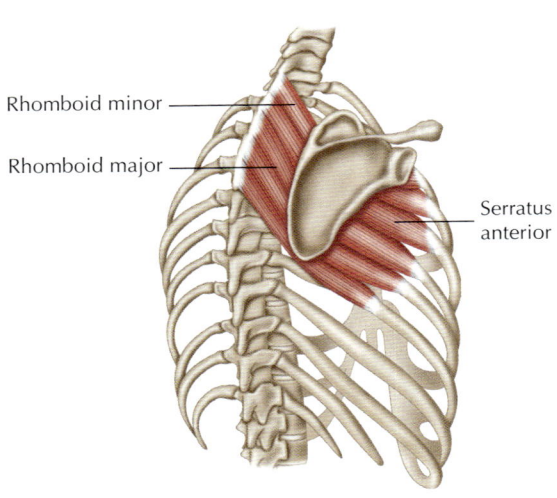

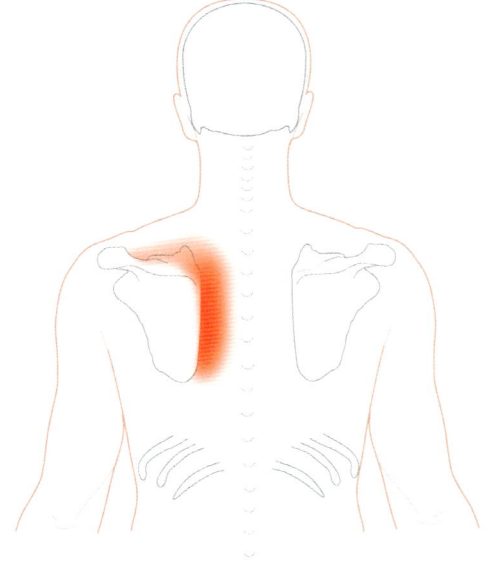

TrPs in the rhomboid major and minor and associated attachments have similar referral patterns

Greek, *rhomboeides*, parallelogram shaped, with only opposite sides and angles equal.

Origin
Spines of C7–T5 and supraspinous ligaments.

Insertion
Lower half of the posteromedial border of the scapula, from the root of the inferior angle to the upper part of the triangular area at the base of the scapular spine.

Nerve
Dorsal scapular nerve C4, C5.

Action
Retracts the scapula. Adducts, elevates, and internally rotates the scapula.

Kinetic System Comment
A hypertonic rhomboid will have a marked effect on the positioning of the scapula by lifting and retracting it. This will consequently inhibit the neural status of the serratus anterior, in turn affecting the external oblique, and so on along the chain. Force couple actions will be out of sequence, setting up the ideal environment for strain and overuse injury. When the serratus anterior is hypertonic, the rhomboids become inhibited, and the scapula will sit wide and drop.

Myofascial Trigger Point Comment
Pain is experienced around the vertebral border of the scapula, especially at night when at rest. The scalenes are primary sponsors of referred pain in this area and are worth treating when patients present with this pain pattern.

PECTORALIS MINOR

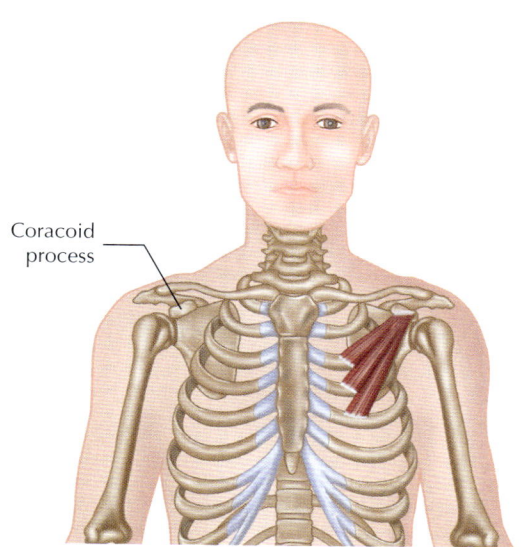

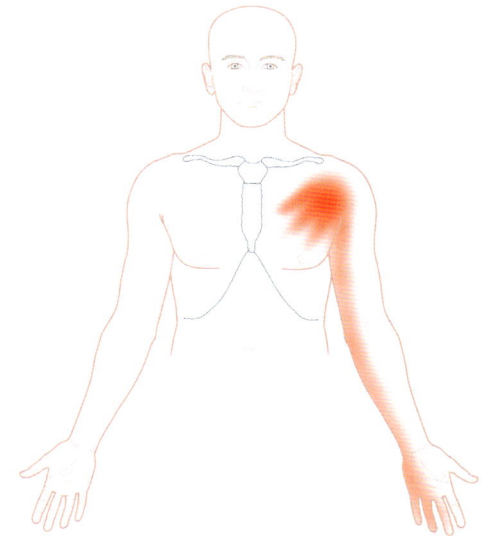

Latin, *pectoralis*, relating to the chest; *minor*, smaller.

Origin
Third, fourth, and fifth ribs.

Insertion
Medial and upper surface of the coracoid process of the scapula.

Nerve
Medial pectoral nerve, with fibers from a communicating branch of lateral pectoral nerve C6–8, T1.

Action
Elevates the ribs if the scapula is fixed, protracts the scapula (assists the serratus anterior), and stiffens to support abduction and flexion at the shoulder joint.

Kinetic System Comment
Pectoralis minor provides the tension to protract the scapula against the posterior ribcage, providing a relationship with the axial skeleton so that some movement can efficiently occur at the glenohumeral joint, e.g., lateral arm raise.

Myofascial Trigger Point Comment
Anterior chest pain is reported, with referred pain down the medial side of the arm and extending into the third to fifth digits. This pain can be mistaken for signs of heart disease but is most often mistaken for carpal tunnel syndrome because of restricted blood vessels and compressed nerves. Pectoralis minor is frequently a part of a double-crush (with the scalenes) or treble-crush problem, where all the muscles involved must be cleared of myofascial trigger points before homeostasis is restored.

SUPRASPINATUS

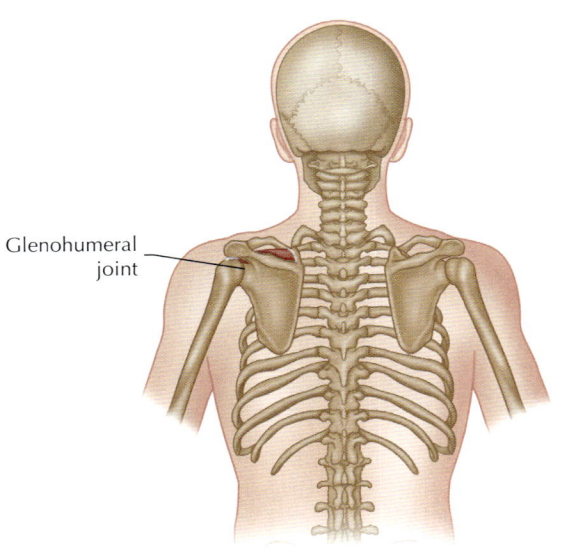

Glenohumeral joint

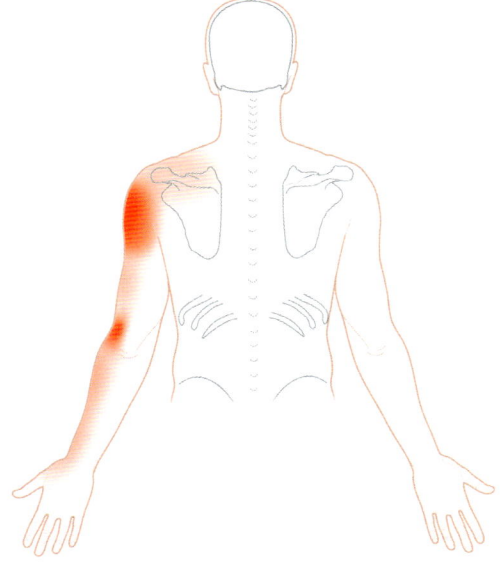

Referral pattern from the upper supraspinatus and attachment areas

Latin, *supra*, above; *spina*, spine.

Origin
Medial three-quarters of the supraspinous fossa of the scapula, and upper surface of the spine (bipennate).

Insertion
Superior facet on the greater tuberosity of the humerus, and capsule of the shoulder joint.

Nerve
Suprascapular nerve C5, C6.

Action
Abducts the arm, weak external rotator, and stabilizes the glenohumeral joint.

Kinetic System Comment
Supraspinatus works in conjunction with the deltoid to produce abduction at the glenohumeral joint. Because of its insertion superiorly onto the greater

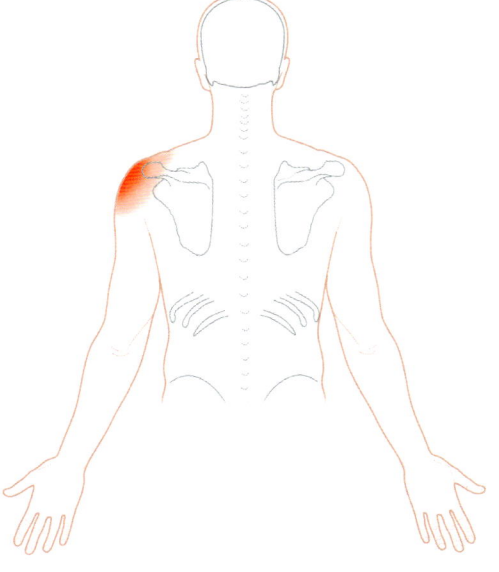

This referral pattern is from TrPs in the area of the supraspinatus tendon attachment to the glenohumeral joint

tuberosity, the muscle pulls the humeral head into the glenohumeral joint, thereby providing the stability needed while the deltoid (pulling halfway down the humerus) abducts the arm.

Myofascial Trigger Point Comment
Deep pain is reported in the lateral shoulder, forearm, and wrist. Radiating pain into the lateral epicondyle can lead to a misdiagnosis of tennis elbow (lateral epicondylitis), while the shoulder pain can be mistaken for bursitis. Difficulty combing the hair or raising the arm in flexion are signs of the presence of myofascial trigger points.

INFRASPINATUS

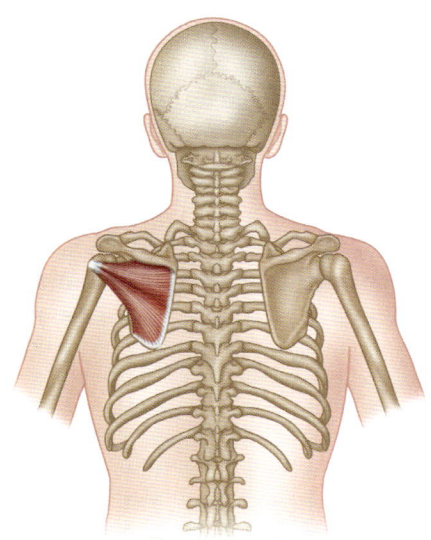

Latin, *infra*, below; *spina*, spine.

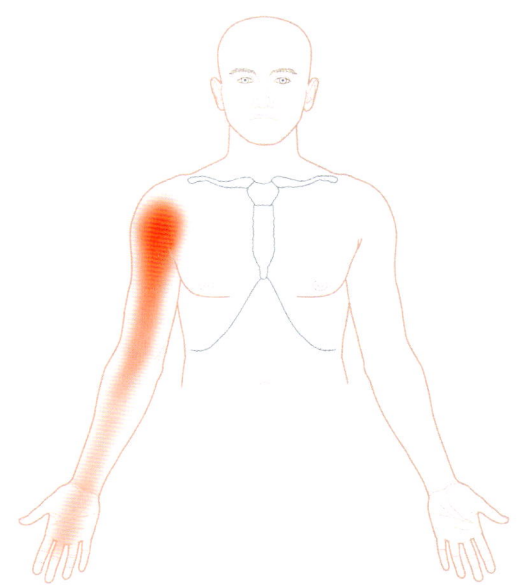

Common infraspinatus TrP referral patterns from the main portion of the muscle

Origin
Medial three-quarters of the infraspinous fossa of the scapula, and fibrous intermuscular septa.

Insertion
Middle facet of the greater tuberosity of the humerus, and capsule of the shoulder joint.

Nerve
Suprascapular nerve C5, C6.

Action
Laterally rotates the arm and stabilizes the shoulder joint.

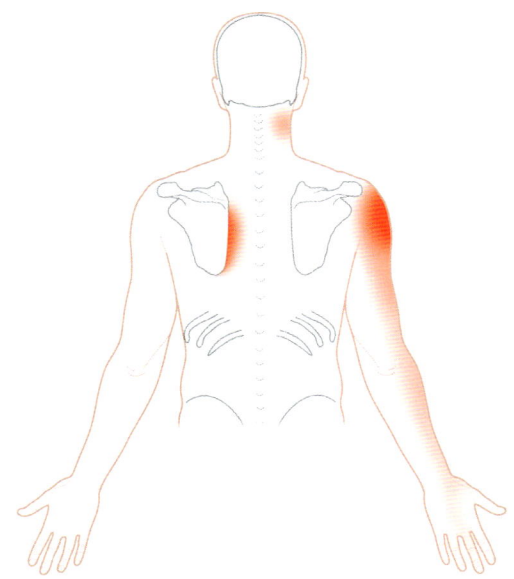

Common infraspinatus TrP referral patterns from the main portion of the muscle. TrPs in the attachment tendon of the infraspinatus cause a referral pattern along the interior shoulder blade edge, adjacent to and sometimes including the area of the TrP

Kinetic System Comment

Infraspinatus is an important muscle in scapula positioning because it decelerates internal rotation and shoulder flexion. Like all the rotator cuff (SITS) muscles, infraspinatus relies on an efficient core (lumbopelvic-hip complex) to translate forces needed from the lower limbs to the upper limbs.

Myofascial Trigger Point Comment

Deep shoulder joint pain is felt, as well as pain in the biceps brachii and down the side of the shoulder, radiating as far as the thumb. Severe pain in the anterior deltoid and bicipital groove are a common aspect of these myofascial trigger points, with pain also experienced in the posterior neck. Combined with other SITS muscles, these myofascial trigger points can cause symptoms mistaken for adhesive capsulitis (frozen shoulder syndrome).

TERES MINOR

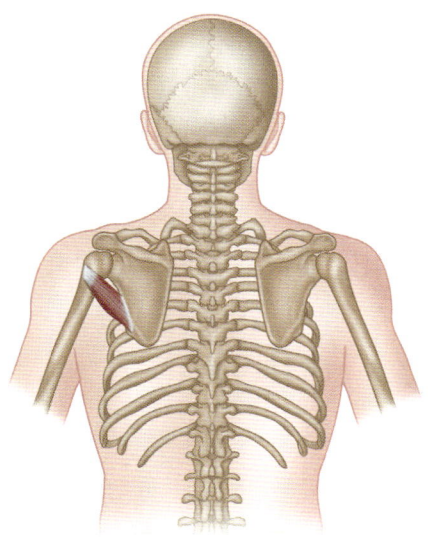

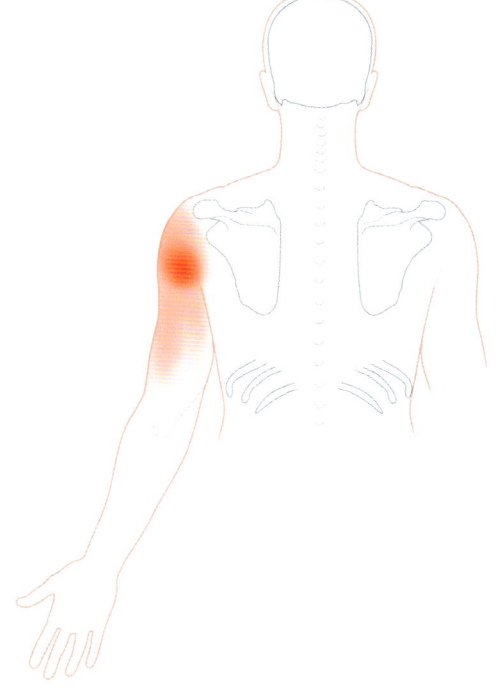

Latin, *teres*, rounded, finely shaped; *minor*, smaller.

Origin
Middle third of the lateral border of the scapula, above the teres major.

Insertion
Inferior facet of the greater tuberosity of the humerus (below infraspinatus) and capsule of the shoulder joint.

Nerve
Axillary nerve C5, C6 (from posterior cord of the brachial plexus).

Action
Laterally rotates the arm and stabilizes the shoulder joint.

Kinetic System Comment
Teres minor decelerates internal rotation of the shoulder joint. Inhibition in this muscle due to short/spastic subscapularis, latissimus dorsi, teres major, and pectoralis major sets up the ideal conditions for repetitive stress in sports, such as swimming and rugby, and in any activity involving acceleration through internal/external rotation and flexion/extension of the shoulder complex.

Myofascial Trigger Point Comment
Numbness or tingling will be felt in the fourth and fifth digits of the same arm, as well as pain in the posterior shoulder at the greater tuberosity. Teres minor myofascial trigger points are often sponsored by the subscapularis.

SUBSCAPULARIS

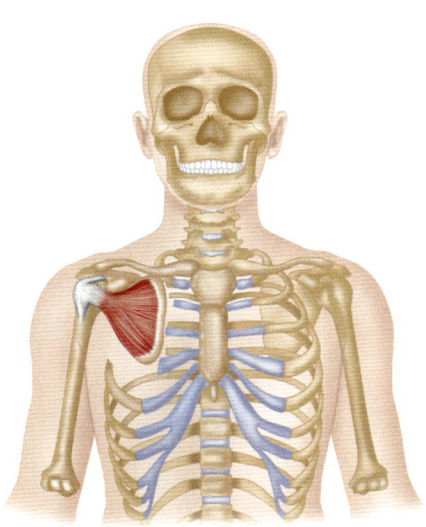

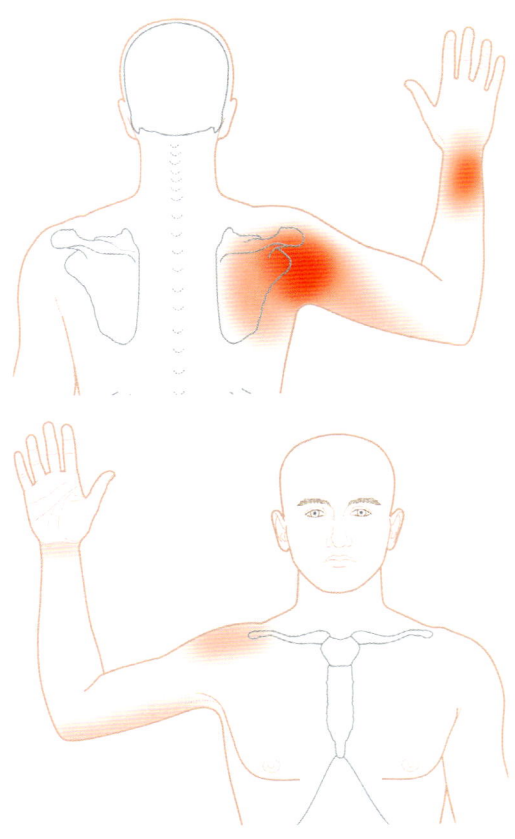

Latin, *sub*, under; *scapular*, relating to the shoulder blade.

Origin
Medial two-thirds of the subscapular fossa.

Insertion
Lesser tuberosity of the humerus, upper medial lip of the bicipital groove, and capsule of the shoulder joint.

Nerve
Upper and lower subscapular nerve C5, C6 (from posterior cord of the brachial plexus).

Action
Medially rotates the arm and stabilizes the shoulder joint.

Kinetic System Comment
Subscapularis eccentrically decelerates external rotation of the glenohumeral joint. This muscle has proved itself time and again to be worthy of special treatment focus in frozen shoulder and carpal tunnel syndrome complaints.

Myofascial Trigger Point Comment
Deep pain is felt in the posterior shoulder and wrist. Pain can radiate down the front of the arm. Spot tenderness on the lesser tuberosity of the humerus is common. Subscapularis myofascial trigger points are often mistaken for bursitis, adhesive capsulitis, bicipital tendinitis, arthritis, and rotator cuff injury. Pain and stiffness are a result of myofascial trigger points in the subscapularis.

TERES MAJOR

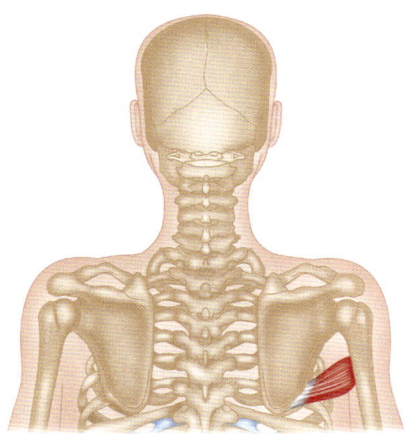

Latin, *teres*, rounded, finely shaped; *major*, larger.

Origin
Dorsal humeral surface of the inferior angle of the scapula, at the level of the lower third portion.

Insertion
Muscle fibers adhere to the fascia of the latissimus dorsi, rising up to attach to the crest of the intertubercular groove.

Nerve
Lower subscapular nerve C5–7 (from posterior cord of the brachial plexus).

Action
This muscle is affectionately known as the "little helper" of "latissimus dorsi". It medially rotates, extends, and adducts the humerus at the glenohumeral joint.

Kinetic System Comment
Teres major helps to eccentrically decelerate flexion, abduction, and external rotation of the humerus.

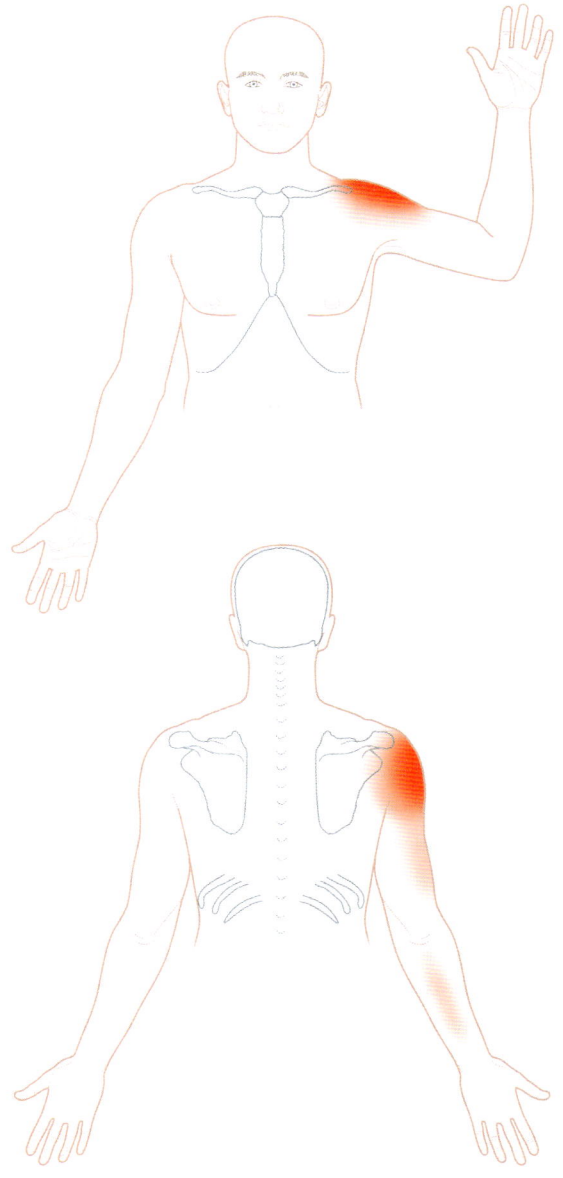

Myofascial Trigger Point Comment
Pain is experienced in the posterior deltoid.

SERRATUS ANTERIOR

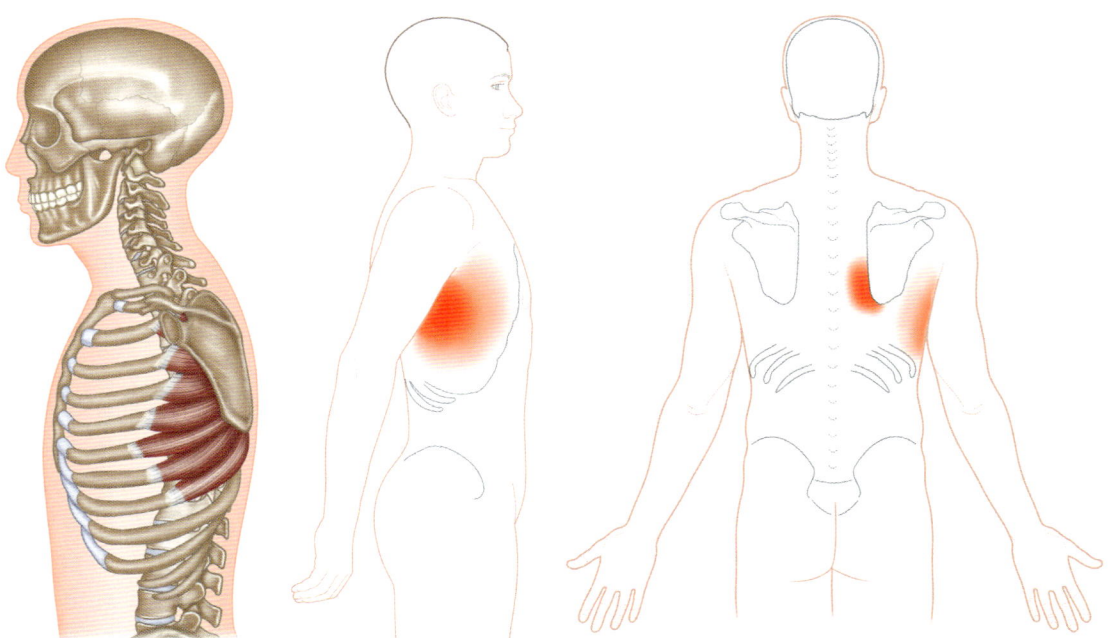

Latin, *serratus*, serrated; *anterior*, at the front.

Origin
Upper eight ribs and anterior intercostal membranes from the midclavicular line. Lower four interdigitate with the external oblique.

Insertion
Inner medial border of the scapula. Slips from ribs 1 and 2: upper angle; 3 and 4: length of the costal surface; 5 to 8: inferior angle.

Nerve
Long thoracic nerve C5–8 (from roots). Slips from ribs 1 and 2: C5; 3 and 4: C6; 5 to 8: C7/8.

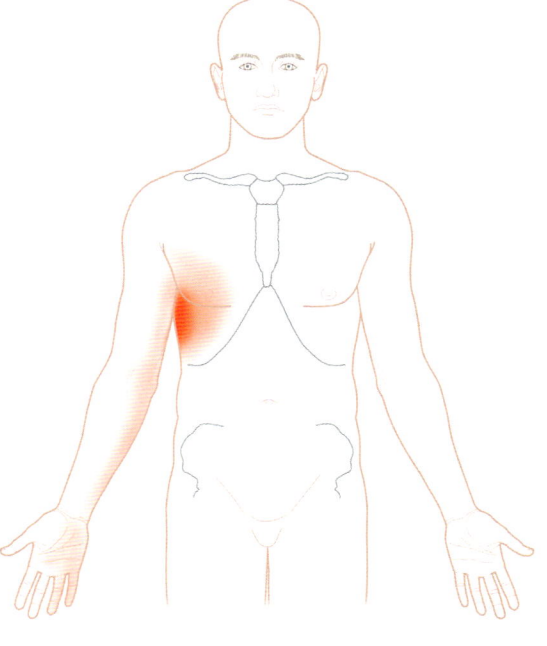

Action

Laterally rotates and protracts scapula.

Kinetic System Comment

Serratus anterior eccentrically decelerates adduction and medial rotation of the inferior angle of the scapula. Actions will change, depending on the origin or insertion being fixed. With the arm static, movement occurs at the ribcage, accelerating or decelerating the ribs as required, e.g., forced exhalation.

Myofascial Trigger Point Comment

Pain will be experienced on the side of the ribcage, travelling into the armpit and posteriorly to the medial aspect of the inferior angle of the scapula. Pain is often mistaken for C8 nerve problems, as pain is referred down the inside of the arm into the palm, fifth digit (little finger), and fourth digit. As this muscle has many digitations, careful assessment is required to locate active central myofascial trigger points.

LEVATOR SCAPULAE

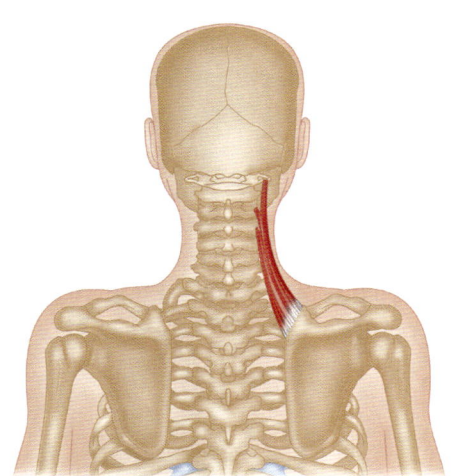 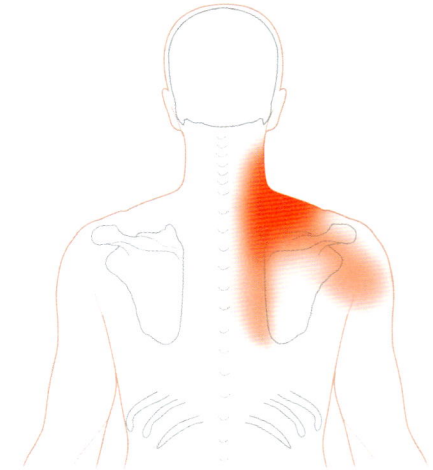

Latin, *levare*, to lift; *scapulae*, of the shoulder blade.

Origin
Posterior tubercles of the transverse processes of C1–4.

Insertion
Upper part of the medial border of the scapula.

Nerve
Dorsal scapular nerve C4, C5, and cervical nerve C3, C4.

Action
Elevates the medial border of the scapula.

Kinetic System Comment
Levator scapulae acts eccentrically to decelerate the downward forces created by the lower fibers of the trapezius and serratus anterior and decelerates contralateral side flexion in the cervical spine.

Myofascial Trigger Point Comment
Almost all neck pain will have myofascial trigger point contributions, and this muscle is commonly involved. Pain will be experienced at the angle of the neck from the superior angle, making its way down to the medial aspect of the inferior angle, with spillover all the way along the medial border of the scapula. Patients often report a stiff neck and reduced range of motion.

PECTORALIS MAJOR

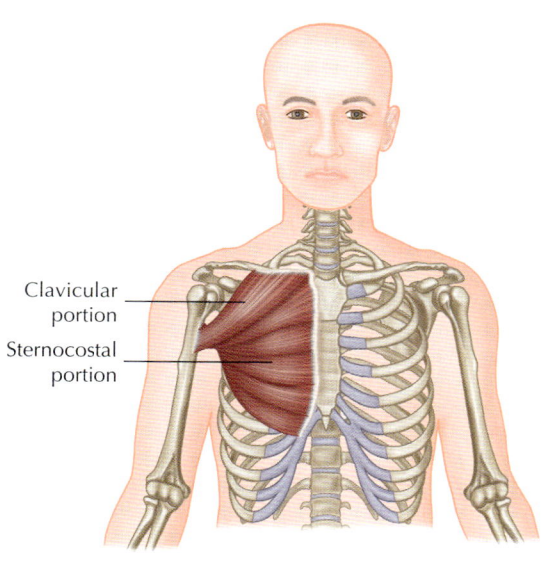

Clavicular portion
Sternocostal portion

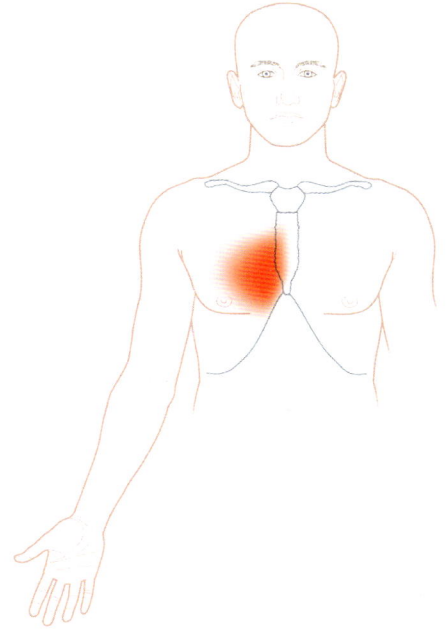

Latin, *pectoralis*, relating to the chest; *major,* larger.

Origin

Medial half of the anterior surface of the clavicle, anterior surface of the manubrium and sternum, and cartilage of the ribs (1–6).

Insertion

By means of a laminated tendon into the lateral crest of the intertubercular groove of the humerus.

Nerve

Medial nerve C6–8, T1.

Action

With the origin fixed, the pectoralis major will adduct and medially rotate the humerus. With the insertion fixed, the muscle can assist in breathing (forced inspiration, as it elevates the chest). It assists in shoulder stabilization during overhead movements.

Kinetic System Comment

This muscle eccentrically decelerates extension, horizontal abduction, external rotation, and retraction of the shoulder joint.

Myofascial Trigger Point Comment

Pectoralis major can develop multiple myofascial trigger points because of its clavicular and sternal fibers, firing pain across the anterior deltoid and down the lateral aspect of the arm into the thumb and fourth and fifth digits. A rare myofascial trigger point can mimic the symptoms of angina pectoris. Pain from these myofascial trigger points can also be felt as interscapular and subscapular pain. Restricted abduction will be evident.

SUBCLAVIUS

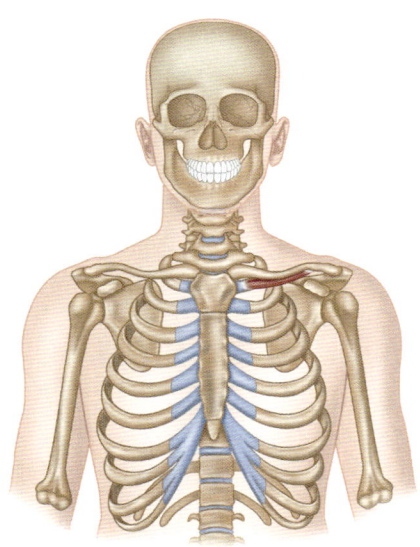

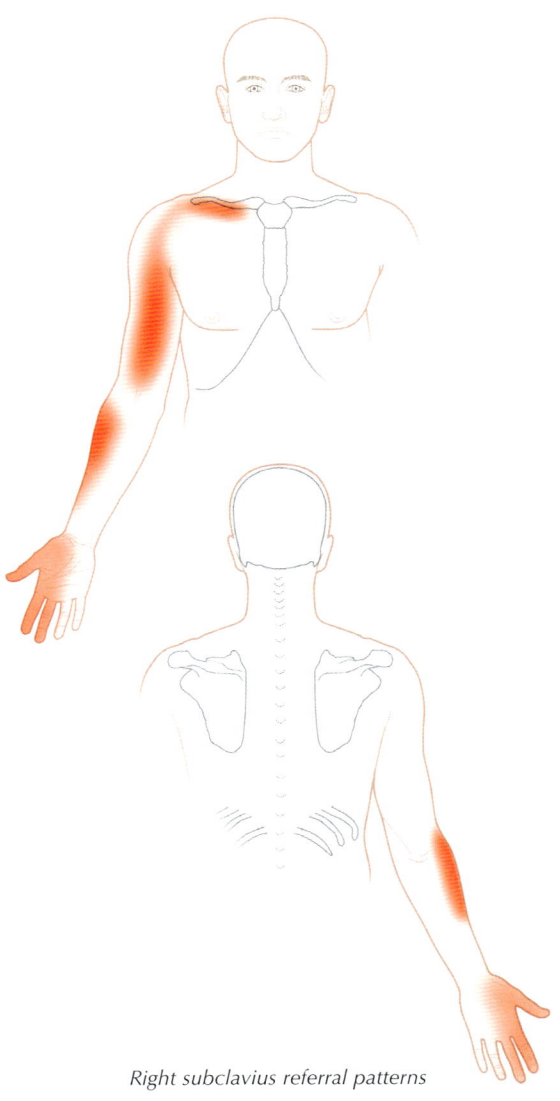

Right subclavius referral patterns

Latin, *sub*, under; *clavis*, key.

Origin
First rib, about its junction of bone and costal cartilage.

Insertion
Undersurface of the clavicle to the subclavian groove.

Nerve
Nerve to subclavius C5, C6.

Action
Pulls the clavicle toward the sternoclavicular joint.

Kinetic System Comment
Weak lumbopelvic-hip musculature can contribute to the formation of myofascial trigger points in subclavius. A change in position of the scapula will compromise this muscle and lead to myofascial trigger point formation.

Myofascial Trigger Point Comment
Pain is referred to the ipsilateral biceps brachii and lateral forearm. Locally, pain will be experienced just below the clavicle and may be felt as pins and needles in the arm, shoulder, and hand. The pain typically bypasses the elbow and wrist, resulting in pain in the radial half of the hand, thumb, and middle finger.

LATISSIMUS DORSI

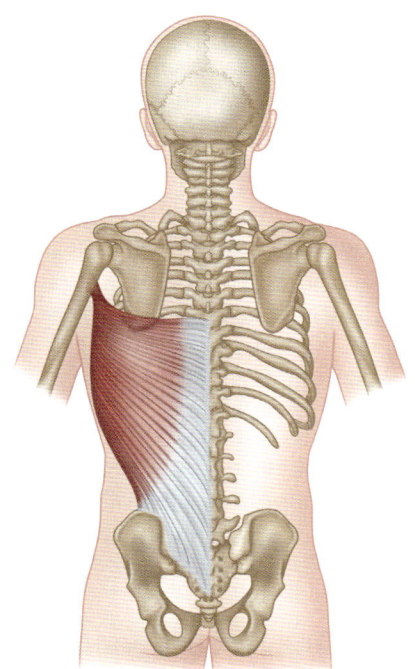

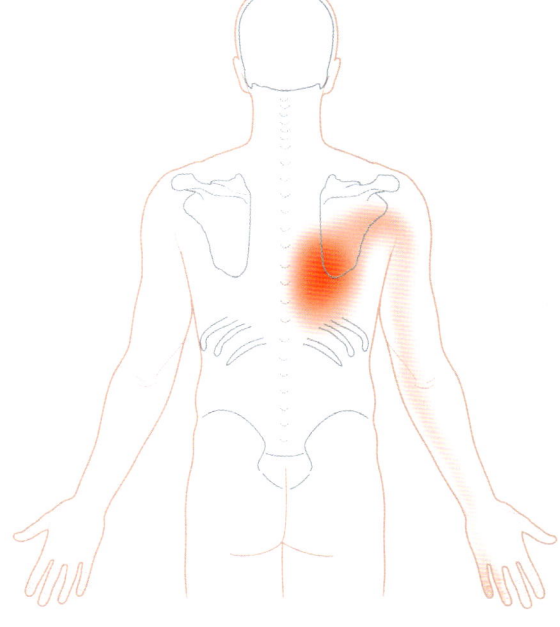

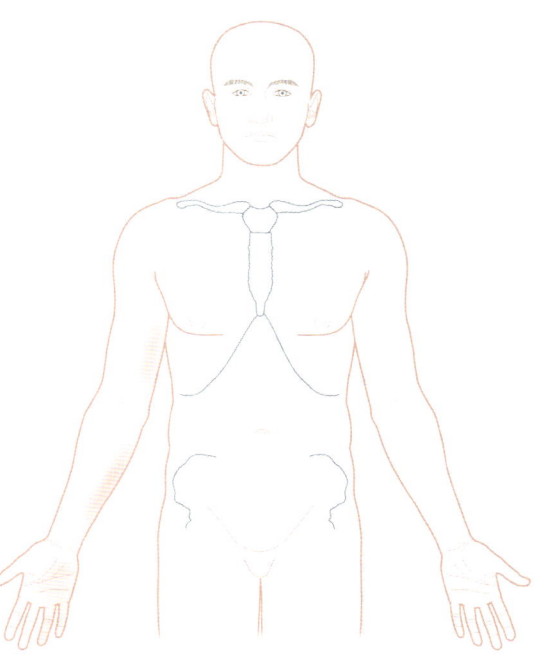

Latin, *latissimus*, widest; *dorsi*, of the back.

Origin
Spinous processes of T6–12, thoracolumbar fascia, iliac crest, and inferior three or four ribs.

Insertion
Intertubercular groove of the humerus.

Nerve
Thoracodorsal nerve C6–8.

Action
Along with its "little helper" (teres major), latissimus dorsi adducts, extends, and medially rotates the humerus in the glenohumeral joint.

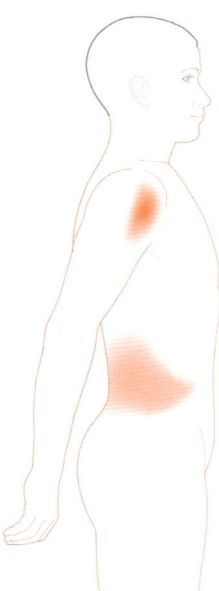

The location of the referral pattern often gives a clue to the location of the latissimus dorsi TrPs

Kinetic System Comment

A neuromuscular efficient core is required for the latissimus dorsi to provide the necessary forces to carry out some function at the glenohumeral joint. Neuromuscular inefficiency sets up the foundation for repetitive stress and associated "frozen shoulder"-type symptoms. The latissimus dorsi decelerates lateral rotation, flexion, and abduction of the humerus in the glenohumeral joint.

When the insertion of latissimus dorsi is fixed, the muscle plays a role in tilting the pelvis in an anterolateral direction. A bilateral contraction leads to hyperextension of the lower back, with accompanying anterior tilting of the pelvis. A muscle this size, covering so much of the posterolateral ribcage, will have an influence on diaphragmatic function. Any movement of the humerus will have an effect that extends into the thoracolumbar fascia and further down the kinetic system.

Concerning satellite myofascial trigger points, consider the following: pectoralis major, teres major, subscapularis, triceps brachii, scalenes, upper rectus abdominis, iliocostalis, serratus anterior, serratus posterior superior and inferior, lower trapezius, and rhomboids.

Myofascial Trigger Point Comment

Latissimus dorsi generates pain in the mid-thoracic area, including the posterolateral abdominal region. Pain of an aching nature is reported in the inferior angle of the scapula and the posterior shoulder. Referred pain travels down the medial aspect of the humerus into the forearm, hand, and fingers.

DELTOID

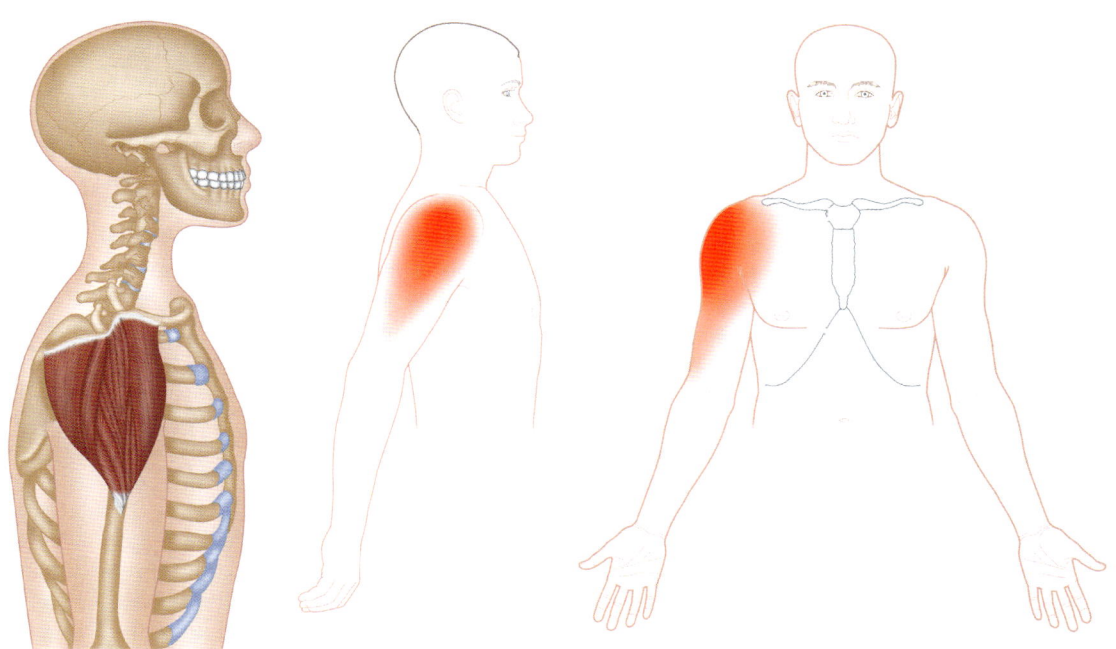

Greek, *deltoeides*, shaped like the Greek capital letter delta (Δ).

Origin
Lateral third of the clavicle, acromion, and spine of the scapula to the deltoid tubercle.

Insertion
Middle of the lateral surface of the humerus (deltoid tuberosity).

Nerve
Axillary nerve C5, C6 (from posterior cord of the brachial plexus).

Action
Abducts the arm, anterior fibers flex and medially rotate, posterior fibers extend and laterally rotate.

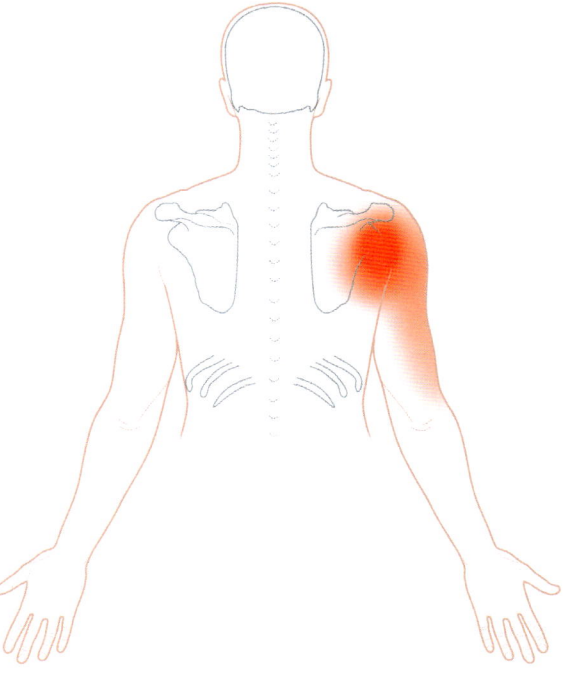

Kinetic System Comment

Deltoid—along with supraspinatus and associated rotator cuff muscles—will regularly develop myofascial trigger points as result of reduced core efficiency. Failure to translate forces from the lower body to the shoulder will result in arthrokinematic stress and the formation of active myofascial trigger points. The restoration of core neuromuscular efficiency will provide a foundation for myofascial trigger point therapy, utilizing fascia-focused therapy and medical exercise.

Myofascial Trigger Point Comment

Pain is felt as a dull ache for the most part, with increased pain on contraction of the muscle or when attempts are made to move the arm. Pain is most often mistaken for bursitis or rotator cuff injury. It is worthwhile checking the muscles that refer pain into the deltoid (SITS, pectorals, and scalenes) as the true source of deltoid pain. Deltoid myofascial trigger points are more often than not "satellite myofascial trigger points".

BICEPS BRACHII

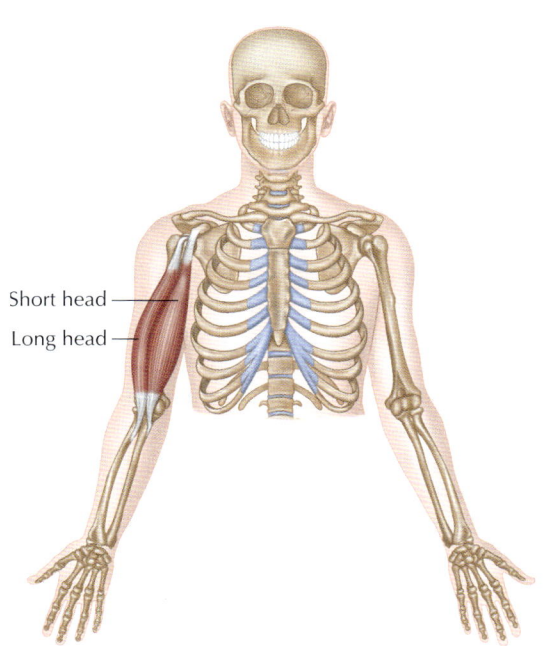

Short head
Long head

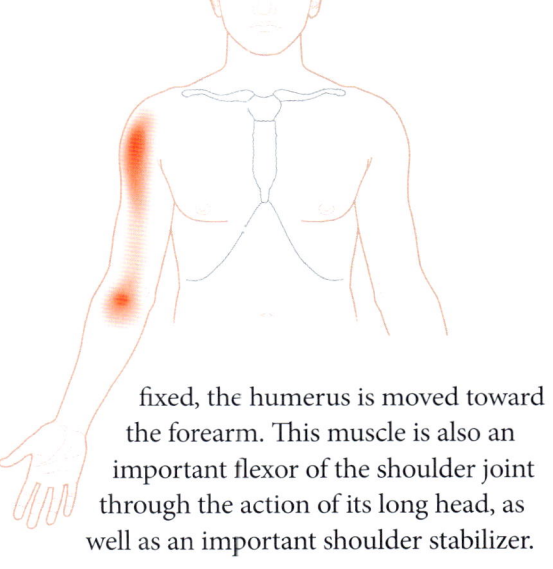

fixed, the humerus is moved toward the forearm. This muscle is also an important flexor of the shoulder joint through the action of its long head, as well as an important shoulder stabilizer.

Latin, *biceps*, two-headed; *brachii*, of the arm.

Origin
Short head: A flat tendon shared with the coracobrachialis, from the apex of the coracoid process of the scapula.
Long head: Supraglenoid tubercle of the scapula, and adjacent glenoid labrum of the glenohumeral joint.

Insertion
Posterior part of the tuberosity of the radius, and aponeurosis of biceps brachii.

Nerve
Musculocutaneous nerve C5, C6

Action
With the origin of the biceps brachii fixed, flexion will occur at the elbow, initiating supination of the forearm. With the insertion

Kinetic System Comment
Biceps brachii decelerates extension and pronation at the elbow and extension at the shoulder joint. It acts as a junction providing myofascial continuity between the thumb and the ribcage (especially obvious when the upper limb is abducted). The muscle plays a vital role in shoulder stability under dynamic conditions and can contract with triceps brachii to stabilize the elbow.

Myofascial Trigger Point Comment
Myofascial trigger points typically evolve in the center of the gaster and refer pain up toward the anterior deltoid and down toward the pronator teres, just distal to the elbow joint. The neuromuscular therapy hypothesis includes weak core stability with poor neuromuscular efficiency, culminating in compensatory myofascial trigger point formation to provide additional tension.

CORACOBRACHIALIS

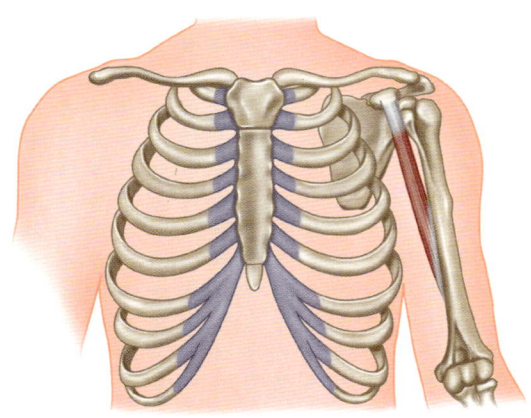

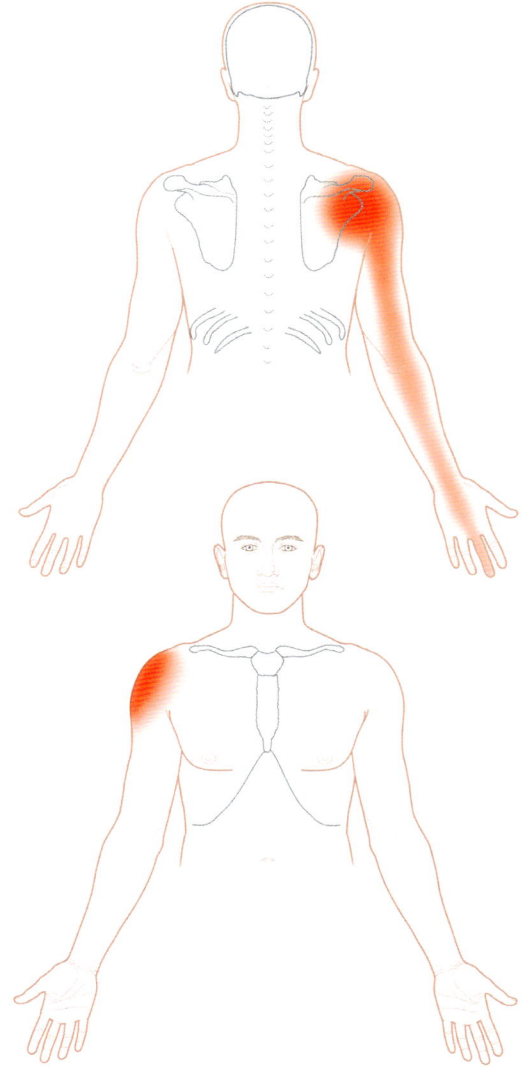

Greek, *korakoeides*, raven-like.
Latin, *brachialis*, relating to the arm.

Origin
Coracoid process of the scapula, along with biceps brachii.

Insertion
Upper half of the medial border of the humerus.

Nerve
Musculocutaneous nerve C5–7 (from lateral cord).

Action
Flexes and weakly adducts the arm.

Kinetic System Comment
Coracobrachialis links the thoracic cage and the scapula with the arm because it shares the tendinous root onto the coracoid process with pectoralis minor. Raising the arm out into abduction, with the hand at the level of the ear, demonstrates the continuity from the pectoralis minor through the coracobrachialis into the periosteum of the upper limb, and traveling on through the brachioradialis all the way to the radial styloid.

Myofascial Trigger Point Comment
Pain and/or numbness can be felt as far away as the posterior surface of the hand and into the middle finger. Pain can be referred to the posterior forearm, triceps brachii, and anterior deltoid.

BRACHIALIS

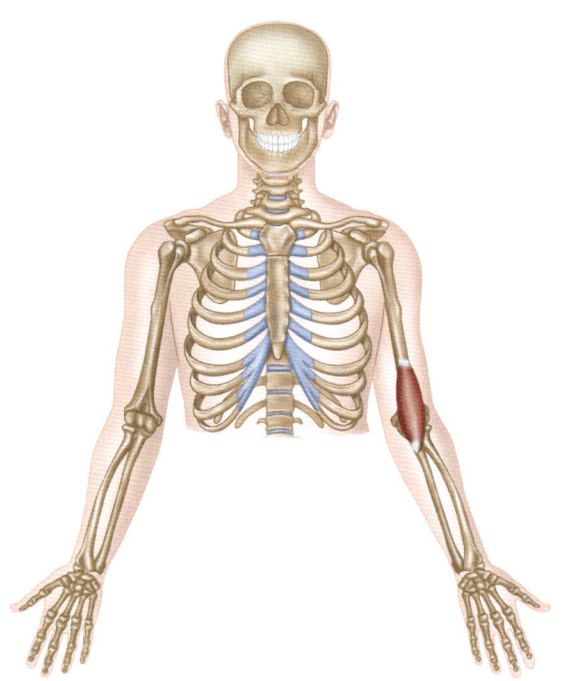

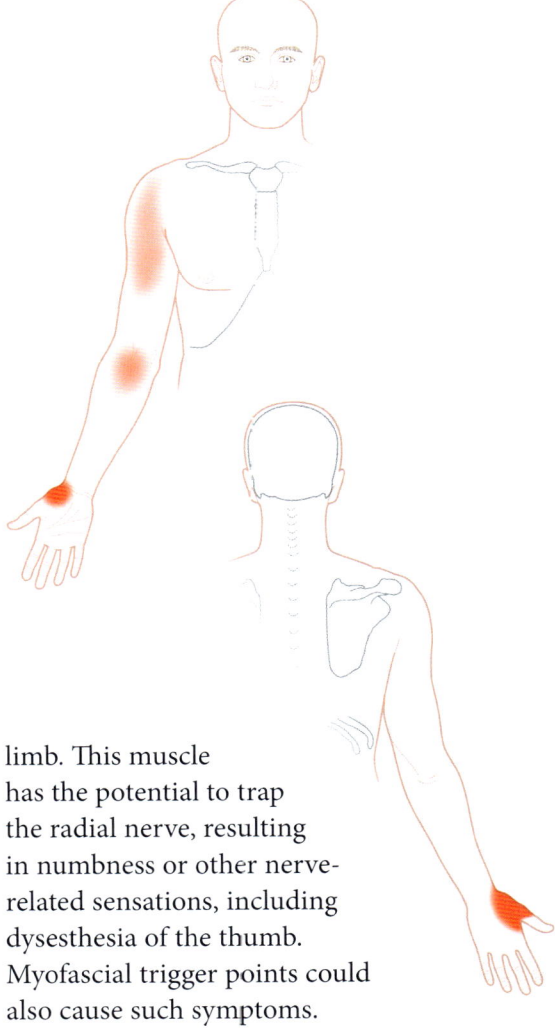

Latin, *brachialis*, relating to the arm.

Origin
Anterior lower half of the humerus, and medial and lateral intermuscular septa.

Insertion
Coronoid process and tuberosity of the ulna.

Nerve
Musculocutaneous nerve C5, C6 (from lateral cord). Also small supply from radial nerve C7.

Action
Flexes the elbow.

Kinetic System Comment
Brachialis is an important link muscle in the chain, connecting the thorax to the upper limb. This muscle has the potential to trap the radial nerve, resulting in numbness or other nerve-related sensations, including dysesthesia of the thumb. Myofascial trigger points could also cause such symptoms.

Myofascial Trigger Point Comment
Pain spreads to the base of the thumb, anterior deltoid, and just below the elbow joint line. Patients often complain of tingling or numbness in the thumb and hand. These problems can be misdiagnosed as carpal tunnel syndrome.

TRICEPS BRACHII

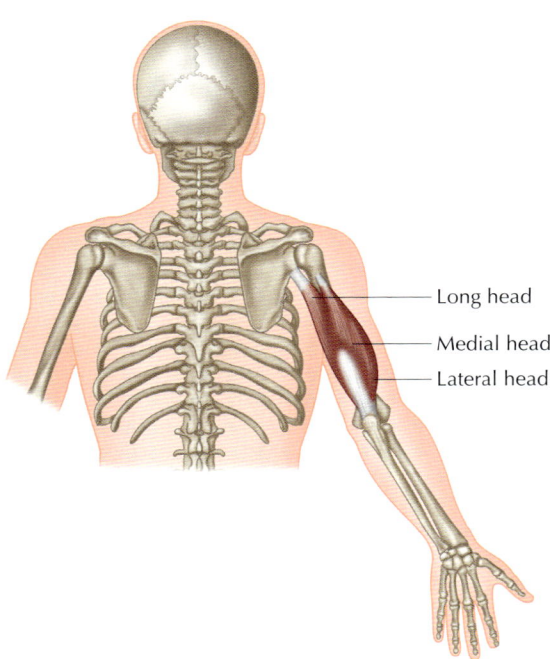

Long head
Medial head
Lateral head

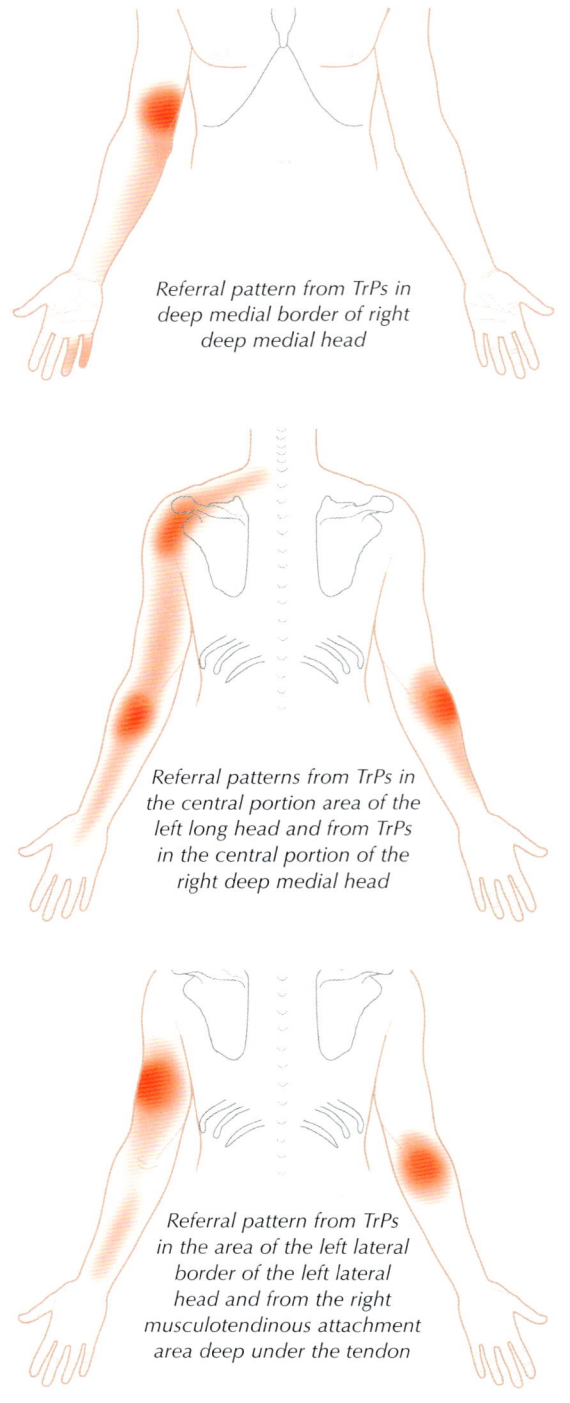

Referral pattern from TrPs in deep medial border of right deep medial head

Referral patterns from TrPs in the central portion area of the left long head and from TrPs in the central portion of the right deep medial head

Referral pattern from TrPs in the area of the left lateral border of the left lateral head and from the right musculotendinous attachment area deep under the tendon

Latin, *triceps*, three-headed; *brachii*, of the arm.

Origin

Long head: Infraglenoid tubercle of the scapula.
Medial head: Lies deep on the lower half of the posterior humerus, inferomedial to the spiral groove and both intermuscular septa.
Lateral head: Upper half of the posterior humerus (linear origin).

Insertion

Posterior part of the upper surface of the olecranon process of the ulna, and posterior capsule.

Nerve

Radial nerve C6–8, T1.

Action

Extends the elbow. The long head stabilizes the shoulder joint. The medial head retracts the capsule of the elbow joint on extension.

Kinetic System Comment

Along with its "little helper," anconeus, triceps brachii assists deceleration of flexion at the glenohumeral joint and the elbow joint. The radial nerve can be irritated by contracture or spasm of the lateral aspect of this muscle.

Myofascial Trigger Point Comment

Pain can be felt in the neck and upper trapezius. Other symptoms can lead to a misdiagnosis of pain felt in the elbow and triceps brachii as tennis or golfer's elbow. Myofascial trigger points in this muscle make it difficult to extend the arm at the elbow. Patients complain that they cannot rest their elbow on any surface, because of the level of sensitivity and pain.

ANCONEUS

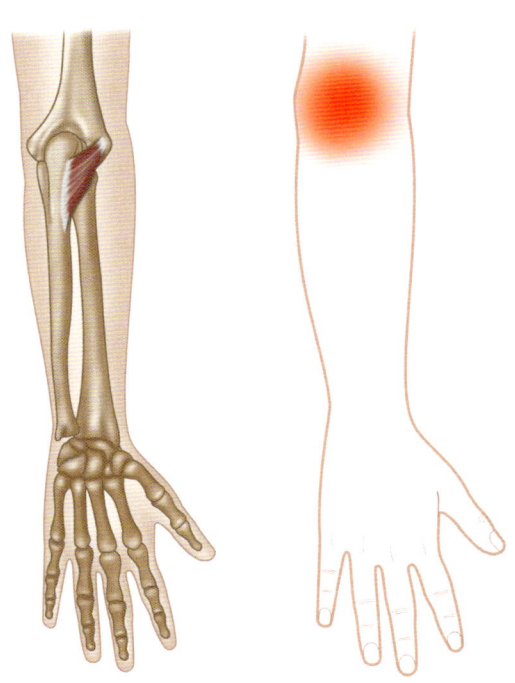

Greek, *agkon*, elbow.

Origin

Smooth surface at the lower extremity of the posterior aspect of the lateral epicondyle of the humerus.

Insertion

Lateral side of the olecranon.

Nerve

Radial nerve C7, C8.

Action

Weak extensor of the elbow and abducts the ulna in pronation.

Kinetic System Comment

Anconeus decelerates elbow flexion and supination. Myofascial trigger points typically evolve due to *active* myofascial trigger points in the more superior and medial muscles of the neck and shoulder. Myofascial trigger points can also evolve here because of gripping too tightly—e.g., a golf club, tennis racket, or writing pen—but reduced core strength must be considered as a causative factor.

Myofascial Trigger Point Comment

Pain from myofascial trigger points in this muscle are often mistaken for tennis elbow. Pain will be experienced when trying to flex the elbow joint and supinate the forearm.

Muscles of the Forearm and Hand

PRONATOR TERES

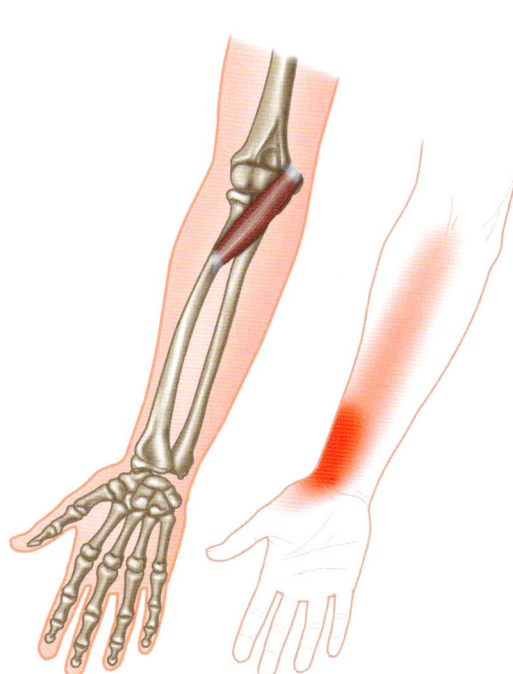

Latin, *pronare*, to bend forward; *teres*, rounded, finely shaped.

Origin
Medial epicondyle of the humerus, and coronoid process of the ulna.

Insertion
Middle of the lateral surface of the radius.

Nerve
Median nerve C6, C7.

Action
Pronates and flexes the forearm at the elbow.

Kinetic System Comment
Decelerates supination and extension of the forearm at the elbow.

Myofascial Trigger Point Comment
Pain is reported on the ulnar side of the forearm and at the base of the thumb. It may be difficult to turn the palm into supination with extension, without pain and stiffness. Patients have difficulty cupping the hand.

FOREARM FLEXORS

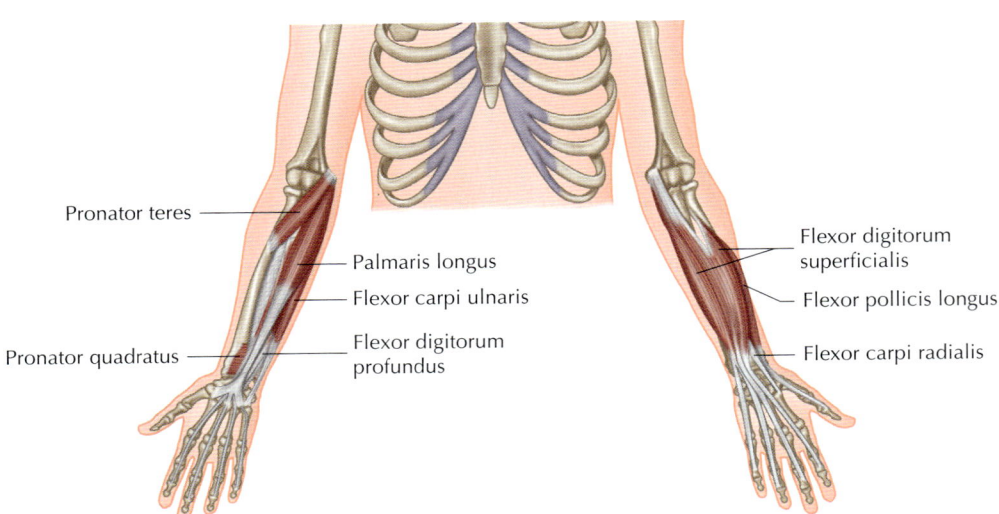

Pronator teres
Palmaris longus
Flexor carpi ulnaris
Pronator quadratus
Flexor digitorum profundus
Flexor digitorum superficialis
Flexor pollicis longus
Flexor carpi radialis

Although the extensor retinaculum is an extensor rather than a flexor, the retinacula are placed together here. TrPs in the extensor retinaculum seem to be more common in computer users. Those in the flexor retinaculum are more common in gymnasts.

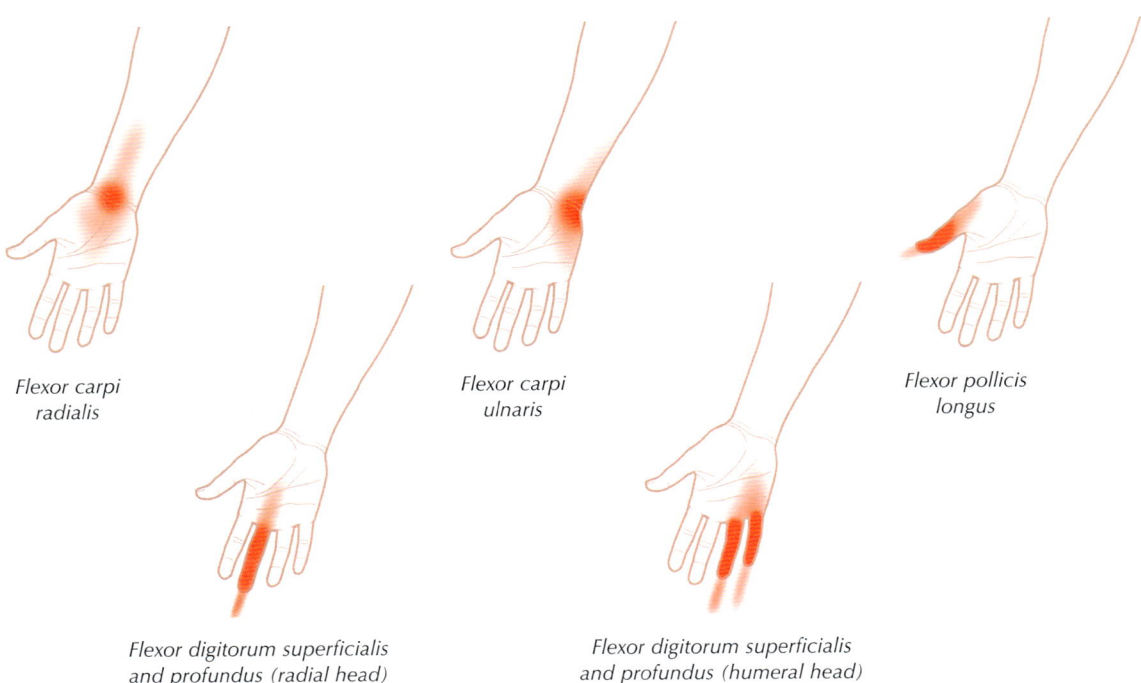

Flexor carpi radialis

Flexor carpi ulnaris

Flexor pollicis longus

Flexor digitorum superficialis and profundus (radial head)

Flexor digitorum superficialis and profundus (humeral head)

Latin, *flectere*, to bend.

Origin
Medial epicondyle of the humerus.

Insertion
Digits of the hand—carpals, metacarpals, and thumb.

Nerve
Radial and ulnar nerves.

Action
Flexion of the wrist and fingers.

Kinetic System Comment
A common theme in this book is the notion that the upper limb relies on forces to be translated from the lower limbs through the core, so that the arms can carry out some function. A lack of core stability will lead to these muscles developing extra stiffness in an effort to provide the forces required when communication has broken down within the kinetic system. Habitual tasks will determine which muscles shorten and which become inhibited; typically, the forearm flexors will shorten, while the extensors will become inhibited.

Treatment of the flexors first can often yield the best results, followed by medical exercise to build extensor endurance and tone.

Myofascial Trigger Point Comment
As there are numerous muscles in this area, various pain pattern behaviors will be influenced by specific muscles. In general, these myofascial trigger points refer pain into the anterior part of the hand and lateral three fingers. Spray and stretch technique is particularly good in the treatment of these muscles and restoration of homeostasis.

ADDUCTOR POLLICIS

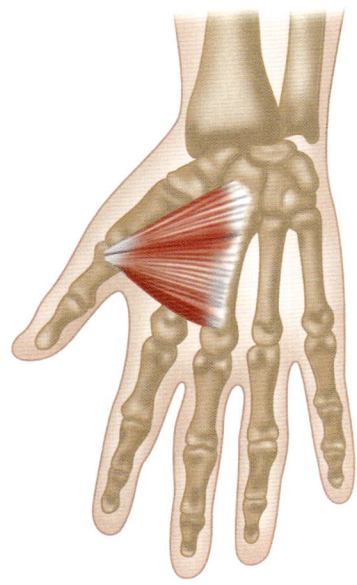

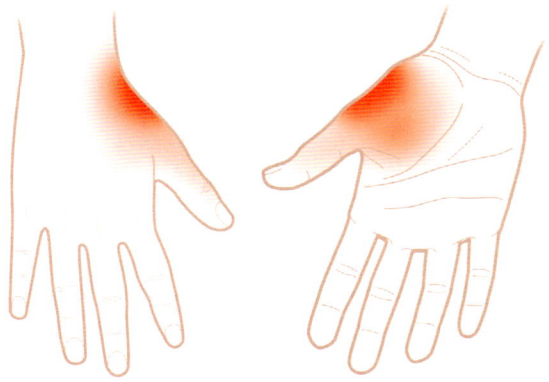

Latin, *adducere*, to lead to; *pollicis*, of the thumb.

Origin
Flexor retinaculum, and tubercles of the scaphoid and trapezium.

Insertion
Lateral side of the base of the proximal phalanx of the thumb.

Nerve
Deep ulnar nerve C8, T1.

Action
Abducts the thumb and helps oppose it.

Kinetic System Comment
Adductor pollicis decelerates abduction of the thumb and extension of the metacarpophalangeal joint of the thumb.

Myofascial Trigger Point Comment
Aching pain is felt on the outside of the thumb and on the hand at the base of the thumb, which has a tendency to lock. Patients find it difficult to control movement of the thumb and have difficulty holding a pen. Difficulty fastening buttons or performing actions that require fine muscle control becomes evident.

Myofascial trigger point pain can be felt in the thumb web space and the thenar eminence. It is worth pointing out at this stage to remember which other muscles refer pain into these areas—the scalenes, brachialis, supinator, extensor carpi radialis longus, and brachioradialis. Remember to check these muscles first (in the order of most medial and superior).

ABDUCTOR POLLICIS LONGUS

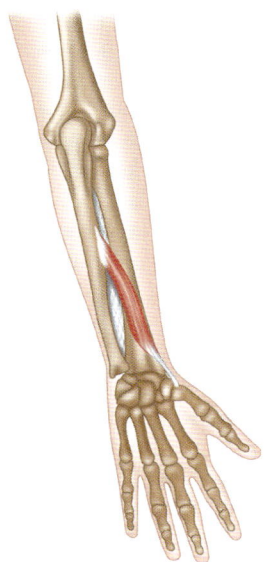
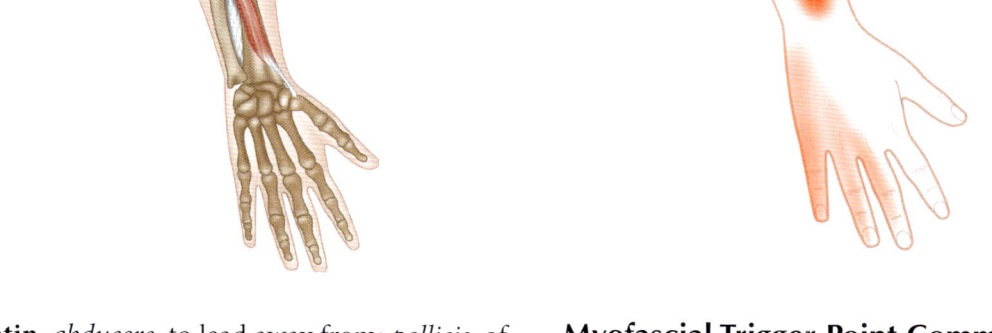

Latin, *abducere*, to lead away from; *pollicis*, of the thumb; *longus*, long.

Origin
Posterior surfaces of the ulna and the radius, and interosseous membrane.

Insertion
Base of the first metacarpal.

Nerve
Posterior interosseous nerve C6–8.

Action
Abducts and extends the thumb at the carpometacarpal joint.

Kinetic System Comment
Decelerates adduction of the thumb.

Myofascial Trigger Point Comment
Abductor pollicis longus is one of a number of muscles that can generate stiffness in the hand and fingers, often mistaken for arthritis. Patients have reported waking from their sleep because of cramping. As a result of inhibitory influences, the fingers and forearm lose local endurance, and fatigue sets in early on. Skilled control of the thumb reduces.

Referred pain patterns of the abductor pollicis longus resemble the C6–8 dermatomes, the superficial radial sensory nerve distribution, and are very similar to the area of pain experienced in de Quervain's tenosynovitis. Identification of abductor pollicis longus myofascial trigger points should be considered in the case of pain of the radial aspect of the wrist and thumb, especially when other neurological abnormalities or inflammatory conditions have been ruled out.

PRONATOR QUADRATUS

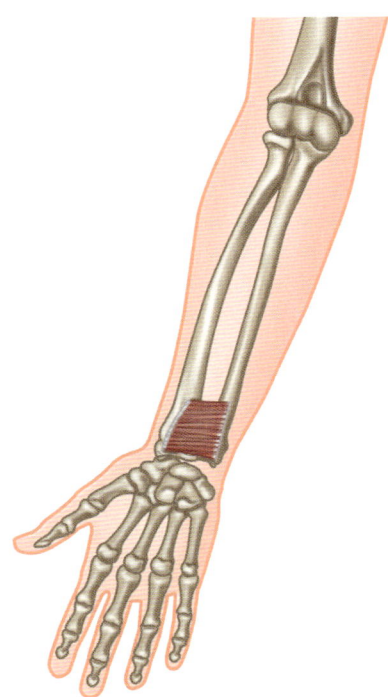

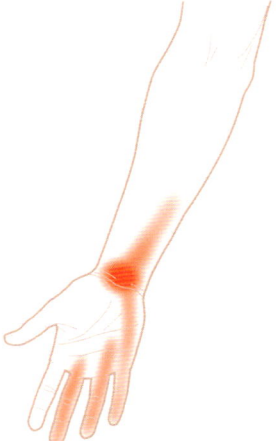

Latin, *pronare*, to bend forward; *quadratus*, squared.

Origin
Distal quarter of the shaft of the ulna.

Insertion
Distal shaft of the radius.

Nerve
Anterior interosseous from median nerve C7, C8, T1.

Action
Pronates the forearm. Deep fibers bind the radius and the ulna together.

Kinetic System Comment
Failure to stabilize the relationship between the radius and the ulna leads to complications along the upper limb fascial sleeve, resulting in shoulder joint and shoulder girdle/neck problems. Attempts to strengthen the forearm through increased weight training or similar will result in compounding the patient's problems. Pronator quadratus must have its myofascial trigger points dealt with before an appropriate course of physical activity with an emphasis on endurance is introduced.

Myofascial Trigger Point Comment
Two main pain patterns are observed. The most common pattern involves pain spreading both distally and proximally along the medial aspect of the forearm. In some cases, the pain area extends to the medial epicondyle proximally and the fifth digit distally. The second main pattern is pain spreading distally to the third and/or fourth digit. The pain patterns originating from the pronator quadratus resemble the C8–T1 dermatomes, and ulnar and median nerve sensory distributions. Therefore, myofascial pain of the pronator quadratus should be considered as a possible cause of pain in the medial forearm and hand, especially when other neurological abnormalities have been ruled out.

ABDUCTOR POLLICIS BREVIS

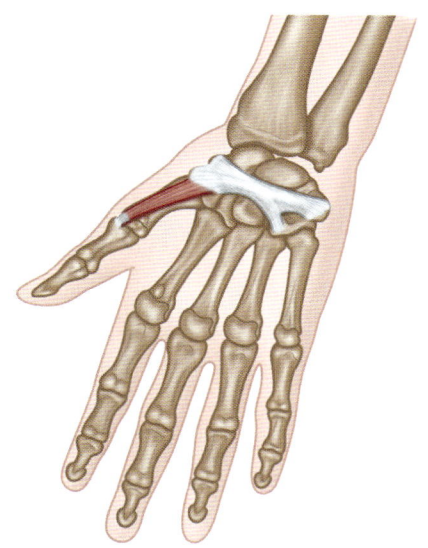 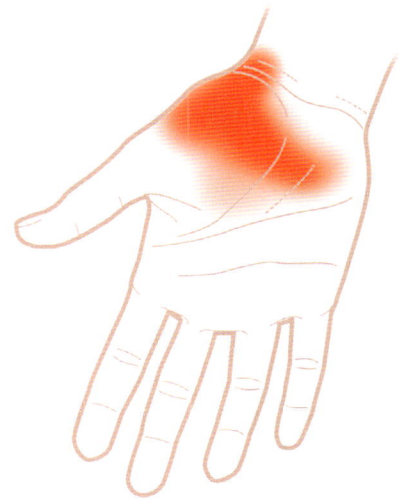

Latin, *abducere*, to lead away from; *pollicis*, of the thumb; *brevis*, short.

Origin
Flexor retinaculum, transverse carpal ligament, and tubercles of the scaphoid and trapezium.

Insertion
Lateral side of the base of the proximal phalanx of the thumb.

Nerve
Recurrent branch of median nerve C7, C8, and T1.

Action
Abducts the thumb and helps to oppose it.

Kinetic System Comment
Decelerates adduction of the thumb.

Myofascial Trigger Point Comment
Patients have reported a loss of grip strength. Pain and sensations are experienced in the palmar aspect of the thumb and wrist (radial side).

ABDUCTOR DIGITI MINIMI

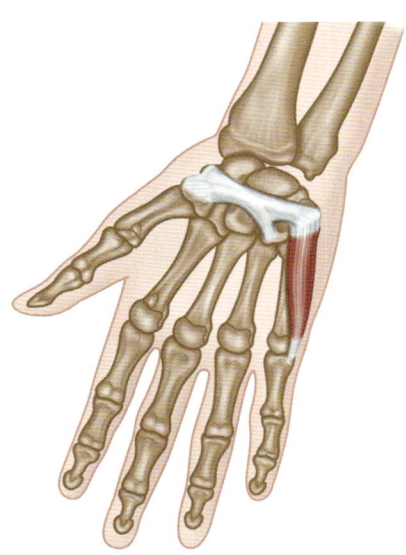

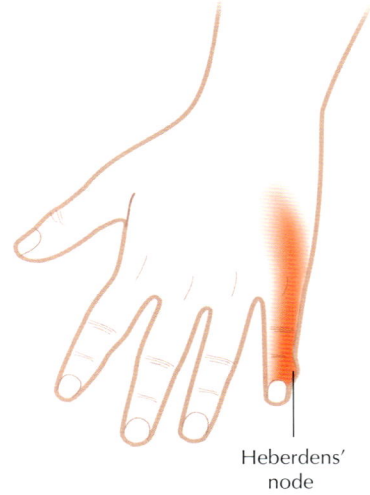

Heberdens' node

Latin, *abducere*, to lead away from; *digiti*, of the finger; *minimi*, of the smallest.

Origin
Pisiform bone, and tendon of the flexor carpi ulnaris.

Insertion
Medial side of the base of the proximal phalanx of the little finger.

Nerve
Deep branch of ulnar nerve C8 and T1.

Action
Abducts the fifth digit (little finger).

Kinetic System Comment
Decelerates adduction of the fifth digit.

Myofascial Trigger Point Comment
As the name of the muscle would suggest, pain and stiffness are felt in the little finger and often described as being an arthritic-type pain.

BRACHIORADIALIS

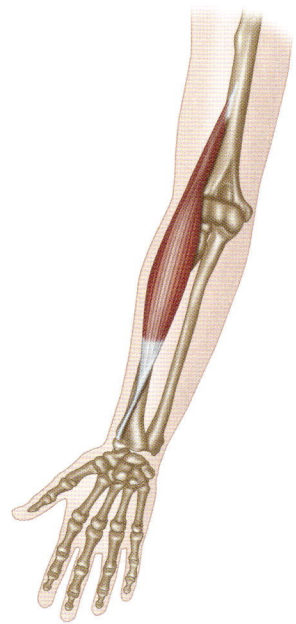

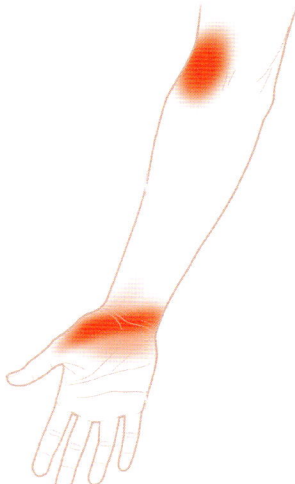

Latin, *brachium*, arm; *radius*, staff, spoke of wheel.

Origin
Proximal two-thirds of the lateral supracondylar ridge of the humerus, and lateral intermuscular septal fascia.

Insertion
Lateral surface of the distal end of the radial styloid process.

Nerve
Radial nerve C5, C6.

Action
Flexes the elbow joint and assists in pronation and supination of the forearm.

Kinetic System Comment
Brachioradialis is an important muscle in joining the forearm and anatomical arm, decelerating extension of the forearm at the elbow. It is a classic example of a "shunt muscle," preventing, as it does, the separation of the elbow joint during rapid movements. Baby or satellite myofascial trigger points should include the supinator, extensor carpi radialis longus, triceps brachii, and extensor digitorum.

Myofascial Trigger Point Comment
This is known as the "politician's myofascial trigger point," as it can be caused by all the shaking hands with so many voters. Pain is referred to the wrist and the base of the thumb in the web space. Also, pain is felt at the lateral epicondyle. A full examination of all the associated muscles in the kinetic system must be carried out, because it is difficult to know for sure which muscle is the major or true source of pain.

EXTENSOR CARPI RADIALIS BREVIS

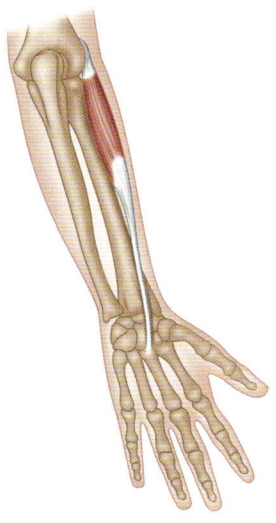
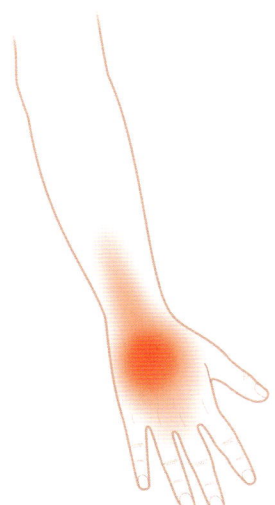

Latin, *extendere*, to extend; *carpi*, of the wrist; *radius*, staff, spoke of wheel; *brevis*, short.

Origin
Lateral epicondyle of the humerus.

Insertion
Posterior base of the third metacarpal bone.

Nerve
Radial nerve C5–8.

Action
Extends the wrist and hand and abducts the hand.

Kinetic System Comment
Decelerates flexion of the wrist and hand and adduction of the hand. Baby or satellite myofascial trigger points to consider include the supinator, brachioradialis, and triceps brachii.

Myofascial Trigger Point Comment
Wrist and hand pain are a common feature of these myofascial trigger points, with noted stiffness in the morning and increased pain on bending the fingers. Difficulty sustaining a grip on handles or golf clubs is reported because of a noticeable increase in weakness of the associated muscles. Changes in sensations include tingling, pins and needles, and numbness. The pain is often mistaken for tendinitis.

EXTENSOR CARPI RADIALIS LONGUS

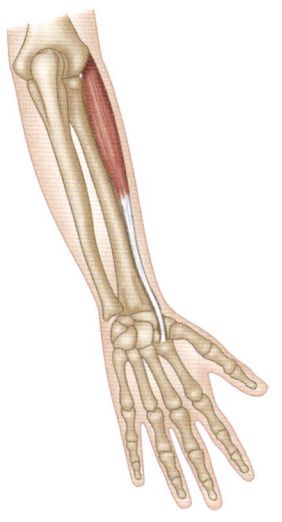

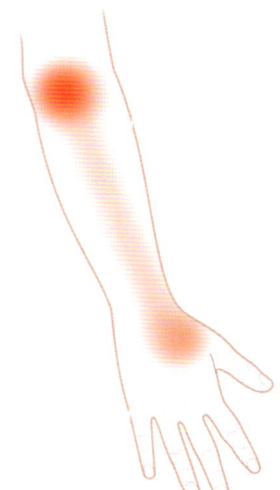

Latin, *extendere*, to extend; *carpi*, of the wrist; *radius*, staff, spoke of wheel; *longus*, long.

Origin
Lateral supracondylar ridge (inferior third) of the humerus, and lateral intermuscular septum.

Insertion
Dorsal base of the second metacarpal.

Nerve
Radial nerve C5–8.

Action
Extends and abducts the hand at the wrist joint.

Kinetic System Comment
Decelerates flexion of the wrist.

Myofascial Trigger Point Comment
Myofascial trigger points in this muscle lead to severe, unrelenting lateral epicondylitis (tennis elbow). Failure to treat these myofascial trigger points will result in the tennis elbow constantly returning—a great example of treating the symptom and not the cause.

My patients complain of an unrelenting burning sensation with a focus on the elbow and referred pain into the wrist and the fleshy part between the thumb and the second digit, known as the "anatomical snuffbox."

EXTENSOR CARPI ULNARIS

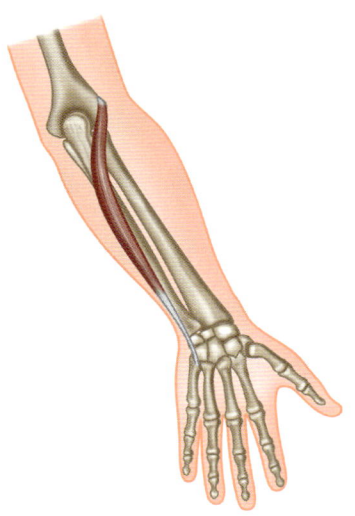

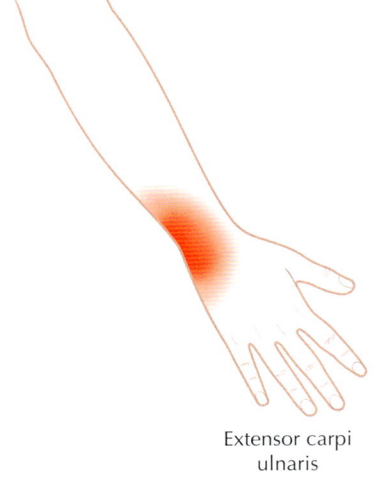

Extensor carpi
ulnaris

Latin, *extensor*, "to extend"; *carpi*, "of the wrist"; *ulnaris*, "of the elbow."

Origin
Lateral epicondyle of humerus and posterior border of ulna.

Insertion
Base of the fifth metacarpal.

Nerve
Posterior interosseous (radial) nerve, C6–C8.

Action
Extends and adducts the hand at the wrist joint.

Kinetic System Comment
Decelerates flexion and abduction of the hand at the wrist. Baby or satellite myofascial trigger points for consideration should include extensor digitorum and brachioradialis.

Myofascial Trigger Point Comment
Pain is referred to the ulnar aspect of the posterior wrist and is often mistaken for a wrist sprain. Sensations include burning or numbness.

EXTENSOR DIGITORUM

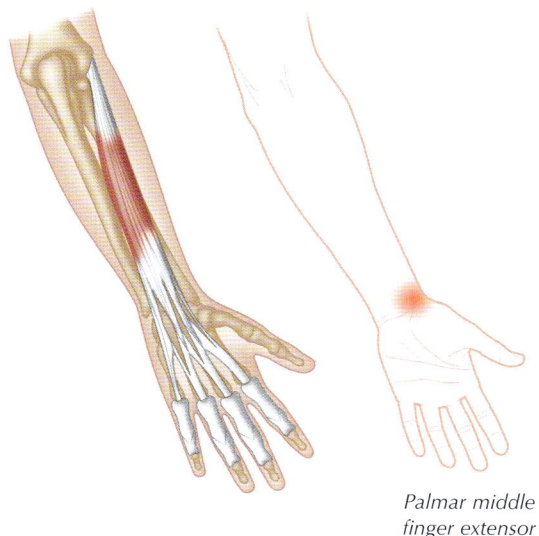

Palmar middle finger extensor

Latin, *extendere*, to extend; *digitorum*, of the fingers/toes.

Origin
Lateral epicondyle of the humerus.

Insertion
Extensor expansions of the medial four digits.

Nerve
Posterior interosseous nerve C6–8.

Action
Extends the medial four digits (not the thumb) at the metacarpophalangeal joints. Extends the hand at the wrist joint.

Kinetic System Comment
Decelerator of the fingers, hands, and wrist through flexion. A good assessment is the finger flexion test, where the patient is asked to touch the pads of their fingers, i.e., fingertips, to the palmar pads while the metacarpophalangeal joints are held straight. All fingers should touch the palmar surface; failure to do so would demonstrate shortness in the muscle(s), most likely requiring treatment. Extensor digitorum is responsible for satellite myofascial trigger points in supinator, brachioradialis, extensor carpi radialis longus, and extensor carpi ulnaris.

Myofascial Trigger Point Comment
Pain, stiffness, cramping, and weakness are the common sensations reported, with pain traveling down the forearm to the posterior part of the hand into the middle finger. Pain can be confused with lateral epicondylitis, C7 radiculopathy, and de Quervain's stenosing tenosynovitis. All the associated muscles—such as the extensor indicis, digitorum, and digiti minimi—must be considered and appropriately treated when pain in the fingers is the chief complaint.

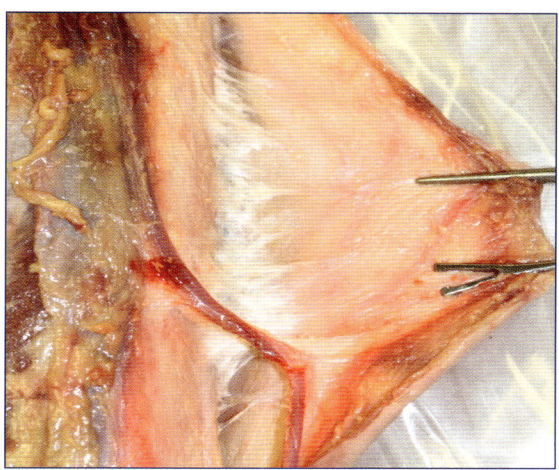

Here the forearm flexors reflect the close relationship of the forearm muscles. Note the ulnar nerve and artery on the medial aspect of the forearm. The deep fascia is clearly seen running in every direction. (Photograph: J. Sharkey 2010.)

FLEXOR CARPI ULNARIS

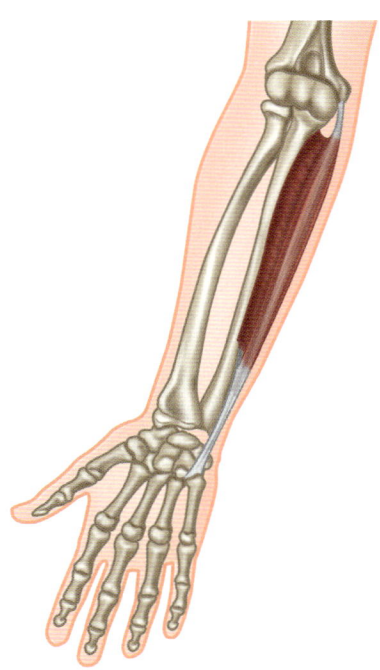

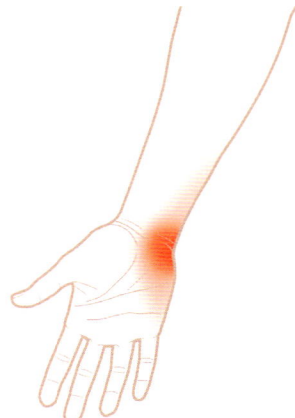

Latin, *flectere*, to bend; *carpi*, of the wrist; *ulnaris*, relating to the elbow/arm.

Origin
Humeral head: Medial epicondyle of the humerus.
Ulnar head: Olecranon process, and proximal posterior ulna.

Insertion
Base of the second metacarpal/pisiform bone, and a portion of the third metacarpal (hamate) and fifth metacarpal bones.

Nerve
Ulnar nerve C7, C8, T1.

Action
Both flexes and abducts the wrist and provides weak pronation of the forearm and elbow flexion.

Kinetic System Comment
Decelerates flexion and abduction of the wrist and hand and extension of the forearm at the elbow.

Myofascial Trigger Point Comment
Numbness and burning sensations can be experienced in the third to fifth digits. Pain is reported on the medial aspect (little-finger side) of the wrist as a sharp pain that can spread across the wrist joint, giving rise to a misdiagnosis of carpal tunnel or wrist sprains, medial epicondylitis, ulnar neuropathy, carpal tunnel syndrome, Charcot arthropathy, rheumatoid arthritis, osteoarthritis, C5 radiculopathy, peripheral neuropathy, Dupuytren's contracture, diabetic neuropathy, polyneuropathy, systemic lupus erythematosus, complex regional pain syndrome (reflex sympathetic dystrophy), and systemic infections or inflammation.

Of course, these must be ruled out by a primary medical practitioner, and so if in doubt, refer.

SUPINATOR

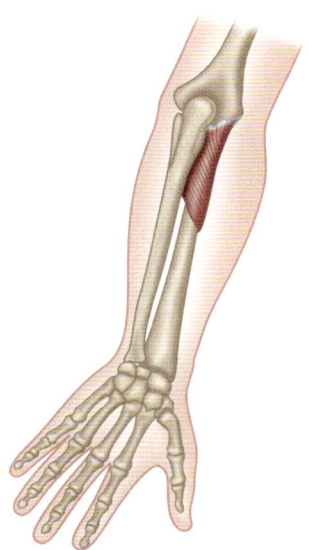

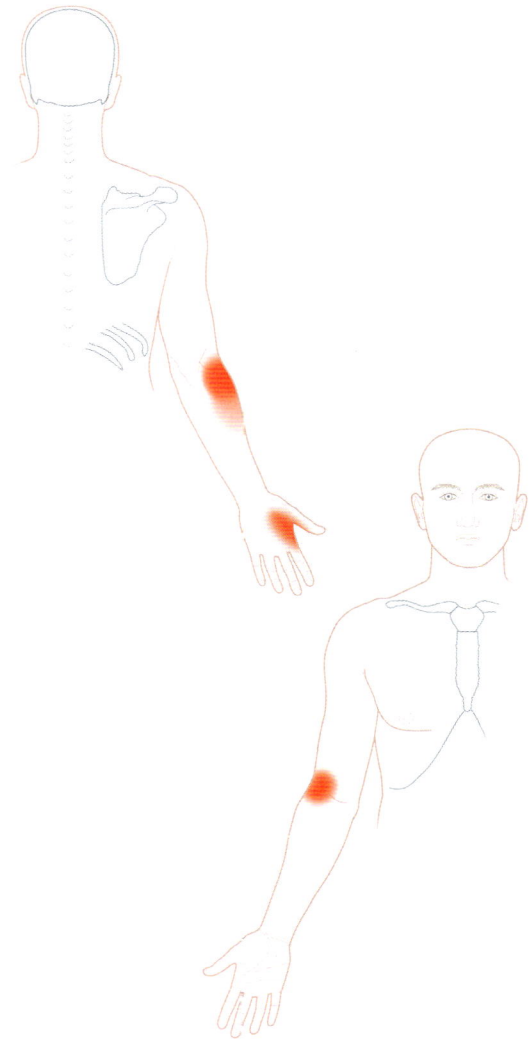

Latin, *supinus*, lying on the back.

Origin
Lateral epicondyle of the humerus, radial collateral ligament of the elbow joint, and annular ligament of the radius, including the superior crest of the ulna.

Insertion
Lateral upper one-third of the radius.

Nerve
Deep branch of radial nerve C5–7.

Action
Supinates the forearm and the hand.

Kinetic System Comment
Supinator is associated with deceleration of the elbow during extension. When the forearm is held between supination and pronation, the supinator will decelerate elbow extension.

Myofascial Trigger Point Comment
Supinator is a lateral elbow pain generator. The muscle sneaks pain down into the web of the thumb on the dorsal side. Changes in sensations include, but are not limited to, numbness and weakness in the hand (which may be due to compression of the deep branch of the radial nerve—the posterior interosseous nerve) and in the fingers.

OPPONENS POLLICIS

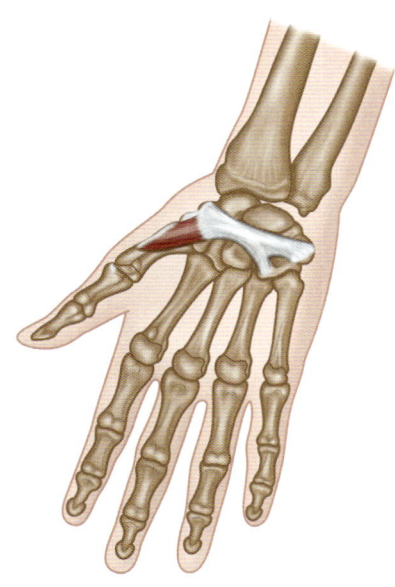

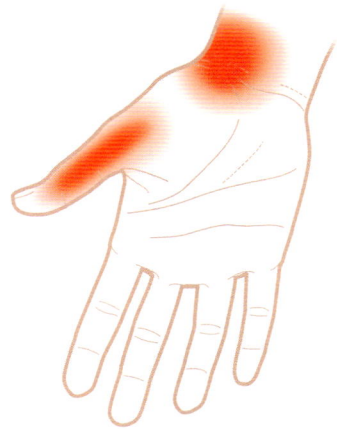

Problems with this muscle may lead to what Travell and Simons say patients refer to as a "clumsy thumb."

Latin, *opponens*, opposing; *pollicis*, of the thumb.

Origin
Flexor retinaculum, and tubercles of the scaphoid and trapezium.

Insertion
Lateral side of the first metacarpal.

Nerve
Median nerve C6–8, T1.

Action
Moves the first metacarpal laterally, opposing the thumb, toward the center of the palm and rotating it medially.

Kinetic System Comment
Opponens pollicis decelerates adduction and extension on the return from opposition.

Myofascial Trigger Point Comment
Pain refers to the palmar surface of both the thumb and the wrist. It has been reported that many patients can identify a specific point on the radial side of the palmar aspect of the wrist as being the source of the pain.

Pain has been mistaken for C6 or C7 radiculopathy, carpal tunnel syndrome, de Quervain's stenosing tenosynovitis, carpometacarpal dysfunction, osteoarthritis, articular dysfunction, paronychia (ingrown thumbnail), bone cancer, bone fracture, strain/sprain, rheumatoid arthritis, Dupuytren's contracture, ganglion cyst, mixed connective tissue disease, Raynaud's phenomenon, frostbite, diabetic neuropathy, systemic infections or inflammation, nutritional inadequacy, metabolic imbalance, and toxicity and side effects of medications.

PALMARIS LONGUS

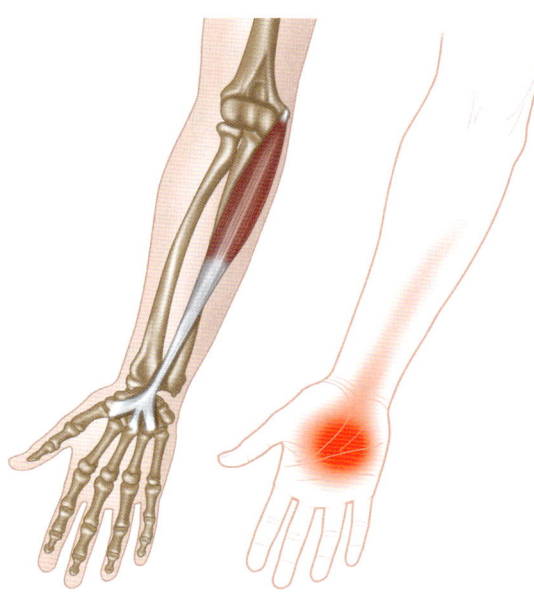

Latin, *palmaris*, relating to the palm; *longus*, long.

Palmaris longus is a meaty muscle with a substantial gaster and long tendon. It is interesting to note how the red muscle fibers run along the entire (or almost) length of this tendon (see image below). It is also worth noting the fascial slips attaching this muscle to neighboring fasciae and perimysial tissues.

Origin
Medial epicondyle of the humerus.

Insertion
Distal half of the flexor retinaculum, palmar aponeurosis, and transverse carpal ligament.

Nerve
Median nerve C7, C8, T1.

Action
Flexes the hand at the wrist, stiffens the aponeurosis of the palm, and assists in pronation and flexion of the forearm.

Kinetic System Comment
Decelerates extension of the hand at the wrist while decelerating supination of the hand against gravity and extension of the forearm at the elbow.

Myofascial Trigger Point Comment
A focal point of pain from the palmaris longus is experienced as a needle-like sensation, rather than the deep aching pain of myofascial trigger points in many other muscles. Pain can extend to the base of the thumb and the distal crease of the palm. A residue of this pain can travel to the distal volar forearm.

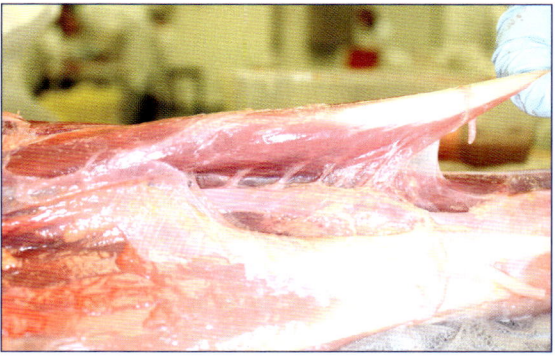

Palmaris longus (Photograph: J. Sharkey, 2010).

Muscles of the Hip and Thigh

GLUTEUS MAXIMUS

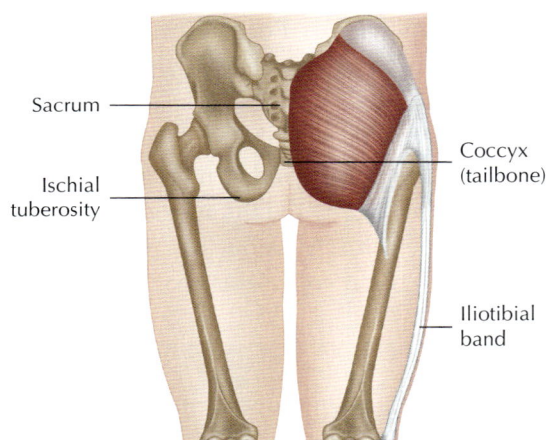

Sacrum

Ischial
tuberosity

Coccyx
(tailbone)

Iliotibial
band

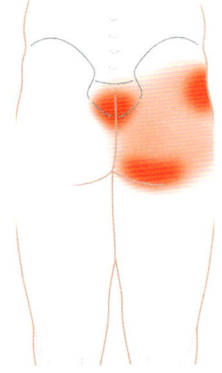

*Referral pattern of TrPs in the lower midportion of
the muscle, over the ischial tuberosity midpoint*

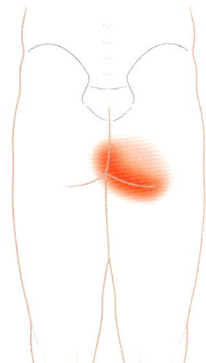

*Referral pattern of TrPs in the lower area of
the interior edge (medial inferior) of the muscle*

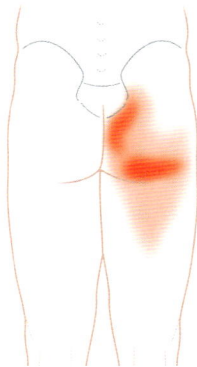

*Referral pattern of TrPs along the sacrum area
(superior medial) of the muscle*

Greek, *gloutos*, buttock. **Latin**, *maximus*, biggest.

Origin

Gluteal surface of the ilium behind the posterior gluteal line, posterior border of the ilium, aponeurosis of the erector spinae, sacrotuberous ligament, and gluteal aponeurosis.

Insertion

Iliotibial tract of the fascia lata, and gluteal tuberosity of the femur by means of a broad aponeurosis.

Nerve

Inferior gluteal nerve L5, S1, S2.

Action

Laterally rotates and extends the hip joint and assists in adduction at the hip joint. Eccentrically, the gluteus maximus contracts to decelerate hip flexion, adduction, and internal rotation.

Kinetic System Comment

Gluteus maximus plays a significant role in stabilizing both the sacroiliac joint and the knee joint. It does so by means of superior fibers, which attach to the aponeurosis of the sacrotuberous ligament, and inferior fibers, which attach anteriorly to the iliotibial tract, providing tension down to the knee. Weak gluteal muscles have wide-reaching implications up and down the kinetic system.

Myofascial Trigger Point Comment

It is hypothesized that gluteal myofascial trigger points could be a result of inhibition in the gluteal muscles caused by spasm in the psoas muscles, gluteus medius, and gluteus minimus. The formation of these myofascial trigger points provides much-needed tension for sacroiliac support. Pain is often felt in the lower back and mimics bursitis of the hip, with pain experienced at the site of the coccygeal bone and of the gluteal crease.

Weakness in gluteus maximus can be resolved by finding which myofascial trigger points are referring the inhibition to it. Gluteus maximus requires specific retraining following appropriate treatment, and commonly causes abnormal gait, which can aggravate many other types of problems, including in the knee.

GLUTEUS MEDIUS

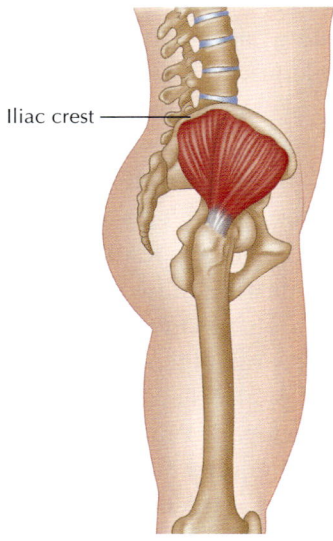

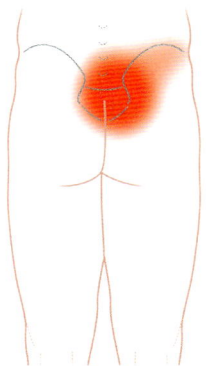

Referral pattern of TrPs usually found under the front portion of the muscle along and under the iliac crest

TrPs in the gluteus medius often occur in a line along and below the iliac crest

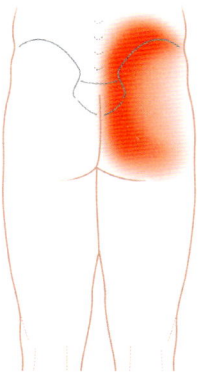

Referral pattern of TrPs usually found under the back portion of the muscle close to the sacrum, along and under the iliac crest

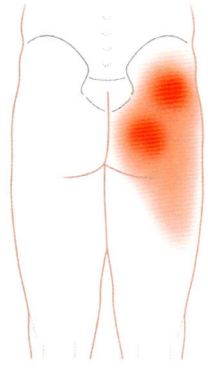

Referral pattern of TrPs usually found under the middle portion of the muscle along and under the iliac crest

Insertion
Posterolateral surface of the greater trochanter of the femur.

Nerve
Superior gluteal nerve L4, L5, S1.

Greek, *gloutos*, buttock. **Latin**, *medius*, middle.

Origin
Outer surface of the ilium, between the posterior and middle gluteal lines.

Action
Abducts and both externally/internally rotates the hip. Tilts the pelvis when walking.

Kinetic System Comment

Gluteus medius is a crucial muscle in offering stability to the lateral line. Weakness leads to lower back pain for runners and creates undue knee stress, which is often mistaken for discogenic problems and sacroiliac dysfunction. The one-leg standing test (Stork test) will often result in the patient being unable to stabilize the iliofemoral relationship on the frontal plane, because gluteus medius is required to eccentrically contract or decelerate the movement. This can be evident as an exaggerated lateral hip-sway during walking, which results from over-pronation of the foot, dropped arch, rotation of the second toe (Morton's foot), and medial rotation of the tibia/femur.

Baby or satellite myofascial trigger points include the quadratus lumborum, piriformis, gluteus minimus, gluteus maximus, and tensor fasciae latae.

Myofascial Trigger Point Comment

Lower back pain is felt above and below the belt line. Pain in the hips makes it difficult to sleep in comfort and leads to disturbed sleep patterns. This muscle is a major generator of lower back and hip pain, as well as being responsible for complaints of a burning sensation along the posterior superior iliac spine (PSIS) and sacroiliac joint. Pain is often mistaken for lumbago-type pain, with discomfort (such as tenderness) into the buttocks and superior thigh.

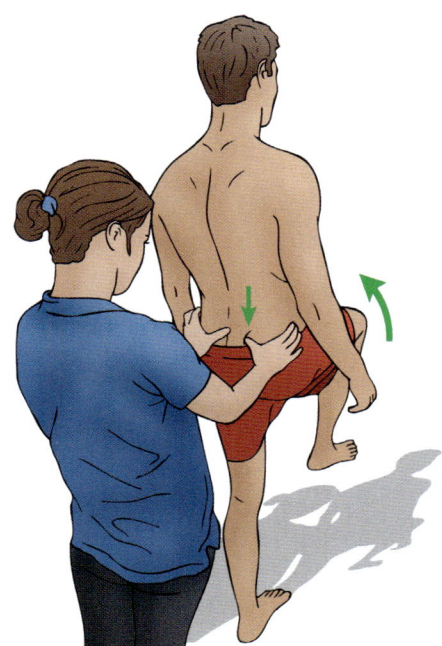

Stork test.

GLUTEUS MINIMUS

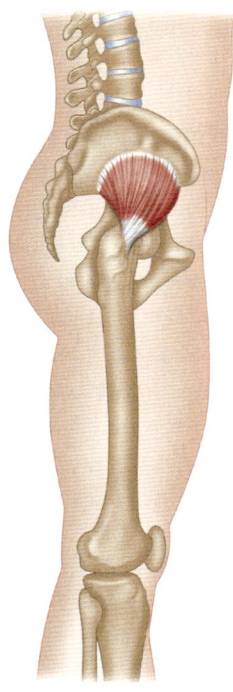

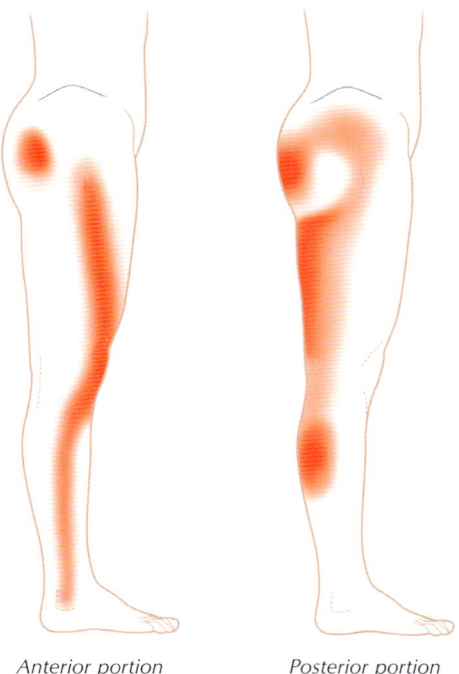

Anterior portion   *Posterior portion*

Greek, *gloutos*, buttock. **Latin**, *minimus*, smallest.

Origin
Outer surface of the ilium, between the middle and inferior gluteal lines.

Insertion
Anterior surface of the greater trochanter of the femur.

Nerve
Superior gluteal nerve L4, L5, S1.

Action
Abducts and medially rotates the hip. Assists in tilting the pelvis when walking.

Kinetic System Comment
Acts to decelerate external rotation and adduction of the femur in the hip joint.

Myofascial Trigger Point Comment
Pain is experienced in the posterior and/or lateral thigh as well as deep in the buttocks. Numbness can be another symptom, and pain can refer as far as the lateral ankle. Such pain and discomfort can be mistaken for sciatic pain.

TENSOR FASCIAE LATAE

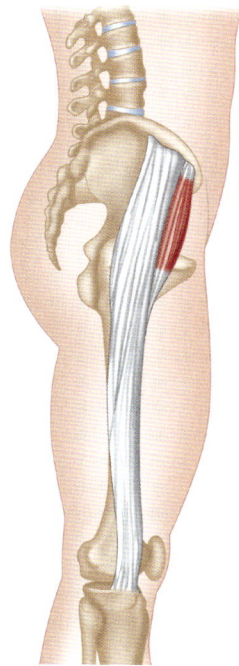

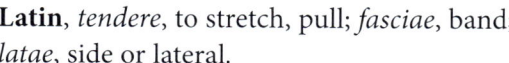

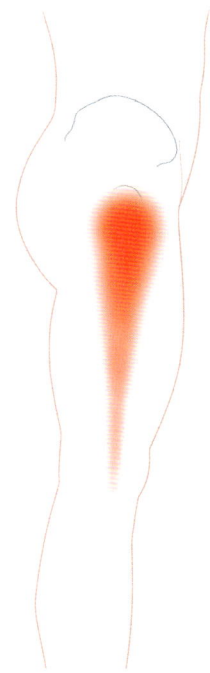

Latin, *tendere*, to stretch, pull; *fasciae*, band; *latae*, side or lateral.

Origin
Anterior superior iliac spine, outer lip of the anterior iliac crest, and fascia lata.

Insertion
Iliotibial tract.

Nerve
Superior gluteal nerve L4, L5, S1.

Action
Assists in stabilizing and steadying the hip and knee joints by putting tension on the iliotibial tract of fascia.

Kinetic System Comment
Tensor fasciae latae is a vitally important structure in providing stability through the knee and pelvis. This muscle is a junction for several chains, including the spiral and lateral chains. The anteromedial fibers are responsible for flexion of the thigh, while the posterolateral fibers provide stability to the knee. Tensor fasciae latae assists various muscles, including the gluteus medius and minimus, rectus femoris, iliopsoas, pectineus, and sartorius.

Myofascial Trigger Point Comment
Pain is felt at the level of the greater trochanter in the hip joint. Walking and running activities make the pain more intense. Pain can refer midway down the lateral thigh and can cause additional knee pain.

PIRIFORMIS

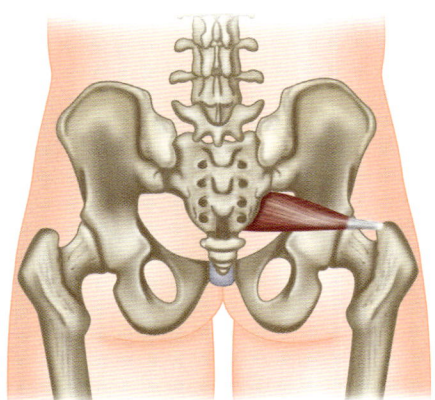

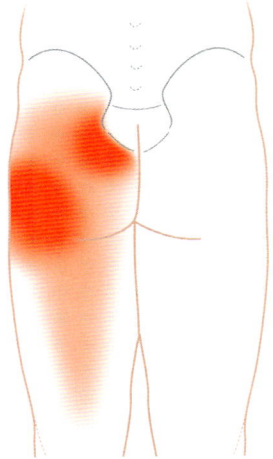

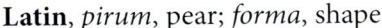

Latin, *pirum*, pear; *forma*, shape.

Origin
Second to fourth costotransverse joints of the anterior sacrum. Small number of fibers arise from the superior border of the greater sciatic notch.

Insertion
Superior border of the greater trochanter of the femur.

Nerve
Ventral rami of lumbar nerve L5, and sacral nerves S1, S2.

Action
Laterally rotates the hip and abducts the thigh when the hip is flexed.

Kinetic System Comment
Piriformis eccentrically contracts to decelerate internal rotation and hip adduction when the hip is flexed. A short piriformis can cause the sacrum to tilt, giving the appearance of a short-leg discrepancy, and result in a rotation or twisting of the sacrum in the sacroiliac joint, setting up additional sacroiliac stress. If not corrected in a timely fashion, this is a recipe for shoulder injury.

Myofascial Trigger Point Comment
Pain is felt in the buttock, hip, and base of the spine, including the sacral base and at times into the upper hamstrings.

GEMELLI

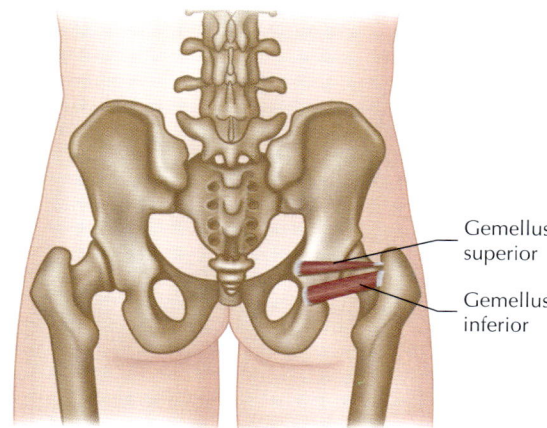

Gemellus superior

Gemellus inferior

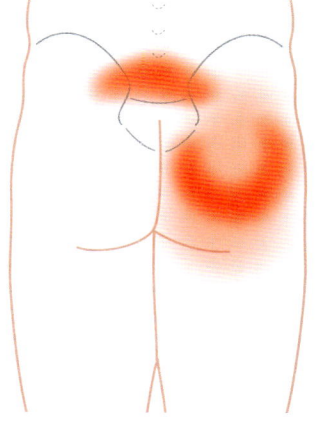

Latin, *gemellus*, twin/double.

Origin

Inferior: Upper border of the ischial tuberosity.
Superior: Spine of the ischium.

Insertion

Middle part of the medial aspect of the greater trochanter of the femur (inferior and superior).

Nerve

Nerve to quadratus femoris L4, L5, S1 (inferior). Nerve to obturator internus L5, S1, S2 (superior).

Action

Laterally rotates and stabilizes the hip.

Kinetic System Comment

Any pain in the pelvic area will result in either an apprehension of movement or a reluctance to move. This often results in postural adaptations and changes in muscle synergies to carry out some function.

Myofascial Trigger Point Comment

Intrapelvic pain is felt, with difficulty sitting for even short periods of time. Intense and unrelenting pain can be referred into the base of the spine and into the gluteal area. The gemelli are difficult to treat with finger applications but myofascial trigger points can be treated successfully with dry needling.

OBTURATOR INTERNUS

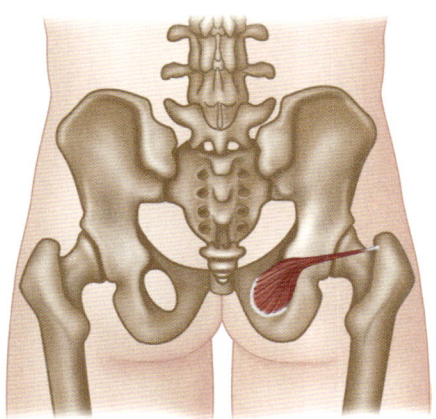

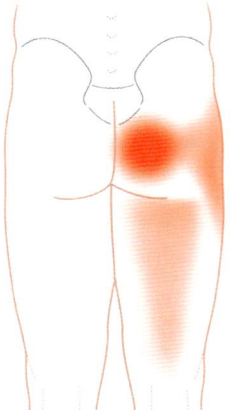

Latin, *obturare*, to obstruct; *internus*, internal.

Origin
Pelvic surface of the obturator membrane, and bony margin of the obturator foramen.

Insertion
Anterior part of the medial surface of the greater trochanter of the femur.

Nerve
Branch of ventral rami of lumbar nerve L5, and sacral nerves S1, S2.

Action
Laterally rotates the extended thigh at the hip, stabilizes the hip, and produces horizontal extension. Abducts the flexed thigh.

Kinetic System Comment
Eccentric contraction of obturator internus decelerates internal rotation of the femur, while pulling the head of the femur into the acetabulum to fix the femoral head during abduction. It eccentrically controls the head of the femur on returning from adduction.

Myofascial Trigger Point Comment
Local pain is experienced deep within the pelvic basin and out as far as the anterior medial portion of the greater trochanter.

OBTURATOR EXTERNUS

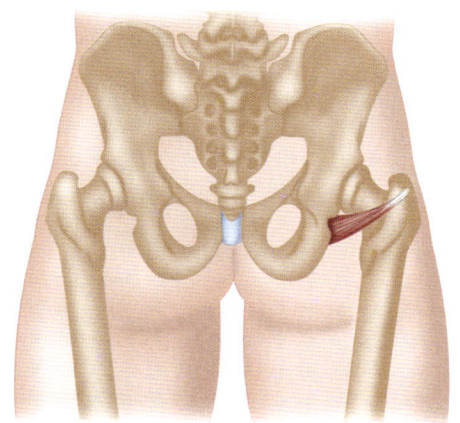

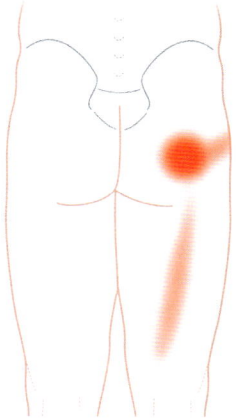

Latin, *obturare*, to obstruct; *externus*, external.

Origin
Rami of the pubis, and ischium.

Insertion
Trochanteric fossa of the femur.

Nerve
Posterior division of obturator nerve L3, L4.

Action
Laterally rotates and stabilizes the hip.

Kinetic System Comment
Eccentric contraction of obturator externus decelerates medial or internal rotation and abduction of the femur.

Myofascial Trigger Point Comment
Local pain is experienced deep within the pelvic basin and out as far as the posterior portion of the greater trochanter. If resisted, medial rotation causes an increase in pain (sometimes the pain shoots down the medial aspect of the femur).

I have found that myofascial trigger points housed in the obturator externus may well be the culprit. Resisted medial rotation may therefore be a worthwhile test to perform.

QUADRATUS FEMORIS

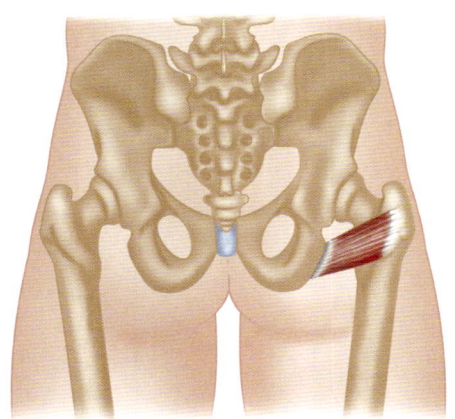

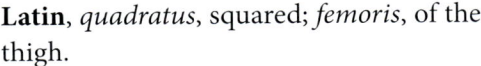

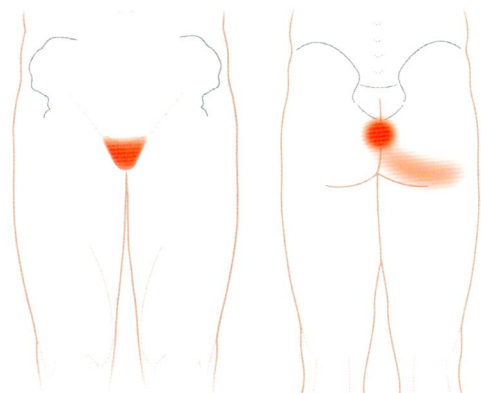

Latin, *quadratus*, squared; *femoris*, of the thigh.

Origin
Lateral border (superior aspect) of the ischial tuberosity.

Insertion
Quadrate tubercle of the femur, and a vertical line below this to the level of the lesser trochanter.

Nerve
Nerve to quadratus femoris L4, L5, S1.

Action
Laterally rotates and stabilizes the hip.

Kinetic System Comment
Quadratus femoris eccentrically decelerates medial rotation of the femur at the hip.

While most therapists immediately target the piriformis for an externally rotated lower limb, I encourage you pay more attention to quadratus femoris.

Myofascial Trigger Point Comment
Pain is felt locally in the posterior pubis and lower gluteal area. Difficulty sleeping and walking downstairs are reported.

ADDUCTOR LONGUS

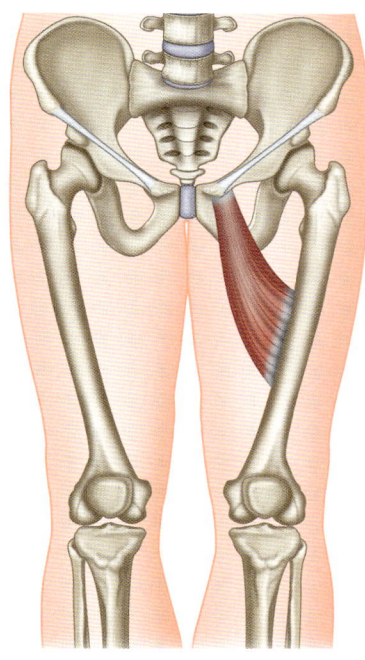

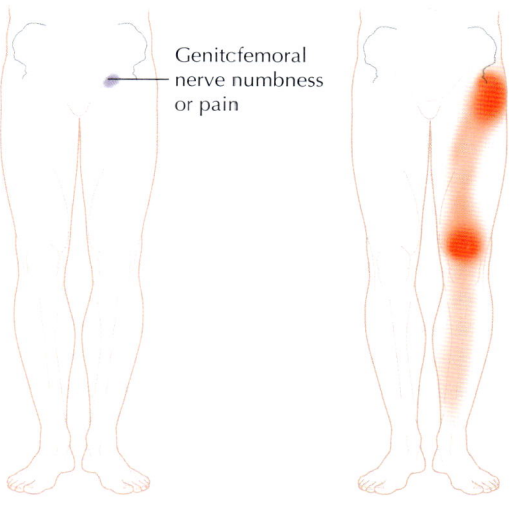

Genitcfemoral nerve numbness or pain

Latin, *adducere*, to lead to; *longus*, long.

Origin
Anterior of the pubis in an angle between the crest and the symphysis.

Insertion
Middle third of the medial lip of the linea aspera.

Nerve
Anterior division of obturator nerve L2–L4.

Action
Adducts the hip joint. Flexes the extended femur at the hip joint. Extends the flexed femur at the hip joint. Assists in lateral rotation of the hip joint.

Kinetic System Comment
Adductor longus decelerates femoral external rotation and abduction of the thigh.

Myofascial Trigger Point Comment
Myofascial trigger points in adductor longus should be considered when patients present with groin pain. Pain can be felt deep in the hip joint, in the inner thigh, and at the medial aspect of the knee. Sensations such as joint stiffness in the hip are reported, restricting the range of motion in all directions.

ADDUCTOR MAGNUS

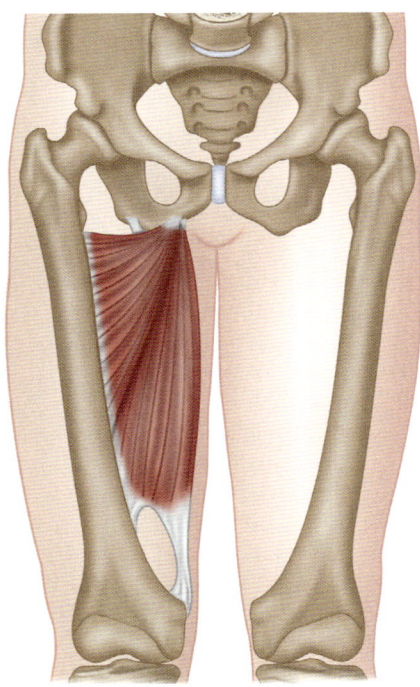

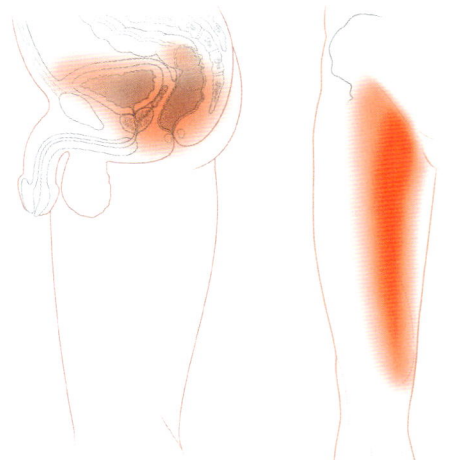

Pelvic referral pattern for TrPs in the high adductor magnus

Latin, *adducere*, to lead to; *magnus*, large.

Origin

Anterior fibers: Inferior or anterior ramus of the pubis, in the angle between the crest and the symphysis.
Posterior fibers: Ischial tuberosity.

Insertion

Entire length of the femur, extending from the gluteal tuberosity along the linea aspera, medial supracondylar line, and adductor tubercle on the medial condyle of the femur.

Nerve

Tibial portion of sciatic nerve L4, L5, S1.
Posterior division of obturator nerve L2–4.

Action

Upper fibers of the adductor magnus adduct and laterally rotate the hip joint. Vertical fibers from the ischium may assist in weak extension of the hip joint.

Kinetic System Comment

Adductor magnus decelerates femoral external rotation and abduction of the thigh.

Myofascial Trigger Point Comment

Pain referred from adductor magnus can manifest itself in many ways, including deep pelvic pain, and pubic, bladder, rectal, or vaginal pain. This pain can often be mistaken for serious visceral or gynecological pathology. When pathology is not clear, myofascial trigger points should be investigated as the root cause of this severe pain.

ADDUCTOR BREVIS

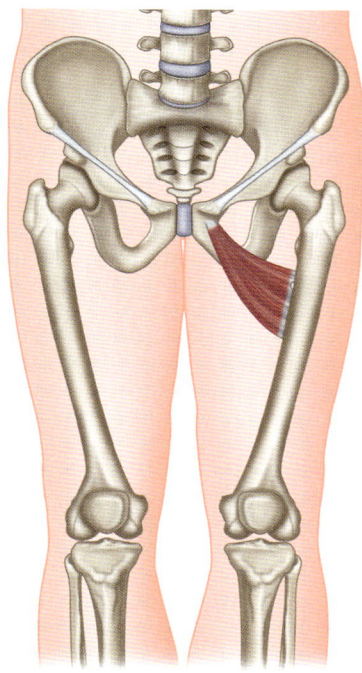

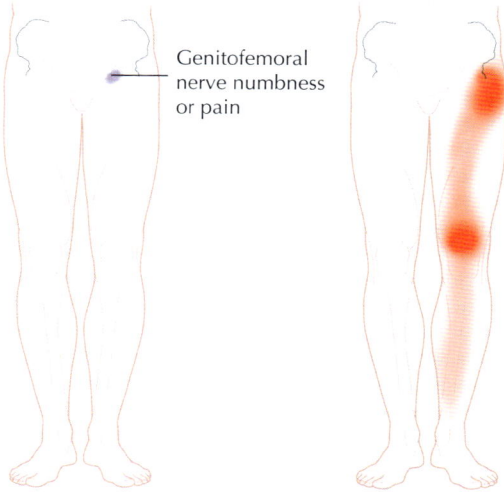

Genitofemoral nerve numbness or pain

Latin, *adducere*, to lead to; *brevis*, short.

Origin
Outer surface of the inferior ramus of the pubis.

Insertion
On a line extending from the lesser trochanter to the upper part of the linea aspera.

Nerve
Anterior division of obturator nerve L2–4.

Action
Adducts the hip joint. Flexes the extended femur at the hip joint. Extends the flexed femur at the hip joint. Assists in lateral rotation of the hip joint.

Kinetic System Comment
Adductor brevis decelerates femoral external rotation and abduction of the thigh.

Myofascial Trigger Point Comment
Pain is felt deep in the hip, predominantly on the medial side of the thigh and referring to the medial aspect of the knee joint, which can be mistaken for arthritic pain.

GRACILIS

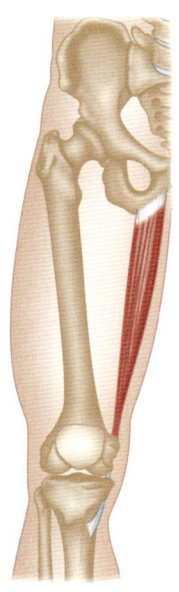

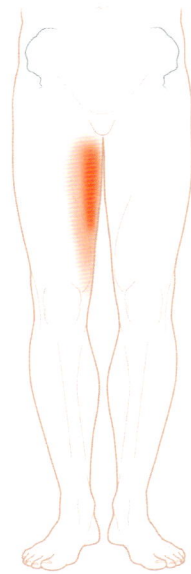

Latin, *gracilis*, slender, delicate.

Origin
Anterior lower half of the symphysis pubis, and medial margin of the inferior ramus of the pubis.

Insertion
Front and medial surface of the shaft of the tibia, just below the condyle.

Nerve
Anterior division of obturator nerve L2–4.

Action
Adducts the hip joint. Flexes the knee joint. Medially rotates the knee joint when flexed.

Kinetic System Comment
Gracilis decelerates femoral external rotation and abduction of the thigh.

Myofascial Trigger Point Comment
Myofascial trigger points can not only refer pain but also produce changes in sensation; gracilis is a good example of that. Patients complain of a hot and stinging feeling on the inner thigh, just superficial to the skin.

PECTINEUS

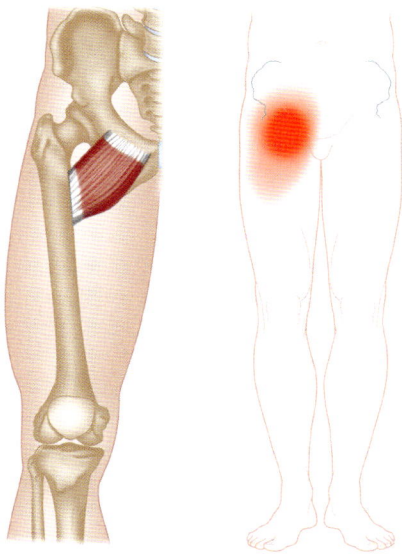

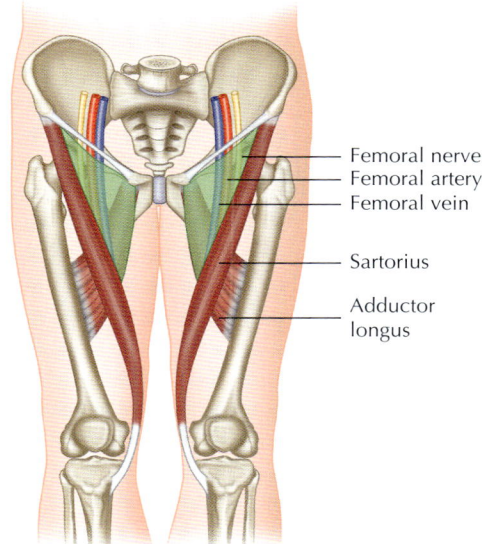

Femoral triangle.

Latin, *pecten*, comb; *pectinatus*, comb shaped.

Origin
Pectineal line of the pubis, between the iliopubic eminence and the pubic tubercle.

Insertion
Pectineal line of the femur, from the lesser trochanter to the linea aspera.

Nerve
Femoral and obturator nerves L2–4.

Action
Adducts the hip joint. Flexes the hip joint.

Kinetic System Comment
Pectineus decelerates femoral external rotation and abduction of the thigh.

Myofascial Trigger Point Comment
Pain is felt deeply in the groin as a sharp pain within the femoral triangle. Similar to the adductor muscle group, the pain is sometimes felt in the joint itself.

HAMSTRINGS

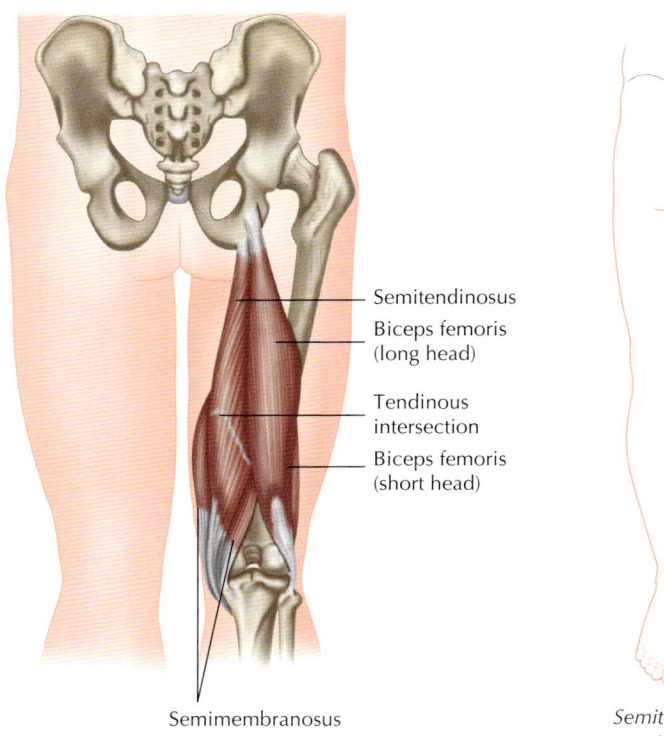

Semitendinosus
Biceps femoris (long head)
Tendinous intersection
Biceps femoris (short head)

Semimembranosus

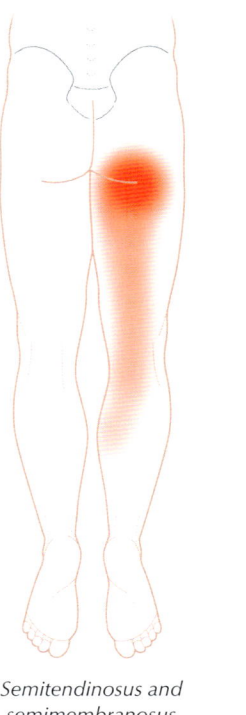
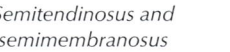

Semitendinosus and semimembranosus

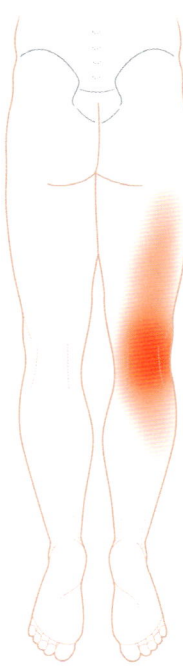

Biceps femoris

German, *hamme*, back of leg. **Latin**, *stringere*, to draw together.

Origin

Hamstrings arise from the ischial tuberosity. Biceps femoris blends a long head with the sacrotuberous ligament, and its short head attaches in the linea aspera and intermuscular septum.

Insertion

Semitendinosus and semimembranosus attach to the posteromedial tibia by means of the tibial condyle (semimembranosus) and the medial surface of the tibia, including the deep fascia (semitendinosus). Biceps femoris inserts on the lateral aspect of the fibula head and the lateral condyle of the tibia.

Nerve

Sciatic nerve L4, L5, S1–3.

Action

Hamstrings flex the knee joint. Semimembranosus and semitendinosus only medially rotate the knee joint, and assist in medial rotation of the hip joint when the knee is flexed. Biceps femoris laterally rotates the knee joint and assists in lateral rotation of the hip joint when the knee is flexed.

Kinetic System Comment

Hamstrings eccentrically contract during gait to decelerate extension of the knee joint and hip flexion, while also playing a very important role in pelvic stability and decelerate internal rotation on heel-strike. They disappear under gluteus maximus and provide force closure of the sacroiliac joint through the coupled action of the force provided by the contralateral latissimus dorsi. This force is transmitted through the sacrotuberous ligament and further up to the thoracolumbar fascia.

Myofascial Trigger Point Comment

Typically, pain is referred up toward the gluteal muscles, with some residual pain spreading down just below and behind the knee into the medial gaster of the gastrocnemius. This pain can often be mistaken for sciatic pain. Weak inhibited gluteal muscles, including gluteus medius, can lead to myofascial trigger points forming in the hamstrings and lumbar erector muscles, including the quadratus lumborum. Ultimately, the hamstrings are trying to be gluteal muscles, while the lumbar muscles are trying to be hamstrings.

SARTORIUS

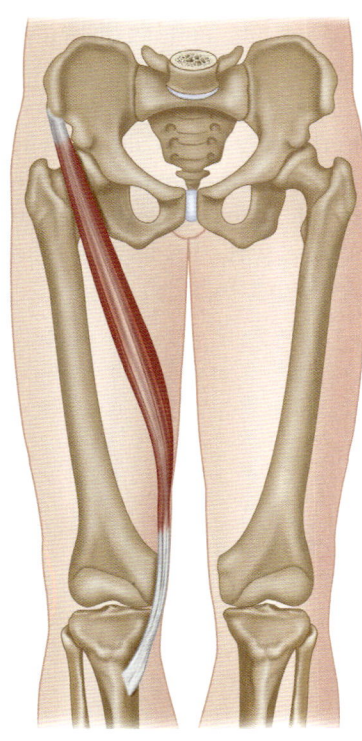

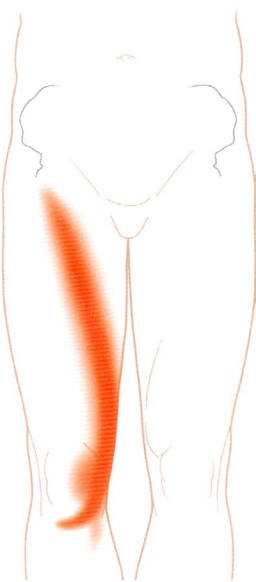

Latin, *sartor*, tailor.

Origin
Anterior superior iliac spine (ASIS).

Insertion
Superior aspect of the medial surface of the tibial shaft, near the tibial tuberosity.

Nerve
Anterior branch of femoral nerve L2–4.

Action
Flexes and laterally rotates the hip joint and flexes the knee (tailor's muscle).

Kinetic System Comment
Decelerates extension and medial rotation at the hip joint and extension at the knee. Muscles with baby or satellite myofascial trigger points to consider include rectus femoris, vastus medialis, pectineus, and the adductors.

Myofascial Trigger Point Comment
A severe burning or sharp tingling pain or sensation is experienced along the anterior but mostly medial aspect of the thigh and kneecap. Typically, this is not felt as a deep knee pain. Be sure to test for chondromalacia patellae (runner's knee).

QUADRICEPS

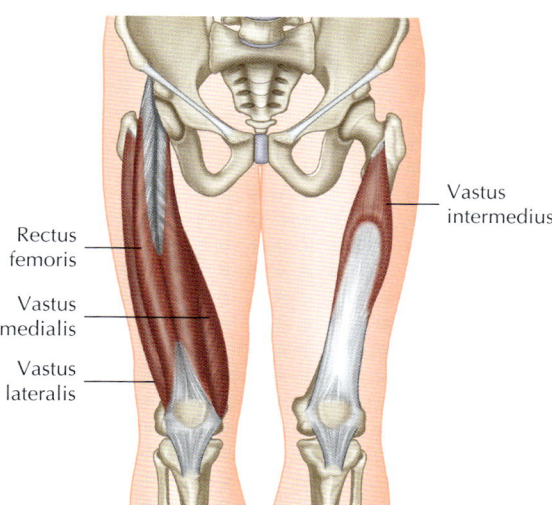

Rectus femoris

Vastus medialis

Vastus lateralis

Vastus intermedius

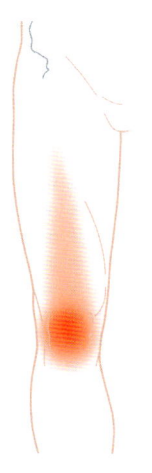 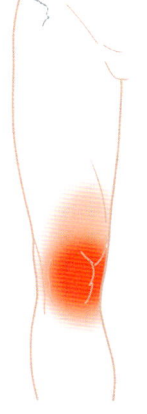 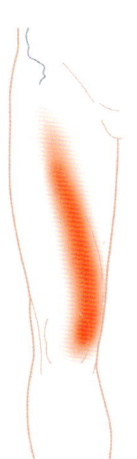

Referral pattern of rectus femoris

Referral pattern of TrPs in the lower muscle

Referral pattern of TrPs in the upper muscle

Latin, *quadriceps*, four-headed.

Some anatomists consider the vastus medialis obliquus fibers to be a separate and functionally distinct structure. These oblique fibers attach to the tendon of the rectus femoris and the medial border of the patella, and to the anterior medial condyle of the tibia. It is interesting to note that the expansions which pass across the knee joint to attach to the tibia replace the joint capsule in this region, and then fuse with the deep fascia embracing the tibial tuberosity.

Origin

Rectus femoris: Anterior inferior iliac spine (AIIS), and groove above the rim of the acetabulum.

Vastus medialis: Anterior intertrochanteric line, medial lip of the linea aspera, and proximal aspect of the medial supracondylar line. It is interesting to note the attachment into the tendons of the adductor longus and magnus and into the medial intermuscular septum.

Vastus lateralis: Intertrochanteric line and greater trochanter, gluteal tuberosity and lateral lip of the linea aspera, and lateral intermuscular septum.

Vastus intermedius: Anterior lateral surface of the proximal two-thirds of the femur, distal half of the linea aspera, and lateral intermuscular septum.

Articularis genu: Two slips from the anterior femur below the vastus intermedius (pulls the capsule superiorly).

Insertion

All the quadriceps wrap up the patella (sesamoid bone), with each having a unique and specific line of pull or directional force acting on the patella. They share a common tendon (patellar tendon or ligament) and attach to the tibial tuberosity.

Nerve

Femoral nerve L2–4.

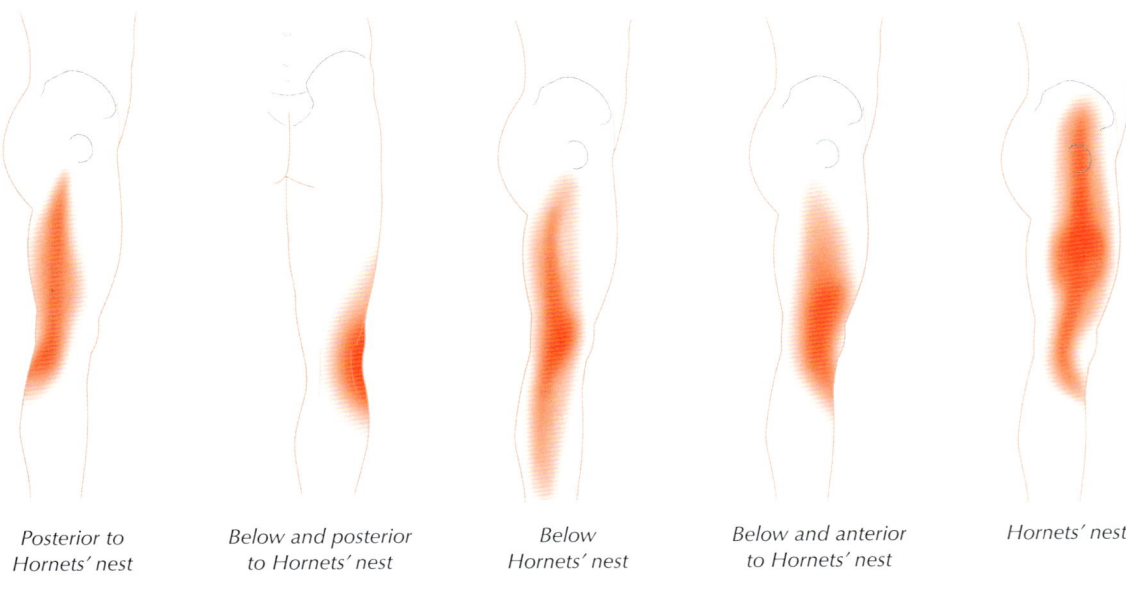

Posterior to Hornets' nest *Below and posterior to Hornets' nest* *Below Hornets' nest* *Below and anterior to Hornets' nest* *Hornets' nest*

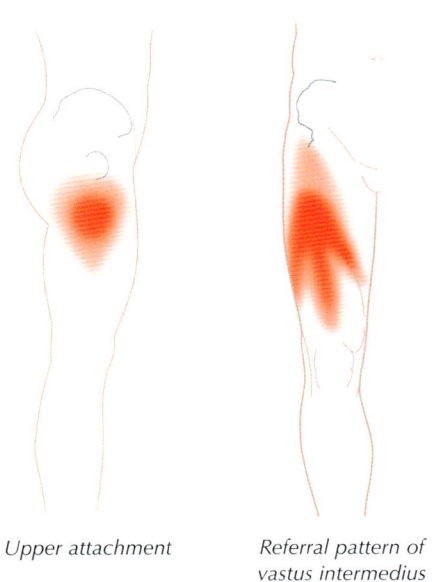

Upper attachment *Referral pattern of vastus intermedius*

Action
Extend the knee joint. Rectus femoris additionally flexes the hip joint.

Kinetic System Comment
Quadriceps have a significant impact on pelvic rotation (anterior), kneecap tracking, and knee positioning, and shortness of them can ultimately influence head and neck positioning, cause knee pain, and affect foot and ankle movement. Eccentric contraction decelerates knee flexion, adduction, and internal rotation during heel-strike of the gait cycle. Rectus femoris eccentrically decelerates hip extension and knee flexion during gait. The interrelationship of all the quadriceps muscles provides dynamic stability to the knee.

Myofascial Trigger Point Comment
A multitude of myofascial trigger points have been identified within the quadriceps group. It may seem strange, but typical pain involves a deep toothache-like pain (vastus medialis) in the knee joint, or on the lateral or medial aspect of the thigh, including the knee.

My tip, based on clinical experience with knee pain, is to check for myofascial trigger points in the muscles of the soft palate of the mouth if no success is achieved with treatment and/or exercise.

Muscles of the Leg and Foot

GASTROCNEMIUS

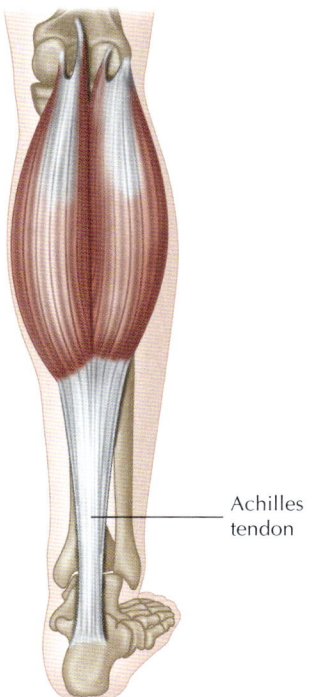

Achilles
tendon

Greek, *gaster*, belly; *kneme*, lower leg.

Origin
Medial and lateral condyles of the femur
(posteriorly), capsule of the knee joint, and
oblique popliteal ligament.

Insertion
Posterior surface of calcaneus.

Nerve
Tibial nerve S1, S2.

Action
When we run or walk, gastrocnemius provides
considerable forces, enough to propel our
bodies in jumping. A powerful plantar flexor,
the muscle contracts eccentrically to assist
in decelerating femoral internal rotation and
assists in external rotation of the knee during
the push-off phase of gait and aids knee flexion
during the swing phase.

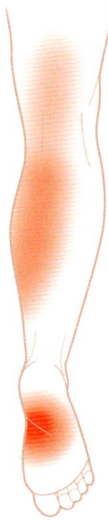

This referral pattern is from TrPs in the area of the upper medial head

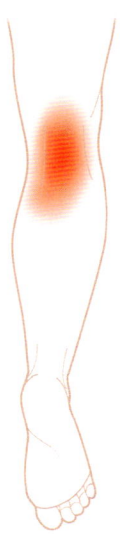

This referral pattern is from TrPs in the extreme upper medial head and its tendon attachment

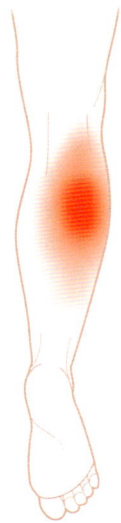

This referral pattern is from TrPs in the area of the middle lateral head

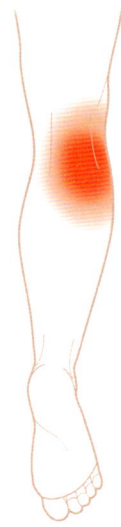

This referral pattern is from TrPs in the area of the upper medial head and its tendon attachment

Kinetic System Comment

The relationship with the heads of gastrocnemius and tendons of the hamstrings must be considered when participating in machine-based exercise. A shared fascia with the plantar muscles of the foot can highlight the need for balance, both up and down the kinetic system. Eccentrically, the muscle decelerates ankle extension in gait.

Myofascial Trigger Point Comment

Several myofascial trigger points can form in this muscle, referring pain and a sense of stiffness or tension into the medial plantar aspect of the foot, and diffuse pain spread over one or both of the gasters. Pain can also refer up into the medial hamstrings. Typically, individuals will try to statically stretch the symptoms away; this will irritate the muscle spindle response and serve only to compound the symptoms. The posterior kinetic system should be assessed to identify short hypertonic muscles and myofascial migration.

TIBIALIS ANTERIOR

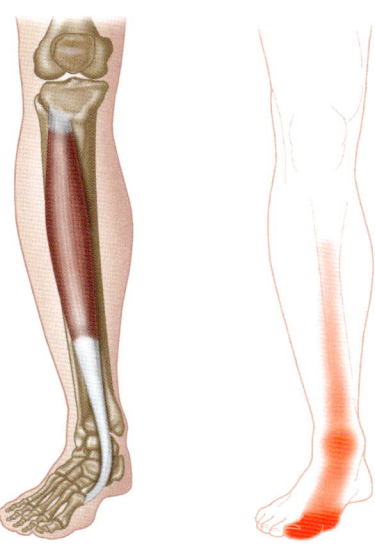

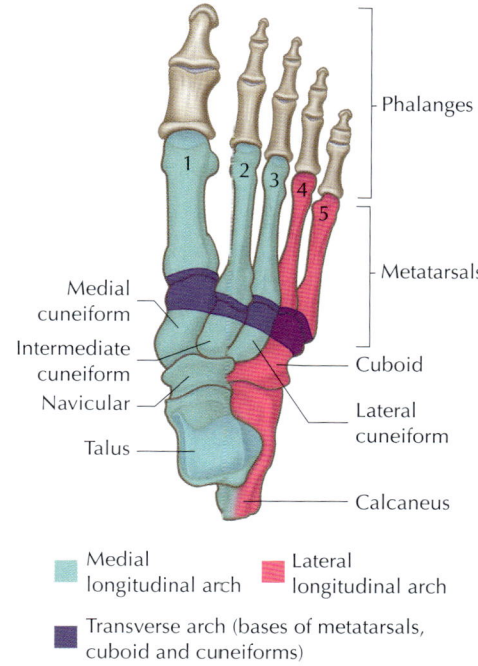

Phalanges

1 2 3 4 5

Medial cuneiform

Intermediate cuneiform

Navicular

Talus

Metatarsals

Cuboid

Lateral cuneiform

Calcaneus

Medial longitudinal arch

Lateral longitudinal arch

Transverse arch (bases of metatarsals, cuboid and cuneiforms)

Foot arches.

Latin, *tibialis*, relating to the shin; *anterior*, at the front.

Origin
Lateral condyle and proximal two-thirds of the lateral surface of the tibia, interosseous membrane, deep fascia, and lateral intermuscular septum.

Insertion
Medial and plantar surface of the medial cuneiform bone, and base of the metatarsal bone.

Nerve
Deep fibular nerve L4, L5, S1.

Action
Dorsiflexes the ankle joint and assists in inverting the foot. When contracting eccentrically, decelerates plantar flexion at heel-strike and eversion of the mid-foot in mid-stance. Offers dynamic stabilization to the mid-tarsal joint and accelerates supination of the foot before heel-strike.

Kinetic System Comment
As a result of reciprocal inhibition, tibialis anterior can become weak, long, and tight, predisposing the foot to over-pronation and eversion (flat foot). Short, spastic, or contractured fibulares will facilitate this inhibition, thereby reducing soft tissue support to all three foot arches.

Myofascial Trigger Point Comment
Myofascial trigger points in tibialis anterior refer down into the great toe. Pain can also be experienced in the ankle (anteromedially) as the muscle tendon passes the retinaculum. Fallen arches in the foot place eccentric loads on tibialis anterior, while hypercontracted fibulares will increase inhibition in this muscle—all in all, a recipe for myofascial trigger point evolution.

A Few Words to Identify Other Muscles Involved with Plantar Flexion

Flexor digitorum longus and flexor hallucis longus are deep muscles of the posterior compartment of the lower limb, attaching all the way down to the toes. Plantar flexion also involves the tibialis posterior. Together these muscles are called Tom, Dick, and Harry.

The plantaris is a muscle with a small gaster, yet it has the longest tendon in the human body. Situated on the lateral condyle of the femur, it runs down to attach to the calcaneus, sharing the common calcaneal tendon with gastrocnemius and soleus.

FLEXOR DIGITORUM LONGUS

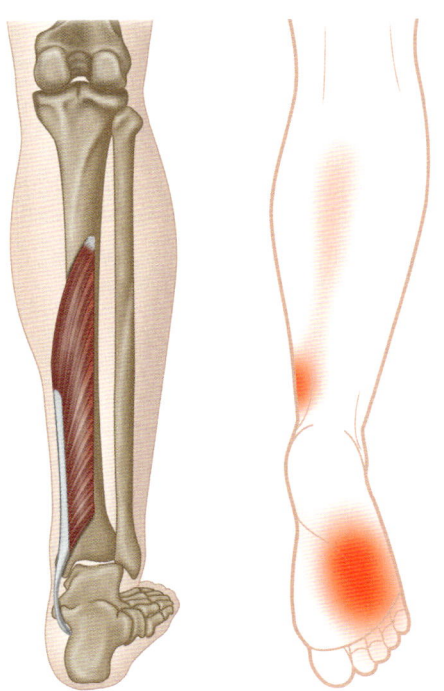

Latin, *flectere*, to bend; *digitorum*, of the toes; *longus*, long.

Origin
Medial part of the posterior surface of the tibia, below the soleal line.

Insertion
Bases of the distal phalanges of the second through fifth toes.

Nerve
Tibial nerve L5, S1, S2.

Action
Flexes all the joints of the lateral four toes (enabling the foot to firmly grip the ground when walking). Helps to plantar flex and invert the ankle joint.

Kinetic System Comment
Decelerates toe extension, foot dorsiflexion, and ankle eversion. An inhibited flexor digitorum longus can predispose the ankle or knee to soft tissue insult or lead to insult further up the kinetic system.

Myofascial Trigger Point Comment
Flexor digitorum longus, accompanied by associated plantar muscles, causes pain and/or weakness in the foot and toes, with pain experienced particularly on the top or dorsal aspect of the foot and at times spreading to the anterior aspect of the tibia.

FLEXOR HALLUCIS LONGUS

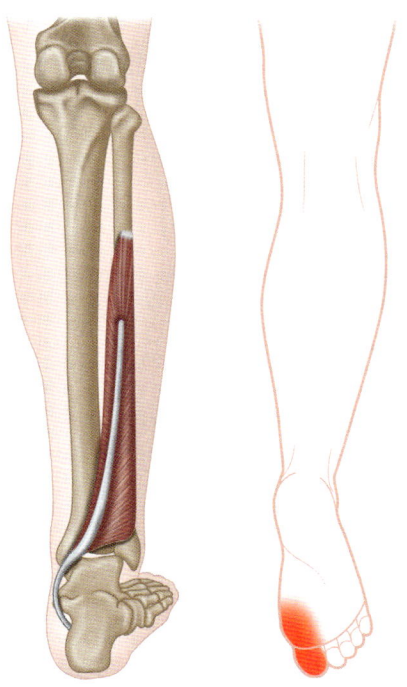

Latin, *flectere*, to bend; *hallucis*, of the great toe; *longus*, long.

Origin

Lower two-thirds of the posterior surface of the fibula, interosseous membrane, and adjacent intermuscular septum.

Insertion

Base of the distal phalanx of the great toe.

Nerve

Tibial nerve L5, S1, S2.

Action

Flexes all the joints of the great toe, playing a vital role in the final propulsive thrust of the foot during walking. Assists in plantar flexion and inversion of the ankle joint.

Kinetic System Comment

All foot and anatomical leg kinematic problems, structural or soft tissue related, can have adverse effects further up the kinetic system, resulting in strain and eventually the formation of myofascial trigger points.

Myofascial Trigger Point Comment

Pain is referred to the great toe, mainly contained on the plantar surface, and is often mistaken for gout, as the pain is often described as a burning sensation, accompanied by stiffness.

EXTENSOR HALLUCIS LONGUS

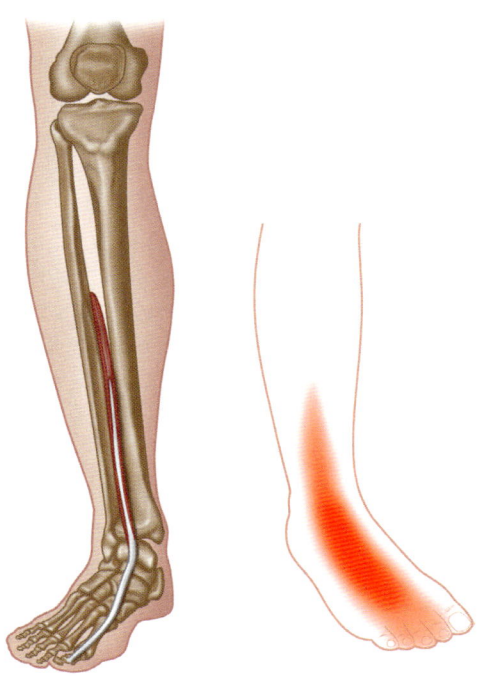

Latin, *extendere*, to extend; *hallucis*, of the great toe; *longus*, long.

Origin
Middle half of the anterior surface of the fibula, and adjacent interosseous membrane.

Insertion
Base of the distal phalanx of the great toe.

Nerve
Deep fibular nerve L4, L5, S1.

Action
Extends all the joints of the great toe. Dorsiflexes the ankle joint. Assists in inversion of the ankle joint.

Kinetic System Comment
Extensor hallucis longus is prone to spastic activity, which can lead to internal rotation of the fibula, resulting in kinematic changes up and down the kinetic system.

Myofascial Trigger Point Comment
Pain and tenderness are experienced primarily on the plantar surface of the foot, with spillover pain on the plantar surface of the great toe. Often mistaken for gout or arthritis, this pain can be sharp and stinging, and can occasionally radiate up the kinetic system for a short distance but does not extend to the heel.

TIBIALIS POSTERIOR

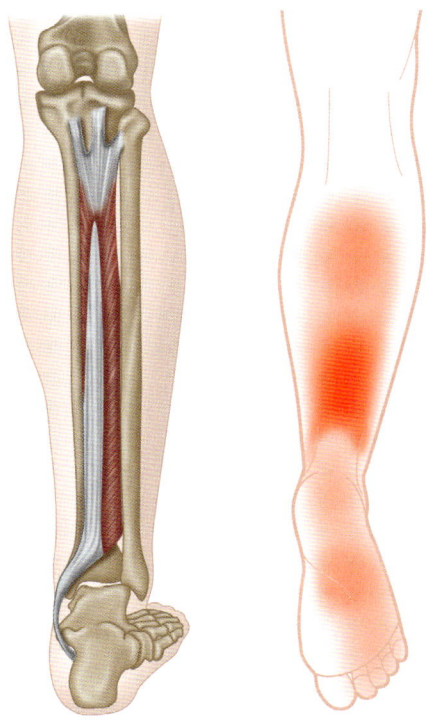

Latin, *tibialis*, relating to the shin; *posterior*, at the back.

Origin
Upper half of the lateral aspect of the posterior surface of the tibia, most of the interosseous membrane, and posterior fibula and fascia covering it posteriorly.

Insertion
Tuberosity of the navicular and plantar surface of the medial cuneiform. Tendinous expansions attach to the plantar surfaces of all the tarsal bones (except the talus), to the tip of the sustentaculum tali, and to the bases of the middle three metatarsals.

Nerve
Branch of the tibial nerve L4, L5, S1.

Action
Plantar flexes and inverts (supinates) the ankle. Eccentrically, decelerates subtalar joint pronation as it controls subtalar eversion and internal rotation of the tibia, and dynamically stabilizes the talonavicular joint. In the push-off phase of gait, assists in plantar flexion and inversion.

Kinetic System Comment
Tibialis posterior dives deep into the sole of the foot, the foundation upon which we all stand. Due to reciprocal inhibition, tibialis posterior can neurologically weaken, leading to compromised arch support. This can have implications further up the chain for links such as popliteus, posterior intermuscular septum, adductor magnus, and the core musculature.

Myofascial Trigger Point Comment
Most people will mistake the myofascial trigger points in tibialis posterior for Achilles tendinitis, plantar fasciitis, or shin splints. Pain is felt on the medial tibia or in the sole of the foot, at the level of the arch, when walking. Clients will often present with a pronated foot. A functional kinetic system assessment is required, with appropriate activity to improve core stability and kinetic system integrity.

POPLITEUS

When the feet are fixed (closed-chain kinetics), laterally rotates the femur on the tibia and flexes the knee joint. Eccentrically, decelerates tibial rotation internally and femoral rotation externally (screw-home effect). Its function in posterolateral stability is significant.

Some anatomical papers describe a common idea of popliteus as a retractor of the lateral meniscus.

Kinetic System Comment

Machine-based exercise, such as prone leg curls, can overstress the popliteus, causing spasm and diminished screw-home capability. This, in turn, can lead to inhibition of the piriformis and deep hip rotators, with hyperextension at the knee. Shortness of popliteus can be confirmed by observing slight flexion and internal rotation of the anatomical leg.

Myofascial Trigger Point Comment

Popliteus is a muscle that takes a lot of stressful abuse, and eventually myofascial trigger points can form, causing pain in the back of the knee. At night the pain reduces or ceases completely. Stiffness in the knee joint is often evident in the morning, with reduced ability to fully extend the anatomical leg.

On assessment, the foot can appear as if the leg has turned in (medial rotation at the knee). This is often a result of heavy squat exercises in the absence of appropriate neuromuscular stability at the joints and within the core.

Latin, *poples*, the ham.

Origin

Anterior aspect of the lateral condyle of the femur, and oblique popliteal ligament of the knee joint. The muscle is anchored to the lateral condyle of the femur by a strong tendon, which passes into the capsule of the knee joint and can include the lateral meniscus.

Insertion

Posterior surface of the posterior side of the proximal tibia, above the soleal line.

Nerve

Tibial nerve L4, L5, S1.

Action

Medially rotates the tibia on the femur and flexes the knee (non-weight bearing).

FIBULARIS LONGUS

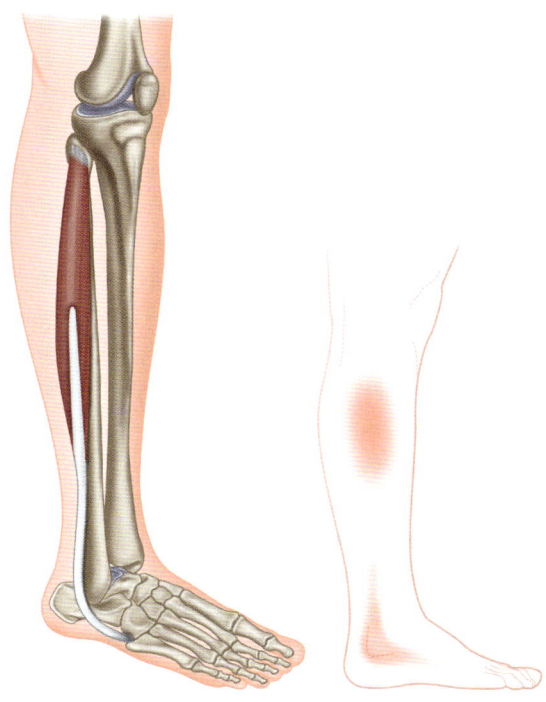

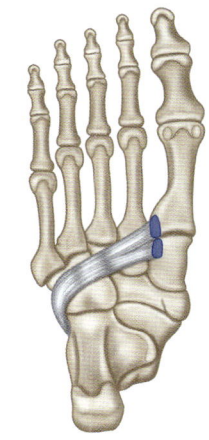

*Insertion on base of first metatarsal
(plantar view, right foot)*

Latin, *fibula*, pin/buckle; *longus*, long. **Greek**, *perone*, pin/buckle.

Origin
Lateral condyle of the tibia (in conjunction with the extensor digitorum longus), upper two-thirds of the lateral surface of the fibula, intermuscular septa, and deep fascia.

Insertion
Plantar and lateral surface of the medial cuneiform, and base of the first metatarsal.

Nerve
Superficial fibular nerve L4, L5, S1.

Action
A foot evertor, fibularis longus assists in plantar flexing the ankle joint. Depresses the head of the first metatarsal. Eccentrically, decelerates ankle dorsiflexion and inversion of the subtalar joint during the push-off phase of gait.

Kinetic System Comment
Fibularis longus forms a sling or stirrup for the foot arches, offering an opposing force to tibialis anterior. Further up the kinetic system, the muscle can affect the function of biceps femoris, sacrotuberous ligament, erector spinae, multifidus, etc.

Myofascial Trigger Point Comment
Along with fibularis brevis, myofascial trigger points refer pain down the leg over, above, and behind the lateral malleolus. Pain can also be felt over the anterolateral aspect of the ankle and the outside of the calcaneus.

Many individuals with these myofascial trigger points complain of numbness or pins and needles in the toes, especially the third, fourth, and great toes.

PLANTARIS

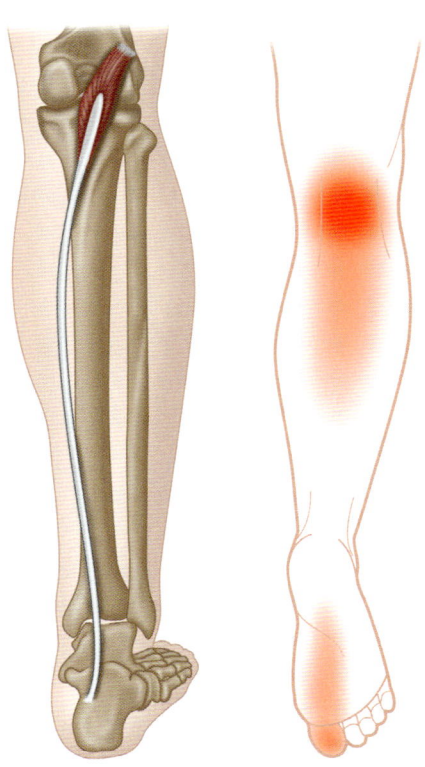

Latin, *plantaris*, relating to the sole.

Plantaris is a short, slender muscle and has the longest tendon in the body. Its origin is on the lateral supracondylar ridge, popliteal surface, and joint capsule. Inserting into the medial surface of the calcaneus, this muscle is a weak flexor of the knee and plantar flexes the ankle in the push-off phase of gait.

Plantaris is absent in about 10% of the population.

Origin

Inferior aspect of the lateral supracondylar line of the distal femur, and oblique ligament of the knee.

Insertion

Middle third of the posterior surface of the calcaneus, medial to the Achilles tendon.

Nerve

Tibial nerve L4, L5, S1.

Action

Plantar flexes the foot at the ankle, inverts the ankle, and assists in flexion at the knee.

Kinetic System Comment

Plantaris is a weak contributor to decelerating extension of the knee joint and decelerating eversion and dorsiflexion at the ankle.

Myofascial Trigger Point Comment

The pain from myofascial trigger points in plantaris mimics many pain syndromes firing into the posterior knee and down the medial aspect of the triceps surae into the heel, and sometimes into the ball of the foot and the great toe.

The therapist must rule out the possibility of S1 or S2 radiculopathy, rupture of the plantaris, popliteus tendinitis, tenosynovitis, popliteal artery aneurysm, Baker's cyst, deep vein thrombosis (DVT), intermittent claudication, peripheral vascular disease (PVD), avulsion of the popliteus tendon, muscle strain, posterior compartment syndrome, popliteal lymphedema, systemic infections or inflammation, nutritional inadequacy, metabolic imbalance, and toxicity and possible side effects of medications.

SOLEUS

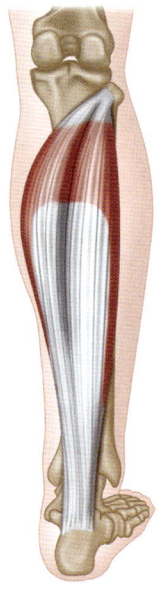

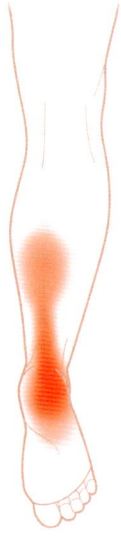

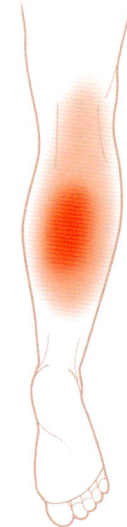

Referral pattern of TrPs in the area of the muscle slightly above a hand's width higher than the ankle crease

Referral pattern of TrPs in the gastrocnemius muscle bellies above the tendons

Latin, *solea*, leather sole/sandal/sole (fish).

Lying deep to gastrocnemius, soleus is a broad, flat muscle resembling a flatfish.

Origin
Soleal line on the medial border of the tibia, posterior surface of the upper third of the fibula, and the fibrous arch between.

Insertion
By means of the calcaneal tendon to the middle part of the posterior surface of the calcaneus (heel bone).

Nerve
Tibial nerve L5, S1, S2.

Action
Plantar flexes the ankle, along with the gastrocnemius and plantaris.

Kinetic System Comment
From a dynamic postural viewpoint, soleus prevents the body falling forward at the ankle joint during standing. In gait, the muscle eccentrically decelerates subtalar joint pronation and internal rotation of the lower leg at heel-strike. It also decelerates dorsiflexion of the foot. Spasm or myofascial trigger points in soleus can be the origin of tight hamstrings, lower back pain, and even headaches.

Myofascial Trigger Point Comment
Soleus typically refers pain into the posterior aspect and plantar surface of the heel and to the distal end of the Achilles tendon. A rare myofascial trigger point spreads pain to the ipsilateral sacroiliac joint and can also refer pain to the jaw in extreme cases.

ABDUCTOR HALLUCIS

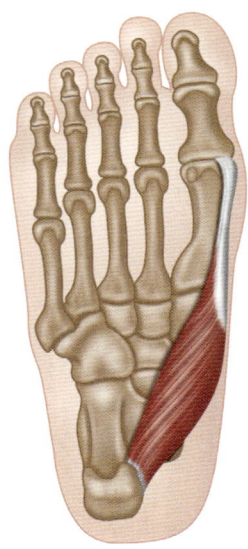
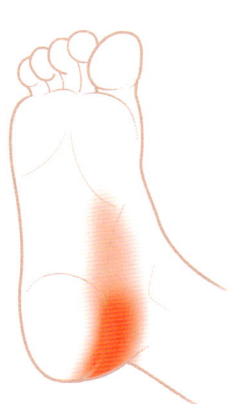

Latin, *abducere*, to lead away from; *hallucis*, of the great toe.

Origin
Along medial tuberosity of the calcaneal bone, flexor retinaculum, and plantar aponeurosis.

Insertion
By means of outer edge of the medial sesamoid, onto medial base of the proximal phalanx of the great toe (hallux).

Nerve
Medial plantar nerve L4, L5, S1.

Action
Abducts and flexes the metatarsophalangeal joint. Assists in adducting the forefoot.

Kinetic System Comment
Working with flexor hallucis brevis and longus and adductor hallucis longus (to control the great toe), abductor hallucis belongs to the first layer of muscles on the foot. It decelerates adduction of the hallux at the metatarsophalangeal joint (eccentric control toward the anatomical axis of the foot). Failure to do this leads to increasing pronation of the great toe and to the progression of the deformity.

Myofascial Trigger Point Comment
Pain is felt in the medial and posterior portions of the heel as well as in the instep. This pain can be experienced as a burning sensation on heel-strike and toe-off. Patients tend to limp into the clinic. Experience leads me to look at the footwear of a patient, which is often too small or fits poorly.

Be sure to rule out contributions from the possibility of L4 radiculopathy, S2 sciatic nerve lesion, Achilles tendinitis, plantar fasciitis, bone spur, pes cavus, pes planus (flat feet), bunions, congenital hypertrophy, Morton's foot syndrome, diabetic neuropathy, polyneuropathy, reflex sympathetic dystrophy, bone fracture, sprain/strain, tarsal tunnel syndrome, callus, involvements of blisters, bursitis, osteoarthritis, and rheumatoid arthritis. If in doubt, refer.

ADDUCTOR HALLUCIS

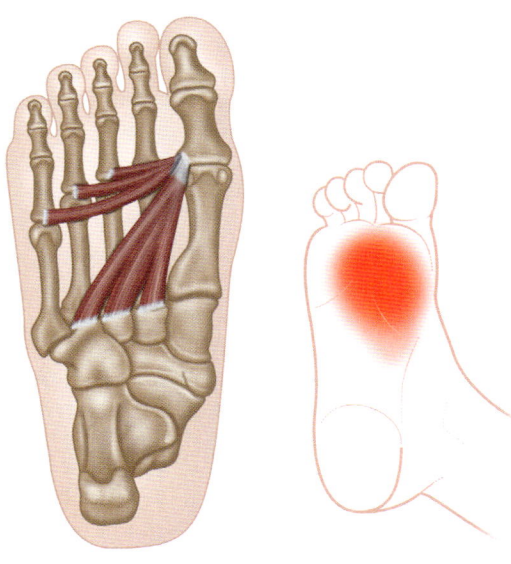

Latin, *adducere*, to lead to; *hallucis*, of the great toe.

Origin

Two heads (oblique and transverse) attach the adductor hallucis to the bases of the second to fourth metatarsal bones, plantar metatarsophalangeal ligaments of the third to fifth toes, and deep transverse metatarsal ligament.

Insertion

Lateral side of the base of the proximal phalanx.

Nerve

Lateral plantar nerve S1, S2.

Action

Adducts and assists in flexing the metatarsophalangeal joint of the great toe.

Kinetic System Comment

Implicated as a major deforming factor in hallux valgus, adductor hallucis decelerates movement of the proximal phalanx away from the second toe as well as the lateral sesamoid, thus reducing further pronation. Failure to do so adequately is a potent cause of the more severe problem of hallux valgus deformity.

Myofascial Trigger Point Comment

The referral pattern is local, with pain felt on the distal sole under the metatarsal heads. Patients often report numbness. A frequently used patient description is a feeling of "fullness" in the area.

Abbreviations

AC	acromioclavicular	**EMG**	electromyography
ACh	acetylcholine	**FIPAT**	Federative International Programme for Anatomical Terminology
AChE	acetylcholinesterase		
ACTs	active cyrotherapy techniques	**GH**	glenohumeral
AIIS	anterior inferior iliac spine	**GIRD**	glenohumeral internal rotation deficit
ASIS	anterior superior iliac spine		
ATP	adenosine triphosphate	**GTO**	Golgi tendon organ
CFD	critical fiber distance	**IFAA**	International Federation of Associations of Anatomists
CNS	central nervous system		
CT	connective tissue	**INIT**	integrated neuromuscular inhibition technique
CTR	connective tissue release (= STR)		
DN	dynamic neutral	**IO**	internal oblique
DROM	dynamic range of movement	**LPH**	lumbo-pelvic-hip
ECM	extracellular matrix	**LTR**	local twitch resposne
		MET	muscle energy techniques
		MTrPs	myofascial trigger points

NMTq   neuromuscular techniques

PIR   post-isometric relaxation

PNF   proprioceptive neuromuscular facilitation

PSIS   posterior superior iliac spine

QA   quick-acting (mechanoreceptors)

RCPmi   rectus capitis posterior minor

RI   reciprocal inhibition

ROM   range of motion

RPR   reactive postural responses

SA   slow-acting (mechanoreceptors)

SAID   specific adaptation to imposed demands

SCM   sternocleidomastoid

SCS   strain/counterstrain

SEA   spontaneous electrical activity

SI   sacroiliac

SITS   supraspinatus, infraspinatus, teres minor, and subscapularis

SR   sarcoplasmic reticulum

STR   soft tissue release (= CTR)

TA   transversus abdominis

TBNL   to be named ligament

VAS   visual analog scale (for measuring pain)

References

References Cited and Further Reading

Chaitow, L. 1976. *The Acupressure Treatment of Pain*. London: Thorsons.

———. 1997. Clinical perspective. *Journal of Bodywork and Movement Therapies* **1**(2):70–71.

———. 2006. *Muscle Energy Techniques, Positional Release and Modern Neuromuscular Techniques*. Edinburgh: Churchill Livingstone.

———. 2015. *Positional Release Techniques*. 4th ed. New York: Elsevier.

Chaitow, L., and J. DeLany. 2002. *Clinical Applications of Neuromuscular Techniques*. Edinburgh: Churchill Livingstone.

Clemente, C. M., ed. 1985. *Gray's Anatomy of the Human Body*. 38th ed. Philadelphia, PA: Lea and Febiger.

Donnelly, J. M., ed. 2013. *Travell, Simons and Simons' Myofascial Pain and Dysfunction: The Trigger Point Manual*. 3rd ed. Baltimore, MD: Lippincott, Williams, and Wilkins.

Hsieh, Y.-L., et al. 2007. Dry needling to a key myofascial trigger point may reduce the irritability of satellite myofascial trigger points. *American Journal of Physical Medicine and Rehabilitation* **86**:397–403.

Ingber, D. E. 1998. The architecture of life. *Scientific American* **278**:48–57.

———. 2006. Mechanical control of tissue morphogenesis during embryological development. *International Journal of Developmental Biology* **50**:255–66.

Jarmey, C. 2018. *The Concise Book of Muscles*. 4th ed. Chichester, UK: Lotus.

Jones, L. H. 1981. *Strain and Counterstrain.* Newark, OH: American Academy of Osteopathy.

Journal of Bodywork and Movement Therapy.

Lewit, K., and D. G. Simons. 1984. Myofascial pain: Relief by post-isometric relaxation. *Archives of Physical Medicine and Rehabilitation* **65**(8):452–56.

Myers, T. 2021. *Anatomy Trains: Myofascial Meridians for Manual Therapists and Movement Professionals.* 4th ed. London: Elsevier.

Myers, T., and J. Earls. 2017. *Fascial Release for Structural Balance.* Rev. ed. Chichester, UK: Lotus.

Niel-Asher, N. 2014. *The Concise Book of Trigger Points.* 3rd ed. Chichester: Lotus.

Persaud, T. 1984. *Early History of Human Anatomy: From Antiquity to the Beginning of the Modern Era.* Springfield, IL: Charles C. Thomas.

Shier, I . 2004. Does stretching improve performance? A systematic and critical review of the literature. *Clinical Journal of Sport Medicine* **14**:267–73.

Simons, D. G., J. G. Travell, and L. S. Simons. 1999. *Myofascial Pain and Dysfunction: The Trigger Point Manual.* 2nd ed. Baltimore, PA: Williams and Wilkins.

Travell, J. G., and D. G. Simons. 1983. *Myofascial Pain and Dysfunction: The Trigger Point Manual.* Baltimore, PA: Williams and Wilkins.

Author's Publications

Eyskens, J., J. Sharkey, J. Appleton, L. De Nil, and J. Staring. 2020. Quest for space: Towards a novel approach in treating pain and fatigue on earth. *International Journal of Biomechanics and Movement Science* **2**:002.

Jarmey, C., and J. Sharkey. 2016. *The Concise Book of Muscles.* 3rd ed. Berkeley, CA: North Atlantic Books.

Zheng, N., X.-Y. Yuan, Y.-F. Li, Y.-Y. Chi, H.-B. Gao, X. Zhao, S.-B. Yu, H.-J. Sui, and J. Sharkey. 2014. Definition of the to be named ligament and vertebrodural ligament and their possible effects on the circulation of CSF. *PLoS One* **9**(8):e103451.

Sharkey, J . 2003. Commentary on The stretching debate by Leon Chaitow. *Journal of Bodywork and Movement Therapies* **7**(2): 90–93.

———. 2008. *Concise Book of Neuromuscular Therapy: A Trigger Point Manual.* Chichester, UK: Lotus.

———. 2010. Anatomy of Human Fasciae: A Review of Current Literature. Presentation to the Academic Board of Studies, Dundee University.

———. 2013. *The Concise Book of Dry Needling: A Practitioner's Guide to Myofascial Trigger Point Applications.* Chichester, UK: Lotus.

———. 2013. Contribution to *Travell, Simons and Simons' Myofascial Pain and Dysfunction: The Trigger Point Manual*, 3rd ed., edited by Joseph M. Donnelly. Philadelphia, PA: Wolters-Kluwer.

———. 2015. Biotensegrity in Sport and Movement. Chapter 11 in *Fascia in Sport and Movement*, 2nd ed., edited by R. Schleip, J. Wilke, and A. Baker. Edinburgh: Handspring.

———. 2016. Fascia and the fallacy of biomechanics: A three-part research review and update. *Massage and Myotherapy Journal* **13**(3).

———. 2018. Biotensegrity: Anatomy for the 21st century informing bodywork and movement therapy. *Massage and Myotherapy Journal* **16**(1).

———. 2018. Biotensegrity: Anatomy for the 21st century informing yoga and physiotherapy concerning new findings in fascia research. *Journal of Yoga and Physiotherapy* **6**(1):555680.

———. 2018. Foreword to *Biotensegrity. The Structural Basis of Life*, 2nd ed., by G. Scarr. Edinburgh: Handspring.

———. 2018. Foreword to *Fascia Dysfunction: Manual Therapy Approaches*, edited by L. Chaitow. Edinburgh: Handspring.

———. 2018. Foreword to *Seeking Symmetry: Finding Patterns in Human Health* by N. Galloway. Edinburgh: Handspring.

———. 2019. Foreword to *Spiral Bound: Integrated Anatomy for Yoga* by K. Kirkness with J. Avison. Edinburgh: Handspring.

———. 2019. Stretching: The faux amis of yoga. Appendix B of *Yoga, Fascia, Anatomy and Movement*, 2nd ed., by J. Avison. Edinburgh: Handspring.

———. 2019. Update on fascial nomenclature: An additional proposal by John Sharkey MSc, clinical anatomist. *Journal of Bodywork and Movement Therapies* **23**(1). https://doi.org/10.1016/j.jbmt.2018.11.005.

———. 2020. Biotensegrity: The structure of life. Chapter 8 in *Fascia, Function and Medical Applications*, edited by D. Lesondak and A. M. Akey. Boca Raton, FL: CRC.

———. 2020. A clinical anatomist's experience of scars and adhesions in the cadaver. Chapter 6 in *Scars and Adhesions and the Biotensegral Body: Science, Assessment, Treatment*, edited by J. Trewartha and S. Wheeler. Edinburgh: Handspring.

———. 2020. Should bone be considered fascia: Proposal for a change in taxonomy of bone—a clinical anatomist's view. *International Journal of Biological and Pharmaceutical Sciences Archive* **1**(1). https://doi.org/10.30574/ijbpsa.2021.1.1.0001.

———. 2020. Site specific fascia tuning pegs and places of perilous passage: Myofascial consideration in upper extremity entrapment neuropathies—a clinical anatomist's view. *International Journal of Anatomy and Research* **8**(4.2):7823–28.

———. 2020. Tensegrity informed observations in human cadaveric studies: A clinical anatomist's perspective. *Integrative Journal of Medical Sciences* **7**. https://doi.org/10.15342/ijms.7.260.

———. 2021. Fascia and living tensegrity considerations in: Lower extremity and pelvic entrapment neuropathies. *International Journal of Anatomy and Research* **9**(1.2):7881–85.

———. 2021. Fascia and tensegrity: The quintessence of a unified systems conception. *International Journal of Anatomy and Research* **9**(1.2):7874–80.

———. 2021. Fascia-focused manual therapy interventions: Proposed treatment for post-covid syndrome. *Integrative Journal of Medical Sciences* **8**. https://doi.org/10.15342/ijms.2021.339.

———. 2021. Fascia the universal singularity of biotensegrity: The dark matter of our inner cosmos. *International Journal of Anatomy and Applied Physiology* **7**(2):179–84.

———. 2023. Contribution to *Kinesiology: The Skeletal System and Muscular Function*, 4th ed., by J. Musculino London: Elsevier.

Sharkey, J., and J. Avison. 2015. Biotensegrity: Powering the fabric of human anatomy. *Terra Rosa*, no. 15 (July 2015).

Sharkey, J., and M. Flannigan. 2023. Towards a paramedical interdisciplinary definition of fascia supporting practitioners offering fascia-focused therapies (part 1). *International Journal of Anatomy and Applied Physiology* **9**(1):218–22.

Sharkey, J., and K. Kirkness. 2021. Proposal for a new pedagogical approach in teaching anatomy to medical students, part I: Fascia continuity in the anatomy curriculum. *International Journal of Anatomy and Applied Physiology* **7**(5):205–8.

Starlanyl, D. J., and J. Sharkey. 2013. *Healing through Trigger Point Therapy: A Guide to Fibromyalgia, Myofascial Pain, and Dysfunction*. Berkeley, CA: North Atlantic Books.

Author's Other Scientific Contributions

Keynote speaker (jointly with Professor Carla Stecco of Padua University) at the 19th Congress of the International Federation of Associations of Anatomists (IFAA), London, August 9–11, 2019. Part of a symposium on new research findings concerning fascia.

Fascia Net Plastination Project in conjunction with the Fascia Research Society and the Von Hagen's Plastinarium, Guben, Germany. Part 2, January 2020. Article reference: YJBMT1749.

Research project 2014–21. World's First 3D Printed Model of the Fascia Profunda of Thigh. Supported by the Fascia Research Society and 3D Life Prints, UK.

Index

abduction, 55, 139
acceleration, 104
acetabulum, 56
acetylcholine (ACh), 118, 155
acetylcholinesterase (AChE), 118
acromioclavicular joints (AC joints),
        190
active cryotherapy techniques
        (ACTs), 210–211. *See also*
        patient assessment and
        treatment protocols
active transport, 62. *See also* cellular
        metabolism
acute, 56
adduction, 55, 139
adenosine diphosphate (ADP),
        64, 118
adenosine triphosphate (ATP),
        61, 62. *See also* energy
    role in cellular work, 118
adhesions, 56
ADP. *See* adenosine diphosphate
afferent, 56
agonist, 92, 94
AIIS. *See* anterior inferior iliac spine
allostasis, 64. *See also* cellular level
        organization
alternate nostril breathing, 25
analogous, 56
anatomy, language of, 44.
                See also integrated anatomy

directional terms, 55–56
localization, 55
naming of muscles, 45–46
neutral position, 55
prefixes, suffixes, and
        combining forms, 48–54
regional areas, 58
terms to indicate body areas, 59
animal cell. *See also* cellular level
        organization
    generalized, 60
    vital processes in, 61
antagonist, 92, 94, 121
anterior, 55
    sagittal system, 136–137
    slide test, 168
    tilt, 56
anterior inferior iliac spine (AIIS),
        136
anterior superior iliac spine (ASIS),
        190
aponeurosis, 39, 56, 89, 90, 113, 125
arcade of Struthers, 144
areolar tissue, 75. *See also* connective
        tissue
Arndt-Schultz's law, 193. *See also*
        neuromuscular laws
arthrokinematics, 140. *See also*
        shoulder biomechanics
    factors influencing, 95
    terms, 139

articulation, 56
ASIS. *See* anterior superior iliac
        spine
ATP. *See* adenosine triphosphate
atrophy, 180
avascular necrosis, 74. *See also*
        osseofascial system

balance, 169. *See also* medical
        exercise; myofascial trigger
        points; proprioception
    components of, 171
    dynamic balance, 171
    mechanoreceptor
        function, 170
    motor coordination, 174
    neurological pathways in, 173
    proprioception and, 170, 171
    reactive postural responses, 171
    spinal reflex, 172–173
    static balance, 171
belly. *See* gaster
bird, 204
biophysical dynamics, 107. *See also*
        muscle kinematics
blood, 82. *See also* cardiorespiratory
        system
    anatomy of, 84
    functions of, 82
    pressure, 87
    vessels, 84

test 1 and 2, 168
trapezius–serratus anterior
relationship, 166
shunt muscle, 291
SI joint. *See* sacroiliac joint
simple reflex arc, 201
single drag technique, 196. *See also*
neuromuscular techniques
SITS. *See* scapula and the
rotator cuff
skeletal muscle, 89, 111, 112.
See also muscle(s)
action of muscles, 92–94
aponeurosis, 89, 90
directional force, 89
forms of muscles, 90–91
motor unit of, 119
muscle attachments, 90
muscle fibers, 90
muscle shapes, 91–92
muscle working with origin
fixed and insertion
moving, 90
mylohyoid raphe, 89, 90
normal tendon structure, 89
origins and insertions, 89–90
strap muscle, 91–92
tendon, 89, 90
"tuning peg" power, 91
variations and explanations,
91–92
skeletal system, 66. *See also*
osseofascial system
axial and appendicular
skeleton, 67
skin, 138–139
sleeping, 200
sliding filament theory, 109, 110–111.
See also muscle(s)
G actins, 116
muscle contraction, 114,
116–118
myofibrils, 114
myosin cross-bridges, 115–116
sarcomere, 114, 115
sarcoplasmic reticulum, 114
tropomyosin, 116

troponin, 116
for understanding formation of
MTrPs, 114
slow-adapting (SA), 171
soft-matter materials, 30
soft tissue release (STR), 149, 211.
See also connective tissue
release
somatosensory system, 171
specific adaptation to imposed
demands (SAID), 187
spillover, 201
spinal reflex, 172–173.
See also balance
spiral system, 134. *See also*
myokinetic system and
subsystems
spontaneous electrical activity
(SEA), 156
SR. *See* sarcoplasmic reticulum
stabilizer, 94
stacking, 207–208
"static dynamic", 99
static stretching, 100, 101–102.
See also stretching
"stereotactic approach", 55
sternocleidomastoid (SCM), 134,
178, 234–235
Stork test, 303
STR. *See* soft tissue release
strain, 104, 184
strain/counterstrain (SCS), 200
strap muscle, 91–92. *See also*
skeletal muscle
stress, 104, 184
stretching, 95. *See also* muscle
kinematics
backscratcher, 98
challenges and misconceptions
in fascia and tissue
dynamics, 97
continuity and complexity
of anatomy, 98
contract, 98
dictionary definitions, 96–97
hamstring flexibility, 102
lengthen, 98

mechanical view of human
body, 95, 96
muscle spindles, 99
muscle stretch reflex, 99, 100
patellar tendon stretch, 101
proprioceptive neuromuscular
facilitation, 102–103
reframing concept of stretch in
fascia therapy, 97
sensory and motor cells, 98
static, 100, 101–102
"static dynamic", 99
stroke volume, 87. *See also*
cardiorespiratory system
suboccipitals, 236
subserous fascia, 112
superficial, 56
and deep aponeurotic
expansions, 144
fascia, 35, 37, 38, 39, 112
superior, 56
supination, 139
supine, 58
synergist, 94
synergistic dominance, 107
synovial joints, 69–70, 71. *See also*
osseofascial system

TA. *See* transversus abdominis
tapotement, 192. *See also* massage
target zone, 156. *See also* myofascial
trigger points
tendon, 58, 90, 111, 113. *See also*
muscle(s)
normal tendon structure, 89
tensegrity, 28, 30, 42–43, 123
extramuscular force pathways, 126
fascia, 127
fascia aponeurosis, 125
fascial layers, 125
fascia tuning pegs, 126
icosahedron model, 30, 31,
123, 124
integrated, 123
integration of fascia and, 32
living, 30
model, 124